Cardiovascular Diseases: Pathophysiology, Diagnosis and Treatment

Cardiovascular Diseases: Pathophysiology, Diagnosis and Treatment

Edited by **Janice Hunter**

FOSTER ACADEMICS

New Jersey

Published by Foster Academics,
61 Van Reypen Street,
Jersey City, NJ 07306, USA
www.fosteracademics.com

Cardiovascular Diseases: Pathophysiology, Diagnosis and Treatment
Edited by Janice Hunter

International Standard Book Number: 978-1-63242-444-0 (Hardback)

Printed in China.

Contents

Preface

Cardiovascular diseases are the disorders related to heart and blood vessels. These generally occur due to the formation and development of plaque in walls of the arteries which narrow downs their circumference blocking the passage for blood flow. This book discusses several methods for the diagnosis and treatment of heart diseases with new perspectives and approaches. It includes the pathophysiology and management of cardiovascular diseases. It provides all contemporary topics of relevance and delves into the unexplored aspects of this field. The aim of this book is to present researches that have transformed this discipline and aided its advancement. With state-of-the-art inputs by acclaimed experts of this field, this book targets students and professionals.

After months of intensive research and writing, this book is the end result of all who devoted their time and efforts in the initiation and progress of this book. It will surely be a source of reference in enhancing the required knowledge of the new developments in the area. During the course of developing this book, certain measures such as accuracy, authenticity and research focused analytical studies were given preference in order to produce a comprehensive book in the area of study.

This book would not have been possible without the efforts of the authors and the publisher. I extend my sincere thanks to them. Secondly, I express my gratitude to my family and well-wishers. And most importantly, I thank my students for constantly expressing their willingness and curiosity in enhancing their knowledge in the field, which encourages me to take up further research projects for the advancement of the area.

Editor

1

Cellular Mechanisms of Drosophila Heart Morphogenesis

Georg Vogler and Rolf Bodmer *

Development, Aging and Regeneration Program, Sanford-Burnham Medical Research Institute, 10901 N. Torrey Pines Road, La Jolla, CA 92037, USA; E-Mail: gvogler@sanfordburnham.org

* Author to whom correspondence should be addressed; E-Mail: rolf@sanfordburnham.org

Academic Editor: Silke R. Sperling

Abstract: Many of the major discoveries in the fields of genetics and developmental biology have been made using the fruit fly, *Drosophila melanogaster.* With regard to heart development, the conserved network of core cardiac transcription factors that underlies cardiogenesis has been studied in great detail in the fly, and the importance of several signaling pathways that regulate heart morphogenesis, such as Slit/Robo, was first shown in the fly model. Recent technological advances have led to a large increase in the genomic data available from patients with congenital heart disease (CHD). This has highlighted a number of candidate genes and gene networks that are potentially involved in CHD. To validate genes and genetic interactions among candidate CHD-causing alleles and to better understand heart formation in general are major tasks. The specific limitations of the various cardiac model systems currently employed (mammalian and fish models) provide a niche for the fly model, despite its evolutionary distance to vertebrates and humans. Here, we review recent advances made using the *Drosophila* embryo that identify factors relevant for heart formation. These underline how this model organism still is invaluable for a better understanding of CHD.

Keywords: *Drosophila*; cardiogenesis; morphogenesis; tinman; Cdc42; congenital heart disease; non-muscle myosin; zipper

---

1. Introduction

Congenital heart disease (CHD) is the most frequently diagnosed birth defect, with an incident rate of about 1% among newborns [1,2]. There are several genetic origins of CHD, such as copy-number variation (CNV), which affects gene dosage (as found in DiGeorge Syndrome and Williams–Beuren Syndrome), or mutations that affect a single gene, often a cardiac transcription factor (*i.e.*, NKX2.5, GATA4) or structural components of the contractile apparatus of the cardiomyocytes (such as MYH6; for a review, see [3,4]). However, the underlying genetics of the majority of cases of CHD (which are labeled "sporadic") seems to be more complex and is likely caused by the interaction of independent alleles and loci ("polygenic"). While recent advances in sequencing technology have led to a drastic increase in the data available on genetic variants among patients' genomes, it is still necessary to experimentally validate candidate genes that were computationally derived from such genomic data.

Understanding the biological basis of CHD requires a molecular understanding of the complex development of the heart itself, and despite the great efforts of the scientific community, our understanding of heart morphogenesis is still very incomplete. Current vertebrate models of heart development are mouse, chicken and zebrafish embryos (for reviews, see [5–8]), which are complemented by cell-based assays, including heart tissue engineered from induced pluripotent stem cells (iPSCs) [9]. These models established valuable concepts for the number and origin of cardiac progenitor cells, lineage restriction and the respective contributions of these cells to different regions of the heart. To study the complexity of the heart and heart morphogenesis, it is necessary to combine different approaches to complement the specific shortcomings of each model. This need has spurred the introduction and adoption of other models, such as tunicates [10], which are basic chordates, and even invertebrate model organisms, such as the fruit fly, *Drosophila melanogaster* [11–14].

In the last three decades, the powerful genetic model system, *Drosophila*, has been instrumental in the identification and dissection of the genetics of many developmental processes, including heart development (for a review, see [15]), serving as a pioneer for higher model organisms. *Drosophila* is an extremely versatile model, with a plethora of reagents and genetic tools available, including RNAi lines to tissue-specific targeting of each fly gene [16]. One particular advantage of the fly model is that heart-specific genetic manipulations of critical factors of heart development still allow its survival into adulthood and permit functional analysis, while the same approach in higher model organisms often causes embryonic lethality. In a reverse-genetic screen for genes affecting adult heart function under stress conditions, several members of the CCR4-Not complex were identified to cause dilated cardiomyopathy in the fly, a function that is conserved in a murine model and with implications for human heart disease [17]. One recent example is the role of the YAK/Hippo pathway in mammalian cardiovascular development [18]. Originally identified in Drosophila, YAK/Hippo plays a major role in tissue size control, and recent data show that this function seems to be conserved in mammals. Therefore, lessons learned from *Drosophila* can be (re-)applied to improve our understanding of human heart development and might even be helpful in identifying strategies for preventing and repairing cardiac dysfunction. Here, we review recent advances in the understanding of the molecular-genetic control of heart morphogenesis in *Drosophila*.

2. Genetics of *Drosophila* Heart Formation

2.1. Genetic Control of Cardiac Specification

The embryonic *Drosophila* heart is a simple, tubular organ comprised of two different cell types: the cardioblasts (CBs), which differentiate into contractile cardiomyocytes of the "working myocardium" and ostia cells, that form the inflow tracts of the heart; and pericardial cells (PCs), most of which become nephrocyte-like cells involved in ultrafiltration that line the outside of the heart tube [19,20]. Pericardial cells have a dual role of also serving as ROS-sensors for the myocardium [21]. The precursors of both the CBs and PCs are specified in the dorsal mesoderm, under the influence of ectodermal TGFβ and WNT signaling pathways [22]. This "cardiac mesoderm" contains the heart's founder cells that will divide and give rise to both pure and mixed lineages of CBs and PCs (and somatic muscle cells). At this stage, a number of cell fate decisions are made, leading to the specification of subtypes of CBs and PCs, which is under the control of the Notch signaling pathway and its regulators, such as Sanpodo, Numb and ADAM metalloproteinase-disintegrins [22–26]. The identification of Tinman [27,28], a homeobox transcription factor, led to the identification of its mammalian homologue, Nkx2.5, as the first essential factor for the specification of the cardiogenic region in both flies and vertebrates. The genetics and specification cascade downstream of *tin* function in *Drosophila* has been described in great detail (for a detailed review, see Bodmer and Frasch [15]). Briefly, Tinman and the TBX transcription factor, Dorsocross-1/2/3 [29], induce expression of the GATA4-homologue Pannier in the dorsal mesoderm, where Pannier acts as a permissive factor for CB specification [30]. Later, during development, Tinman is subsequently required for the further specification and differentiation of CBs [31], in part through activation of Mef2 [32]. Other examples of cardiac transcription factors studied in *Drosophila* include HAND [33], Neuromancer1/2-TBX20 [34,35], Tail-up/Islet-1 [36,37] and the COUP transcription factor, Seven-up [38]. This genetic and mutational interrogation of cardiogenesis was recently complemented by ChIP-on-chip studies of whole embryos [39,40], which globally identified the transcriptional activity and regulatory networks controlled by Tinman and several other cardiac transcription factors.

2.2. Genetics of Heart Morphogenesis

Once specified, the cardiac precursor cells migrate towards the dorsal midline, where they undergo changes in cell shape and assemble to form a linear heart tube. While the bilateral origin of the heart precursors and their fusion at the midline resembles early vertebrate heart morphogenesis (*i.e.*, heart cone formation; compare [41,42]), the linear arrangement of ipsilateral CBs along the anterior-posterior axis and the two-cell composition of the cardiac lumen appear to be morphologically distinct and more similar to mammalian blood vessels than the mammalian heart (e.g., developing mouse aorta [43]). In *Drosophila*, the CBs migrate and undergo morphogenesis in about five hours, which is experimentally advantageous, as it allows cell behavior to be studied in real time throughout heart formation. The CBs and heart are also very accessible for confocal time-lapse and fluorescence imaging of stained whole-mount embryos, since these cells are localized just below the epidermis, which is a single-cell layer and, thus, semi-transparent.

Once the CBs have migrated to the midline, they establish dorsal contacts with the contralateral counterpart, then undergo cell shape changes and ventrally contact the other CBs, thereby enclosing a central lumen. This occurs in a "zipper-like" fashion that closes from both the anterior and posterior ends. The *Drosophila* heart tube is compartmentalized along the A/P axis. A cardiac outflow tract (OFT) is already formed anteriorly while the bilateral heart cells are closing [44], whereas the posterior region of the heart, the "heart proper" forms a larger heart lumen. The CBs in this section differentiate into contractile cardiomyocytes and pairs of cells that form inflow tracts (ostia cells; see [45]). The "aortic" region of the heart is located between the OFT and heart proper and is characterized by the much smaller diameter of the heart lumen and the lack of ostia cells. The heart itself is physically connected to a number of other cell types that also directly contribute to heart function, specifically the alary muscle cells [46,47], which may anchor the heart tube to the epidermis, and the nephrocyte-like pericardial cells [21,48–50]. Extracellular matrix proteins, such as laminins and collagens (including Pericardin and Multiplexin), localize in and around the heart and are required for heart assembly and integrity [51–55]. Signaling proteins, such as Integrins [56], as well as G proteins [57], regulate cardiac ECM and cell adhesion directly or indirectly.

Once such pathways are uncovered in *Drosophila*, homologous pathways can be investigated in higher model organisms. For example, studies on the role of the Slit-Robo signaling pathway in *Drosophila* heart morphogenesis have triggered the analysis of homologous genes in vertebrate model organisms. Early on, it was noticed that the ligand Slit is expressed in fly CBs [58]. Subsequent mutational analysis of *slit* and the genes encoding its receptors *robo* and *robo2* revealed that this pathway is indeed critical for maintaining CB chain integrity during migration [59] and for CB cell shape changes during heart morphogenesis [60–62]. In vertebrates, Slit/Robo has been implicated in zebrafish heart tube formation [63], where *slit2* is necessary for the migration of endocardial cells during heart tube formation, and in *robo1/2* and *slit3* mutant mouse models, where the formation of the pericardial and venous return is defective [64]. How the Slit-Robo signaling cascade controls morphogenetic events was first worked out for post-mitotic neurons, as they migrate during *Drosophila* nervous system development: binding of the signaling molecule Slit to its receptor Robo induces recruitment of Son-of-Sevenless, a guanine nucleotide exchange factor (GEF), which, in turn, activates the Rho family of GTPases that control the cytoskeletal changes required for the specific migratory response of the neuronal growth cone [65]. The simple *Drosophila* heart tube is well suited to allow the identification of the factors downstream of Slit-Robo, which, in turn, become candidate genes to be analyzed in higher model organisms. Subsequent analyses of the downstream effectors of Slit-Robo using *Drosophila* will likely reveal additional candidate genes to be tested in these models. For example, the *Drosophila* gene encoding Multiplexin (Mp, a collagen15/18) was recently identified to modify Slit-Robo signaling and potentiating Slit activity, resulting in reduced formation of F-actin and altered heart lumen size [54].

2.3. Analyzing the Actomyosin Network during Drosophila Heart Morphogenesis

Underneath the instructive layer of cardiac transcription factors and signaling molecules are those proteins that transduce these cues into cellular behavior. For example, CB-specific mutation of *tinman* causes misspecification of cells and morphogenetic defects that are a combination of cell fate changes and inappropriate cell behavior [31].

Elucidating how the cells interpret these internal and external cues is fundamental not only for a comprehensive understanding of organogenesis, but it also offers additional, alternate and specific therapeutic avenues by targeting the effector molecules of disease genes. These basic aspects of cell biology are usually studied in cell culture, where high-resolution analysis of cellular effectors is possible. However, cell culture lacks the complexity of differentiated, three-dimensional multicellular environments, which are present in a living embryo. Therefore, the simplicity of the developing *Drosophila* heart is advantageous to analyze cardiac cell biology during heart morphogenesis and to eventually explain how signaling pathways, such as Slit/Robo and Integrin signaling, give rise to specific cardiac phenotypes when mutated.

Members of the small Rho GTPase family are common molecular hubs that control a large variety of cellular responses, such as cell polarization or cytoskeletal organization (for a review, see [66,67]). Interestingly, the small GTPase *Cdc42* was previously identified as a genetic interactor with *tinman* in adult hearts of *Drosophila* and mice [68]. This interaction was also manifest in the *Drosophila* embryo during heart morphogenesis [69], indicating that Tinman might control heart morphogenesis through Cdc42. During heart development, Cdc42 is necessary for Tin-positive cardioblasts to complete dorsal migration [70], and it controls CB cell shape changes during heart lumen formation. Interestingly, both processes appear to be specific for the small Rho-GTPase Cdc42, but not for the other members, such as Rho1 or Rac1 [69].

Lumen formation in *Drosophila* occurs by enclosing of a central lumen, where the CBs actively bend around the luminal space (see Figure 1). Such changes in cell shape are achieved by the activity of the actomyosin network, which has not been studied in detail in the context of *Drosophila* heart formation. Throughout dorsal closure, actomyosin is active in epidermal cells (as "purse-string" actin-myosin cables that pull epidermal sheets towards the midline) and in the cells of the amnioserosa, an extra-embryonic layer that degenerates at late stages of development and, thereby, creates tension by reducing surface area.

Analysis of the expression pattern of the *Drosophila* non-muscle myosin-II *Zipper* (*Zip*) revealed a specific and very dynamic pattern throughout heart morphogenesis [69]. During Stage 15–16, before dorsal closure, Zip repetitively accumulates at the apical side of the CBs, which may be important for apical constriction of CBs to support dorsal closure. During lumen formation, Zip temporarily accumulates at the luminal surface to maintain CB/lumen curvature. In CBs, non-muscle myosin II dynamics is positively regulated by Cdc42 and formin activity, with *Cdc42* also showing genetic interaction with *zip* and the formin, d*DAAM1* [69]. Interestingly, cardiac laterality during zebrafish heart morphogenesis depends on the control of non-muscle myosin-II by BMP signaling [71]. This highlights the need for a better understanding of how the actomyosin network functions *in vivo* and how it is spatio-temporally regulated.

While these aspects of actomyosin regulation might relate to how force generation shapes the heart, Cdc42/formins also control the heart lumen in a more general fashion. The activation of Cdc42 and formins is sufficient to relocate the entire set of known lumen markers, such as Dystroglycan (Dg), Perlecan/Trol, Slit and Multiplexin, to newly formed, ectopic heart lumina. The latter proteins are part of the extracellular matrix (including anchoring proteins, like Dg, or signaling molecules, like Slit; for an overview, see [72]), and they carry out specific functions during heart morphogenesis and lumen formation, including the downregulation of F-actin itself [54]. In addition, Cdc42 controls the migration of Tin-positive cells before dorsal closure and independent of the known Cdc42 downstream effector p21-activated kinase. The number and hierarchy of genes involved in heart morphogenesis that mediate this cellular behavior are still unknown. In addition, the upstream signals controlling CB migration and lumen formation have yet to be identified. While different signaling pathways (Slit-Robo, Netrin-Unc5, Integrins) are required for heart formation, the molecular-genetic pathways mediating the cellular responses have not been found. In fact, neither Slit-Robo, nor Netrin-Unc5 mutants show changes in non-muscle myosin dynamics [69], which indicates that other pathways are involved, as well. Furthermore, the interaction between CBs and the surrounding tissues (amnioserosa, pericardial cells, dorsal ectoderm) is likely to be critical for heart morphogenesis, as well, but to date, very little is known about how these tissues interact. Recent work showed that regulation of lipid phosphates, Wunen and Wunen2, expressed in the developing heart, is necessary for heart morphogenesis [73], as well as for the timing of dorsal closure, which is delayed in *wun/wun2* mutants.

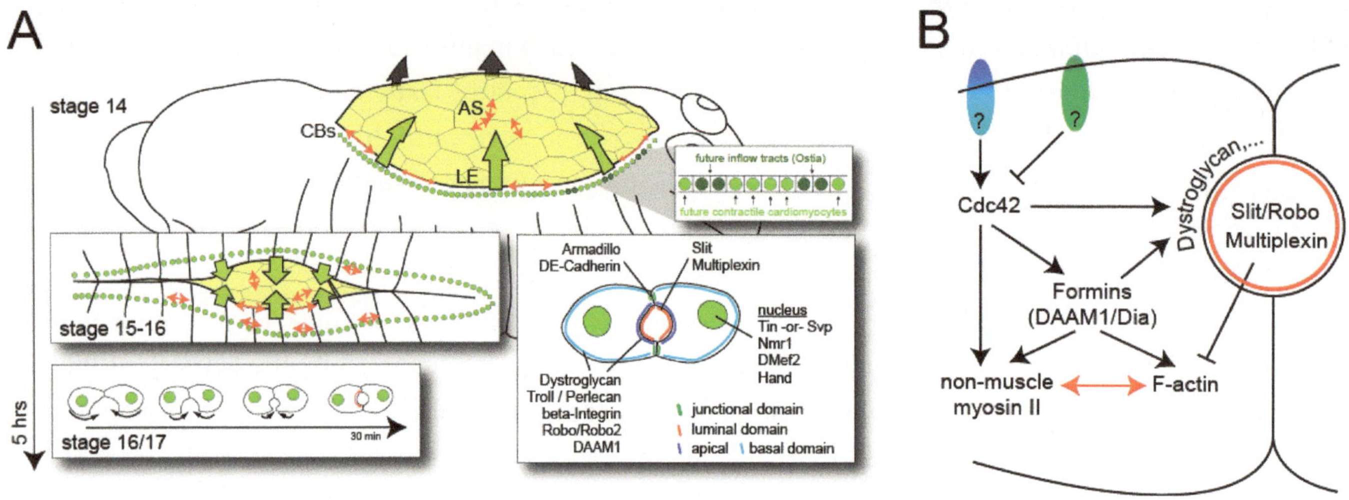

Figure 1. (**a**) Overview of Drosophila heart morphogenesis. Cardioblasts (CBs, green circles) collectively migrate towards the dorsal midline of the embryo. These differentiate later into contractile cardiomyocytes (light green) and ostia cells (dark green). Actomyosin activity can be detected at the edge of the cells of the amnioserosa (AS), at the leading edge of the epidermis (LE) and at the apical side of CBs (red arrows indicate the axis of actomyosin bundles). CB migration is completed within 5 h. Epithelial closure precedes heart closure, and once the CBs make first contact at Stage 16, within 30 min, they actively enclose a central lumen. At that stage, several compartments within the CBs can be identified using several different markers. (**b**) Model showing genetic interactions between Cdc42, formins, actomyosin and the luminal proteins, Slit and Multiplexin. The upstream regulators of Cdc42 (both positive and negative) are yet to be identified.

With the advent of affordable whole-genome sequencing, forward genetic screens (such as EMS screens, e.g., in [74]) to identify new players in heart development or genetic interactors of known cardiac factors become more feasible again. In addition, improved RNAi-based approaches, as well as targeted mutations using CRISPR/Cas9 [75–77] will allow one to model candidate genes identified from human patients in the fly model and to subsequently functionally evaluate these variants and test for genetic interaction. CRISPR/Cas9 also permits rapid analysis of single genes in zebrafish and mouse models (e.g., see [78]), and these model organisms have a much smaller evolutionary distance to humans compared to flies. Genetic variants that might be responsible for CHD might not be present in the fly genome and, therefore, are a limitation to the analysis of potentially disease-causing alleles. However, the study of genetic interaction (*i.e.*, with core cardiac factors) is still a domain of the fruit fly due to the lack of genetic redundancy for the vast majority of *Drosophila* genes compared to vertebrates, which (in addition to many other advantages; see [79]) makes the fruit fly a promising model for CHD research.

3. Conclusions

Drosophila is a powerful tool with which to study the genetic and cellular mechanisms of heart formation. Significant genetic homology between flies and humans means that many of the signaling pathways and gene networks uncovered in the fruit fly are relevant in human patients (for an overview see Table 1). The reverse is likely to also be true. Therefore, the fly heart model can be used to screen through candidate CHD-causing genes.

The interactions of Cdc42 with downstream effectors, such as formins, as well as feedback from ECM and signaling pathways therefore represents an experimental entry point to study the cellular events leading to organ formation. Dysregulation of these pathways is likely to contribute to CHD, while understanding the cellular mechanism of heart morphogenesis is necessary for the repair and the engineering of cardiac tissue [80].

Table 1. List of selected *Drosophila* genes regulating heart development.

***Drosophila* Gene**	**Class**	**Selected Ref.**	**Vertebrate Ortholog(s)**	**Selected Ref.**
Diaphanous	Formin	[69]	DRF3	[10]
Zipper	Non-muscle myosin	[69]	NMHC-II A/B/C	[43,81]
Netrin	Signaling molecule	[82,83]	NET1/3	[84]
Slit	Signaling molecule	[59–62,69,85]	SLIT1/2/3	[64,86]
Decapentaplegic	Signaling molecule	[87]	BMPs	[88]
Wingless	Signaling molecule	[89]	WNTs	[90]
Frazzled	Signaling Receptor	[83]	NEO1	[91]
heartless	Signaling Receptor	[92]	FGFR3/4	[93]
Notch	Signaling Receptor	[25]	NOTCH1/2/3	[94]
Robo1/2/3	Signaling Receptor	[59,61,62,85]	ROBO1/2/3/4	[64]
Unc-5	Signaling Receptor	[82]	UNC5A/B/C/D	[95]
Kuzbanian	ADAM10 metalloprotease	[23]	ADAM10	[96]
Cdc42	Small Rho GTPase	[69,70]	CDC42	[68,97]
Multiplexin	Collagen type XV/XVIII	[54]	COL15/18	[98,99]
dHand	Transcription factor	[33,100,101]	HAND1/2	[102,103]
DMef2	Transcription factor	[32,104,105]	MEF2A/C/D	[106,107]
Dorsocross1/2/3	Transcription factor	[29]	TBX2/3/5	[108–110]
Ladybird-early/late	Transcription factor	[111,112]	Lbx1/2/3	[113]
Neuromancer1/2	Transcription factor	[34,35,114]	TBX20	[115,116]
Pannier	Transcription factor	[30,117,118]	GATA4/6	[119]
Seven-up	Transcription factor	[38,45]	COUP-TF II	[120]
Tail-up	Transcription factor	[36,37,121]	ISL1	[122]
Tinman	Transcription factor	[27,28]	NKX2.5	[123]

Acknowledgments

We thank Leah Cannon for her critical reading of this manuscript. Work in the laboratory of Rolf Bodmer is funded by grants from the National Institutes of Health (RO1 HL054732) to Rolf Bodmer.

Author Contributions

Georg Vogler and Rolf Bodmer wrote the paper.

Conflicts of Interest

The authors declare no conflict of interest.

References

1. Marelli, A.J.; Ionescu-Ittu, R.; Mackie, A.S.; Guo, L.; Dendukuri, N.; Kaouache, M. Lifetime prevalence of congenital heart disease in the general population from 2000 to 2010. *Circulation* **2014**, doi:10.1161/CIRCULATIONAHA.113.008396.
2. Reller, M.D.; Strickland, M.J.; Riehle-Colarusso, T.; Mahle, W.T.; Correa, A. Prevalence of congenital heart defects in metropolitan atlanta, 1998–2005. *J. Pediatri.* **2008**, *153*, 807–813.
3. Pierpont, M.E.; Basson, C.T.; Benson, D.W.; Gelb, B.D.; Giglia, T.M.; Goldmuntz, E.; McGee, G.; Sable, C.A.; Srivastava, D.; Webb, C.L.; *et al.* Genetic basis for congenital heart defects: Current knowledge: A scientific statement from the American heart association congenital cardiac defects committee, council on cardiovascular disease in the young: Endorsed by the american academy of pediatrics. *Circulation* **2007**, *115*, 3015–3038.
4. Fahed, A.C.; Gelb, B.D.; Seidman, J.G.; Seidman, C.E. Genetics of congenital heart disease: The glass half empty. *Circ. Res.* **2013**, *112*, 707–720.
5. Staudt, D.; Stainier, D. Uncovering the molecular and cellular mechanisms of heart development using the zebrafish. *Ann. Rev. Genet.* **2012**, *46*, 397–418.
6. Bruneau, B.G. *Heart Development*; Academic Press: Waltham, MA, USA, 2012; p. 408.
7. Bruneau, B.G. The developmental genetics of congenital heart disease. *Nature* **2008**, *451*, 943–948.
8. Kruithof, B.P.T.; Duim, S.N.; Moerkamp, A.T.; Goumans, M.-J. Tgfβ and BMP signaling in cardiac cushion formation: Lessons from mice and chicken. *Differentiation* **2012**, *84*, 89–102.
9. Alexander, J.M.; Bruneau, B.G. Lessons for cardiac regeneration and repair through development. *Trends Mol. Med.* **2010**, *16*, 426–434.
10. Christiaen, L.; Davidson, B.; Kawashima, T.; Powell, W.; Nolla, H.; Vranizan, K.; Levine, M. The transcription/migration interface in heart precursors of ciona intestinalis. *Science* **2008**, *320*, 1349–1352.
11. Vogler, G.; Bodmer, R.; Akasaka, T. A Drosophila model for congenital heart disease. *Drug Discov. Today Dis. Models* **2009**, *6*, 47–54.
12. Ocorr, K.; Vogler, G.; Bodmer, R. Methods to assess Drosophila heart development, function and aging. *Methods* **2014**, *68*, 265–272.
13. Reim, I.; Frasch, M. Genetic and genomic dissection of cardiogenesis in the Drosophila model. *Pediatr. Cardiol.* **2009**, *31*, 325–334.

14. Medioni, C.; Sénatore, S.; Salmand, P.-A.; Lalevée, N.; Perrin, L.; Sémériva, M. The fabulous destiny of the Drosophila heart. *Curr. Opin. Genet. Dev.* **2009**, *19*, 518–525.
15. Bodmer, R.; Frasch, M. Development and aging of the Drosophila heart. In *Heart Development and Regeneration*; Harvey, R.P., Rosenthal, N., Eds.; Academic Press: Waltham, MA, USA, 2010; pp. 47–86.
16. Mohr, S.E.; Hu, Y.; Kim, K.; Housden, B.E.; Perrimon, N. Resources for functional genomics studies in Drosophila melanogaster. *Genetics* **2014**, *197*, 1–18.
17. Neely, G.G.; Kuba, K.; Cammarato, A.; Isobe, K.; Amann, S.; Zhang, L.; Murata, M.; Elmen, L.; Gupta, V.; Arora, S.; *et al.* A global *in vivo* Drosophila RNAi screen identifies Not3 as a conserved regulator of heart function. *Cell* **2010**, *141*, 142–153.
18. Zhou, J. An emerging role for hippo-yap signaling in cardiovascular development. *J. Biomed. Res.* **2014**, *28*, 251–254.
19. Rizki, T.M. *The Circulatory System and Associated Cells and Tissues*; Ashburner, M., Wright, T.R., Eds.; Academic Press: Waltham, MA, USA, 1978; pp. 397–452.
20. Zhang, F.; Zhao, Y.; Chao, Y.; Muir, K.; Han, Z. Cubilin and amnionless mediate protein reabsorption in Drosophila nephrocytes. *J. Am. Soc. Nephrol.* **2013**, *24*, 209–216.
21. Lim, H.-Y.; Wang, W.; Chen, J.; Ocorr, K.; Bodmer, R. Ros regulate cardiac function via a distinct paracrine mechanism. *Cell Rep.* **2014**, *7*, 35–44.
22. Bryantsev, A.L.; Cripps, R.M. Cardiac gene regulatory networks in Drosophila. *Biochim. Biophys. Acta* **2009**, *1789*, 343–353.
23. Albrecht, S.; Wang, S.; Holz, A.; Bergter, A.; Paululat, A. The adam metalloprotease kuzbanian is crucial for proper heart formation in Drosophila melanogaster. *Mech. Dev.* **2006**, *123*, 372–387.
24. Ward, E.J.; Skeath, J.B. Characterization of a novel subset of cardiac cells and their progenitors in the Drosophila embryo. *Development* **2000**, *127*, 4959–4969.
25. Han, Z.; Bodmer, R. Myogenic cells fates are antagonized by notch only in asymmetric lineages of the Drosophila heart, with or without cell division. *Development* **2003**, *130*, 3039–3051.
26. Park, M.; Yaich, L.E.; Bodmer, R. Mesodermal cell fate decisions in Drosophila are under the control of the lineage genes numb, Notch, and sanpodo. *Mech. Dev.* **1998**, *75*, 117–126.
27. Bodmer, R. The gene Tinman is required for specification of the heart and visceral muscles in Drosophila. *Development* **1993**, *118*, 719–729.
28. Azpiazu, N.; Frasch, M. Tinman and bagpipe: Two homeo box genes that determine cell fates in the dorsal mesoderm of Drosophila. *Genes Dev.* **1993**, *7*, 1325–1340.
29. Reim, I.; Frasch, M. The dorsocross T-box genes are key components of the regulatory network controlling early cardiogenesis in Drosophila. *Development* **2005**, *132*, 4911–4925.
30. Klinedinst, S.L.; Bodmer, R. GATA factor pannier is required to establish competence for heart progenitor formation. *Development* **2003**, *130*, 3027–3038.
31. Zaffran, S.; Reim, I.; Qian, L.; Lo, P.C.; Bodmer, R.; Frasch, M. Cardioblast-intrinsic Tinman activity controls proper diversification and differentiation of myocardial cells in Drosophila. *Development* **2006**, *133*, 4073–4083.
32. Gajewski, K.; Kim, Y.; Lee, Y.M.; Olson, E.N.; Schulz, R.A. D-MEF2 is a target for Tinman activation during Drosophila heart development. *EMBO J.* **1997**, *16*, 515–522.

33. Han, Z.; Yi, P.; Li, X.; Olson, E.N. Hand, an evolutionarily conserved bHLH transcription factor required for Drosophila cardiogenesis and hematopoiesis. *Development* **2006**, *133*, 1175–1182.
34. Miskolczi-McCallum, C.M.; Scavetta, R.J.; Svendsen, P.C.; Soanes, K.H.; Brook, W.J. The Drosophila melanogaster T-box genes midline and H15 are conserved regulators of heart development. *Dev. Biol.* **2005**, *278*, 459–472.
35. Qian, L.; Liu, J.; Bodmer, R. Neuromancer TBX20-related genes (H15/midline) promote cell fate specification and morphogenesis of the Drosophila heart. *Dev. Biol.* **2005**, *279*, 509–524.
36. Tao, Y.; Wang, J.; Tokusumi, T.; Gajewski, K.; Schulz, R.A. Requirement of the LIM homeodomain transcription factor tailup for normal heart and hematopoietic organ formation in Drosophila melanogaster. *Mol. Cell. Biol.* **2007**, *27*, 3962–3969.
37. Mann, T.; Bodmer, R.; Pandur, P. The Drosophila homolog of vertebrate Islet1 is a key component in early cardiogenesis. *Development* **2009**, *136*, 317–326.
38. Lo, P.C.H.; Frasch, M. A role for the coup-tf-related gene seven-up in the diversification of cardioblast identities in the dorsal vessel of Drosophila. *Mech. Dev.* **2001**, *104*, 49–60.
39. Junion, G.; Spivakov, M.; Girardot, C.; Braun, M.; Gustafson, E.H.; Birney, E.; Furlong, E.E.M. A transcription factor collective defines cardiac cell fate and reflects lineage history. *Cell* **2012**, *148*, 473–486.
40. Jin, H.; Stojnic, R.; Adryan, B.; Ozdemir, A.; Stathopoulos, A.; Frasch, M. Genome-wide screens for *in vivo* tinman binding sites identify cardiac enhancers with diverse functional architectures. *PLOS Genet.* **2013**, *9*, e1003195.
41. Rugendorff, A.; Younossi-Hartenstein, A.; Hartenstein, V. Embryonic origin and differentiation of the Drosophila heart. *Roux's Arch. Dev. Biol.* **1994**, *203*, 266–280.
42. Holtzman, N.G.; Schoenebeck, J.J.; Tsai, H.J.; Yelon, D. Endocardium is necessary for cardiomyocyte movement during heart tube assembly. *Development* **2007**, *134*, 2379–2386.
43. Strilić, B.; Kucera, T.; Eglinger, J.; Hughes, M.R.; McNagny, K.M.; Tsukita, S.; Dejana, E.; Ferrara, N.; Lammert, E. The molecular basis of vascular lumen formation in the developing mouse aorta. *Dev. Cell* **2009**, *17*, 505–515.
44. Zikova, M.; da Ponte, J.-P.; Dastugue, B.; Jagla, K. Patterning of the cardiac outflow region in Drosophila. *Proc. Natl. Acad. Sci. USA* **2003**, *100*, 12189–12194.
45. Molina, M.R.; Cripps, R.M. Ostia, the inflow tracts of the Drosophila heart, develop from a genetically distinct subset of cardial cells. *Mech. Dev.* **2001**, *109*, 51–59.
46. LaBeau, E.M.; Trujillo, D.L.; Cripps, R.M. Bithorax complex genes control alary muscle patterning along the cardiac tube of Drosophila. *Mech. Dev.* **2009**, *126*, 478–486.
47. Boukhatmi, H.; Schaub, C.; Bataillé, L.; Reim, I.; Frendo, J.-L.; Frasch, M.; Vincent, A. An Org-1-Tup transcriptional cascade reveals different types of alary muscles connecting internal organs in Drosophila. *Development* **2014**, *141*, 3761–3771.
48. Zhuang, S.; Shao, H.; Guo, F.; Trimble, R.; Pearce, E.; Abmayr, S.M. Sns and Kirre, the Drosophila orthologs of Nephrin and Neph1, direct adhesion, fusion and formation of a slit diaphragm-like structure in insect nephrocytes. *Development* **2009**, *136*, 2335–2344.
49. Weavers, H.; Prieto-Sánchez, S.; Grawe, F.; Garcia-López, A.; Artero, R.; Wilsch-Bräuninger, M.; Ruiz-Gómez, M.; Skaer, H.; Denholm, B. The insect nephrocyte is a podocyte-like cell with a filtration slit diaphragm. *Nature* **2009**, *457*, 322–326.

50. Buechling, T.; Akasaka, T.; Vogler, G.; Ruiz-Lozano, P.; Ocorr, K.A.; Bodmer, R. Non-autonomous modulation of heart rhythm, contractility and morphology in adult fruit flies. *Dev. Biol.* **2009**, *328*, 483–492.
51. Hollfelder, D.; Frasch, M.; Reim, I. Distinct functions of the laminin β LN domain and collagen IV during cardiac extracellular matrix formation and stabilization of alary muscle attachments revealed by ems mutagenesis in Drosophila. *BMC Dev. Biol.* **2014**, *14*, 26.
52. Yarnitzky, T.; Volk, T. Laminin is required for heart, somatic muscles, and gut development in the Drosophila embryo. *Dev. Biol.* **1995**, *169*, 609–618.
53. Chartier, A.; Zaffran, S.; Astier, M.; Sémériva, M.; Gratecos, D. Pericardin, a Drosophila type IV collagen-like protein is involved in the morphogenesis and maintenance of the heart epithelium during dorsal ectoderm closure. *Development* **2002**, *129*, 3241–3253.
54. Harpaz, N.; Ordan, E.; Ocorr, K.; Bodmer, R.; Volk, T. Multiplexin promotes heart but not aorta morphogenesis by polarized enhancement of Slit/Robo activity at the heart lumen. *PLOS Genet.* **2013**, *9*, e1003597.
55. Volk, T.; Wang, S.; Rotstein, B.; Paululat, A. Matricellular proteins in development: Perspectives from the Drosophila heart. *Matrix Biol.* **2014**, *37*, 162–166.
56. Vanderploeg, J.; Vazquez Paz, L.L.; MacMullin, A.; Jacobs, J.R. Integrins are required for cardioblast polarisation in Drosophila. *BMC Dev. Biol.* **2012**, *12*, 8.
57. Yi, P.; Johnson, A.N.; Han, Z.; Wu, J.; Olson, E.N. Heterotrimeric g proteins regulate a noncanonical function of septate junction proteins to maintain cardiac integrity in Drosophila. *Dev. Cell* **2008**, *15*, 704–713.
58. Rothberg, J.M.; Jacobs, J.R.; Goodman, C.S.; Artavanis-Tsakonas, S. Slit: An extracellular protein necessary for development of midline glia and commissural axon pathways contains both EGF and LRR domains. *Genes Dev.* **1990**, *4*, 2169–2187.
59. Qian, L.; Liu, J.; Bodmer, R. Slit and Robo control cardiac cell polarity and morphogenesis. *Curr. Biol.* **2005**, *15*, 2271–2278.
60. Medioni, C.; Astier, M.; Zmojdzian, M.; Jagla, K.; Semeriva, M. Genetic control of cell morphogenesis during Drosophila melanogaster cardiac tube formation. *J. Cell Biol.* **2008**, *182*, 249–261.
61. MacMullin, A.; Jacobs, J.R. Slit coordinates cardiac morphogenesis in Drosophila. *Dev. Biol.* **2006**, *293*, 154–164.
62. Santiago-Martínez, E.; Soplop, N.H.; Patel, R.; Kramer, S.G. Repulsion by Slit and roundabout prevents Shotgun/E-cadherin-mediated cell adhesion during Drosophila heart tube lumen formation. *J. Cell Biol.* **2008**, *182*, 241–248.
63. Fish, J.E.; Wythe, J.D.; Xiao, T.; Bruneau, B.G.; Stainier, D.Y.R.; Srivastava, D.; Woo, S. A Slit/miR-218/Robo regulatory loop is required during heart tube formation in zebrafish. *Development* **2011**, *138*, 1409–1419.
64. Mommersteeg, M.T.M.; Andrews, W.D.; Ypsilanti, A.R.; Zelina, P.; Yeh, M.L.; Norden, J.; Kispert, A.; Chédotal, A.; Christoffels, V.M.; Parnavelas, J.G. Slit-Robo signaling regulates the development of the cardiac systemic venous return and pericardium. *Circ. Res.* **2012**, *112*, 465–475.
65. Yang, L.; Bashaw, G.J. Son of sevenless directly links the Robo receptor to Rac activation to control axon repulsion at the midline. *Neuron* **2006**, *52*, 595–607.

66. Hanna, S.; El-Sibai, M. Signaling networks of Rho GTPases in cell motility. *Cell. Signal.* **2013**, *25*, 1955–1961.
67. Iden, S.; Collard, J.G. Crosstalk between small GTPases and polarity proteins in cell polarization. *Nat. Rev. Mol. Cell Biol.* **2008**, *9*, 846–859.
68. Qian, L.; Wythe, J.D.; Liu, J.; Cartry, J.; Vogler, G.; Mohapatra, B.; Otway, R.T.; Huang, Y.; King, I.N.; Maillet, M.; *et al.* Tinman/Nkx2–5 acts via miR-1 and upstream of Cdc42 to regulate heart function across species. *J. Cell Biol.* **2011**, *193*, 1181–1196.
69. Vogler, G.; Liu, J.; Iafe, T.W.; Migh, E.; Mihály, J.; Bodmer, R. Cdc42 and formin activity control non-muscle myosin dynamics during Drosophila heart morphogenesis. *J. Cell Biol.* **2014**, *206*, 909–922.
70. Swope, D.; Kramer, J.; King, T.R.; Cheng, Y.-S.; Kramer, S.G. Cdc42 is required in a genetically distinct subset of cardiac cells during Drosophila dorsal vessel closure. *Dev. Biol.* **2014**, *392*, 221–232.
71. Veerkamp, J.; Rudolph, F.; Cseresnyes, Z.; Priller, F.; Otten, C.; Renz, M.; Schaefer, L.; Abdelilah-Seyfried, S. Unilateral dampening of BMP activity by nodal generates cardiac left-right asymmetry. *Dev. Cell* **2013**, *24*, 660–667.
72. Brandt, R.; Paululat, A. Microcompartments in the Drosophila heart and the mammalian brain: General features and common principles. *Biol. Chem.* **2013**, *394*, 217–230.
73. Haack, T.; Schneider, M.; Schwendele, B.; Renault, A.D. Drosophila heart cell movement to the midline occurs through both cell autonomous migration and dorsal closure. *Dev. Biol.* **2014**, *396*, 169–182.
74. Reim, I.; Hollfelder, D.; Ismat, A.; Frasch, M. The FGF8-related signals Pyramus and Thisbe promote pathfinding, substrate adhesion, and survival of migrating longitudinal gut muscle founder cells. *Dev. Biol.* **2012**, *368*, 28–43.
75. Harrison, M.M.; Jenkins, B.V.; O'Connor-Giles, K.M.; Wildonger, J. A crispr view of development. *Genes Dev.* **2014**, *28*, 1859–1872.
76. Mohr, S.E.; Smith, J.A.; Shamu, C.E.; Neumüller, R.A.; Perrimon, N. RNAi screening comes of age: Improved techniques and complementary approaches. *Nat. Rev. Mol. Cell Biol.* **2014**, *15*, 591–600.
77. Gratz, S.J.; Cummings, A.M.; Nguyen, J.N.; Hamm, D.C.; Donohue, L.K.; Harrison, M.M.; Wildonger, J.; O'Connor-Giles, K.M. Genome engineering of Drosophila with the CRISPR RNA-guided Cas9 nuclease. *Genetics* **2013**, *194*, 1029–1035.
78. Long, C.; McAnally, J.R.; Shelton, J.M.; Mireault, A.A.; Bassel-Duby, R.; Olson, E.N. Prevention of muscular dystrophy in mice by CRISPR/Cas9-mediated editing of germline DNA. *Science* **2014**, *345*, 1184–1188.
79. Bier, E. Drosophila, the golden bug, emerges as a tool for human genetics. *Nat. Rev. Genet.* **2005**, *6*, 9–23.
80. Xin, M.; Olson, E.N.; Bassel-Duby, R. Mending broken hearts: Cardiac development as a basis for adult heart regeneration and repair. *Nat. Rev. Mol. Cell Biol.* **2013**, *14*, 529–541.
81. Tullio, A.N.; Accili, D.; Ferrans, V.J.; Yu, Z.X.; Takeda, K.; Grinberg, A.; Westphal, H.; Preston, Y.A.; Adelstein, R.S. Nonmuscle myosin II-B is required for normal development of the mouse heart. *Proc. Natl. Acad. Sci. USA* **1997**, *94*, 12407–12412.
82. Albrecht, S.; Altenhein, B.; Paululat, A. The transmembrane receptor uncoordinated5 (UNC5) is essential for heart lumen formation in Drosophila melanogaster. *Dev. Biol.* **2011**, *350*, 89–100.

83. Macabenta, F.D.; Jensen, A.G.; Cheng, Y.-S.; Kramer, J.J.; Kramer, S.G. Frazzled/DCC facilitates cardiac cell outgrowth and attachment during Drosophila dorsal vessel formation. *Dev.Biol.* **2013**, *380*, 233–242.
84. Lai Wing Sun, K.; Correia, J.P.; Kennedy, T.E. Netrins: Versatile extracellular cues with diverse functions. *Development* **2011**, *138*, 2153–2169.
85. Santiago-Martínez, E.; Soplop, N.H.; Kramer, S.G. Lateral positioning at the dorsal midline: Slit and roundabout receptors guide Drosophila heart cell migration. *Proc. Natl. Acad. Sci. USA* **2006**, *103*, 12441–12446.
86. Medioni, C.; Bertrand, N.; Mesbah, K.; Hudry, B.; Dupays, L.; Wolstein, O.; Washkowitz, A.J.; Papaioannou, V.E.; Mohun, T.J.; Harvey, R.P.; *et al.* Expression of Slit and Robo genes in the developing mouse heart. *Dev. Dyn.* **2010**, *239*, 3303–3311.
87. Frasch, M. Induction of visceral and cardiac mesoderm by ectodermal Dpp in the early Drosophila embryo. *Nature* **1995**, *374*, 464–467.
88. Rojas, A.; de Val, S.; Heidt, A.B.; Xu, S.-M.; Bristow, J.; Black, B.L. GATA4 expression in lateral mesoderm is downstream of BMP4 and is activated directly by Forkhead and GATA transcription factors through a distal enhancer element. *Development* **2005**, *132*, 3405–3417.
89. Park, M.; Wu, X.; Golden, K.; Axelrod, J.D.; Bodmer, R. The wingless signaling pathway is directly involved in Drosophila heart development. *Dev. Biol.* **1996**, *177*, 104–116.
90. Ueno, S.; Weidinger, G.; Osugi, T.; Kohn, A.D.; Golob, J.L.; Pabon, L.; Reinecke, H.; Moon, R.T.; Murry, C.E. Biphasic role for WNT/beta-catenin signaling in cardiac specification in zebrafish and embryonic stem cells. *Proc. Natl. Acad. Sci. USA* **2007**, *104*, 9685–9690.
91. Wilson, N.H.; Key, B. Neogenin: One receptor, many functions. *Int. J. Biochem. Cell Biol.* **2007**, *39*, 874–878.
92. Wilson, R.; Vogelsang, E.; Leptin, M. FGF signalling and the mechanism of mesoderm spreading in Drosophila embryos. *Development* **2005**, *132*, 491–501.
93. Marguerie, A.; Bajolle, F.; Zaffran, S.; Brown, N.A.; Dickson, C.; Buckingham, M.E.; Kelly, R.G. Congenital heart defects in Fgfr2-IIIb and Fgf10 mutant mice. *Cardiovasc. Res.* **2006**, *71*, 50–60.
94. Niessen, K.; Karsan, A. Notch signaling in cardiac development. *Circ. Res.* **2008**, *102*, 1169–1181.
95. Navankasattusas, S.; Whitehead, K.J.; Suli, A.; Sorensen, L.K.; Lim, A.H.; Zhao, J.; Park, K.W.; Wythe, J.D.; Thomas, K.R.; Chien, C.-B.; *et al.* The netrin receptor UNC5B promotes angiogenesis in specific vascular beds. *Development* **2008**, *135*, 659–667.
96. Hartmann, D.; de Strooper, B.; Serneels, L.; Craessaerts, K.; Herreman, A.; Annaert, W.; Umans, L.; Lubke, T.; Lena Illert, A.; von Figura, K.; *et al.* The disintegrin/metalloprotease ADAM 10 is essential for notch signalling but not for alpha-secretase activity in fibroblasts. *Hum. Mol. Genet.* **2002**, *11*, 2615–2624.
97. Maillet, M.; Lynch, J.M.; Sanna, B.; York, A.J.; Zheng, Y.; Molkentin, J.D. Cdc42 is an antihypertrophic molecular switch in the mouse heart. *J. Clin. Investig.* **2009**, *119*, 3079–3088.
98. Rasi, K.; Piuhola, J.; Czabanka, M.; Sormunen, R.; Ilves, M.; Leskinen, H.; Rysä, J.; Kerkelä, R.; Janmey, P.; Heljasvaara, R.; *et al.* Collagen XV is necessary for modeling of the extracellular matrix and its deficiency predisposes to cardiomyopathy. *Circ. Res.* **2010**, *107*, 1241–1252.

99. Eklund, L.; Piuhola, J.; Komulainen, J.; Sormunen, R.; Ongvarrasopone, C.; Fássler, R.; Muona, A.; Ilves, M.; Ruskoaho, H.; Takala, T.E.; *et al*. Lack of type XV collagen causes a skeletal myopathy and cardiovascular defects in mice. *Proc. Natl. Acad. Sci. USA* **2001**, *98*, 1194–1199.
100. Lo, P.C.H.; Zaffran, S.; Sénatore, S.; Frasch, M. The Drosophila hand gene is required for remodeling of the developing adult heart and midgut during metamorphosis. *Dev. Biol.* **2007**, *311*, 287–296.
101. Han, Z.; Olson, E.N. Hand is a direct target of tinman and GATA factors during Drosophila cardiogenesis and hematopoiesis. *Development* **2005**, *132*, 3525–3536.
102. Firulli, A.B.; McFadden, D.G.; Lin, Q.; Srivastava, D.; Olson, E.N. Heart and extra-embryonic mesodermal defects in mouse embryos lacking the bHLH transcription factor hand1. *Nat. Genet.* **1998**, *18*, 266–270.
103. Cheng, Z.; Lib, L.; Li, Z.; Liu, M.; Yan, J.; Wang, B.; Ma, X. Two novel hand1 mutations in chinese patients with ventricular septal defect. *Clin. Chim. Acta* **2012**, *413*, 675–677.
104. Cripps, R.M.; Lovato, T.L.; Olson, E.N. Positive autoregulation of the myocyte enhancer factor-2 myogenic control gene during somatic muscle development in Drosophila. *Dev. Biol.* **2004**, *267*, 536–547.
105. Lilly, B.; Zhao, B.; Ranganayakulu, G.; Paterson, B.M.; Schulz, R.A.; Olson, E.N. Requirement of MADS domain transcription factor D-MEF2 for muscle formation in Drosophila. *Science* **1995**, *267*, 688–693.
106. Lin, Q.; Schwarz, J.; Bucana, C.; Olson, E.N. Control of mouse cardiac morphogenesis and myogenesis by transcription factor mef2c. *Science* **1997**, *276*, 1404–1407.
107. Naya, F.J.; Black, B.L.; Wu, H.; Bassel-Duby, R.; Richardson, J.A.; Hill, J.A.; Olson, E.N. Mitochondrial deficiency and cardiac sudden death in mice lacking the MEF2A transcription factor. *Nat. Med.* **2002**, *8*, 1303–1309.
108. Bruneau, B.G.; Nemer, G.; Schmitt, J.P.; Charron, F.; Robitaille, L.; Caron, S.; Conner, D.A.; Gessler, M.; Nemer, M.; Seidman, C.E.; *et al.* A murine model of holt-oram syndrome defines roles of the T-box transcription factor TBX5 in cardiogenesis and disease. *Cell* **2001**, *106*, 709–721.
109. Harrelson, Z.; Kelly, R.G.; Goldin, S.N.; Gibson-Brown, J.J.; Bollag, R.J.; Silver, L.M.; Papaioannou, V.E. TBX2 is essential for patterning the atrioventricular canal and for morphogenesis of the outflow tract during heart development. *Development* **2004**, *131*, 5041–5052.
110. Bakker, M.L.; Boukens, B.J.; Mommersteeg, M.T.M.; Brons, J.F.; Wakker, V.; Moorman, A.F.M.; Christoffels, V.M. Transcription factor TBX3 is required for the specification of the atrioventricular conduction system. *Circ. Res.* **2008**, *102*, 1340–1349.
111. Junion, G.; Bataillé, L.; Jagla, T.; Da Ponte, J.P.; Tapin, R.; Jagla, K. Genome-wide view of cell fate specification: Ladybird acts at multiple levels during diversification of muscle and heart precursors. *Genes Dev.* **2007**, *21*, 3163–3180.
112. Jagla, K.; Jagla, T.; Heitzler, P.; Dretzen, G.; Bellard, F.; Bellard, M. Ladybird, a tandem of homeobox genes that maintain late wingless expression in terminal and dorsal epidermis of the Drosophila embryo. *Development* **1997**, *124*, 91–100.
113. Schäfer, K.; Neuhaus, P.; Kruse, J.; Braun, T. The homeobox gene Lbx1 specifies a subpopulation of cardiac neural crest necessary for normal heart development. *Circ. Res.* **2003**, *92*, 73–80.

114. Reim, I.; Mohler, J.P.; Frasch, M. TBX20-related genes, mid and H15, are required for tinman expression, proper patterning, and normal differentiation of cardioblasts in Drosophila. *Mech. Dev.* **2005**, *122*, 1056–1069.
115. Kirk, E.P.; Sunde, M.; Costa, M.W.; Rankin, S.A.; Wolstein, O.; Castro, M.L.; Butler, T.L.; Hyun, C.; Guo, G.; Otway, R.; *et al.* Mutations in cardiac T-box factor gene TBX20 are associated with diverse cardiac pathologies, including defects of septation and valvulogenesis and cardiomyopathy. *Am. J. Hum. Genet.* **2007**, *81*, 280–291.
116. Hammer, S.; Toenjes, M.; Lange, M.; Fischer, J.J.; Dunkel, I.; Mebus, S.; Grimm, C.H.; Hetzer, R.; Berger, F.; Sperling, S. Characterization of TBX20 in human hearts and its regulation by TFAP2. *J. Cell. Biochem.* **2008**, *104*, 1022–1033.
117. Alvarez, A.D.; Shi, W.; Wilson, B.A.; Skeath, J.B. Pannier and pointedP2 act sequentially to regulate Drosophila heart development. *Development* **2003**, *130*, 3015–3026.
118. Gajewski, K.; Fossett, N.; Molkentin, J.D.; Schulz, R.A. The zinc finger proteins pannier and GATA4 function as cardiogenic factors in Drosophila. *Development* **1999**, *126*, 5679–5688.
119. Zhou, P.; He, A.; Pu, W.T. Regulation of GATA4 transcriptional activity. In *Cardiovascular Development and Disease*; Academic Press: Waltham, MA, USA, 2012; Volume 100, pp. 143–169.
120. Pereira, F.A.; Qiu, Y.; Zhou, G.; Tsai, M.J.; Tsai, S.Y. The orphan nuclear receptor COUP-TFII is required for angiogenesis and heart development. *Genes Dev.* **1999**, *13*, 1037–1049.
121. Zmojdzian, M.; Jagla, K. Tailup plays multiple roles during cardiac outflow assembly in Drosophila. *Cell Tissue Res.* **2013**, *354*, 639–645.
122. Cai, C.-L.; Liang, X.; Shi, Y.; Chu, P.-H.; Pfaff, S.L.; Chen, J.; Evans, S. Isl1 identifies a cardiac progenitor population that proliferates prior to differentiation and contributes a majority of cells to the heart. *Dev. Cell* **2003**, *5*, 877–889.
123. Akazawa, H.; Komuro, I. Cardiac transcription factor Csx/Nkx2-5: Its role in cardiac development and diseases. *Pharmacol. Ther.* **2005**, *107*, 252–268.

2

Targeted *Mybpc3* Knock-Out Mice with Cardiac Hypertrophy Exhibit Structural Mitral Valve Abnormalities

Daniel P. Judge [1,2], Hany Neamatalla [3,4], Russell A. Norris [5], Robert A. Levine [6], Jonathan T. Butcher [7], Nicolas Vignier [8], Kevin H. Kang [7], Quangtung Nguyen [4], Patrick Bruneval [1,9], Marie-Cécile Perier [3], Emmanuel Messas [1,3], Xavier Jeunemaitre [1,3], Annemarieke de Vlaming [5], Roger Markwald [5], Lucie Carrier [10] and Albert A. Hagège [1,3,4,*]

[1] Faculté de Médecine, Université Paris Descartes, Sorbonne Paris Cité, Paris 75005 France; E-Mails: djudge@jhmi.edu (D.P.J.); patrick.bruneval@egp.aphp.fr (P.B.); emmanuel.messas@egp.aphp.fr (E.M.); xavier.jeunemaitre@inserm.fr (X.J.)

[2] Division of Cardiology, Johns Hopkins University, Baltimore, MD 21287, USA

[3] Paris Cardiovascular Research Center, INSERM U970, Paris 75016 France; E-Mails: hnematalla@hotmail.com (H.N.); marie-cecile.perier@inserm.fr (M.-C.P.)

[4] Department of Cardiology, Assistance Publique-Hôpitaux de Paris, Hôpital Européen Georges Pompidou, Paris 75016 France; E-mail: quangtungdhyhn@yahoo.com (Q.N.)

[5] Department of Regenerative Medicine and Cell Biology, Medical University of South Carolina, Charleston, SC 29403, USA; E-Mails: norrisra@musc.edu (R.A.N.); annemarieke.de.vlaming@gmail.com (A.V.); markwald@musc.edu (R.M.)

[6] Cardiac Ultrasound Laboratory, Massachusetts General Hospital and Harvard Medical School, Boston, MA 02114 USA; E-Mail: rlevine@partners.org

[7] Department of Biomedical Engineering, Cornell University, Ithaca, NY 14853 USA; E-Mails: jtb47@cornell.edu (J.T.B.); hk576@cornell.edu (K.H.K.)

[8] INSERM U582, University Pierre et Marie Curie-Paris 6, IFR14, Paris 75005 France; E-Mail: vigniernicolas@yahoo.fr

[9] Institut de recherche des Cordeliers, INSERM U652, Paris 75005, France

[10] Institute of Experimental and Clinical Pharmacology and Toxicology, University Medical Center Hamburg-Eppendorf, Hamburg 20246, Germany; E-Mail: l.carrier@uke.de

* Author to whom correspondence should be addressed; E-Mail: albert.hagege@egp.aphp.fr

Academic Editor: Cheryl L. Maslen

Abstract: *MYBPC3* mutations cause hypertrophic cardiomyopathy, which is frequently associated with mitral valve (MV) pathology. We reasoned that increased MV size is caused by localized growth factors with paracrine effects. We used high-resolution echocardiography to compare *Mybpc3*-null, heterozygous, and wild-type mice (n = 84, aged 3–6 months) and micro-CT for MV volume (n = 6, age 6 months). *Mybpc3*-null mice showed left ventricular hypertrophy, dilation, and systolic dysfunction compared to heterozygous and wild-type mice, but no systolic anterior motion of the MV or left ventricular outflow obstruction. Compared to wild-type mice, echocardiographic anterior leaflet length (adjusted for left ventricular size) was greatest in *Mybpc3*-null mice (1.92 ± 0.08 *vs.* 1.72 ± 0.08 mm, $p < 0.001$), as was combined leaflet thickness (0.23 ± 0.04 *vs.* 0.15 ± 0.02 mm, $p < 0.001$). Micro-CT analyses of *Mybpc3*-null mice demonstrated increased MV volume (0.47 ± 0.06 *vs.* 0.15 ± 0.06 mm^3, $p = 0.018$) and thickness (0.35 ± 0.04 *vs.* 0.12 ± 0.04 mm, $p = 0.002$), coincident with increased markers of TGFβ activity compared to heterozygous and wild-type littermates. Similarly, excised MV from a patient with *MYBPC3* mutation showed increased TGFβ activity. We conclude that MYBPC3 deficiency causes hypertrophic cardiomyopathy with increased MV leaflet length and thickness despite the absence of left ventricular outflow-tract obstruction, in parallel with increased TGFβ activity. MV changes in hypertrophic cardiomyopathy may be due to paracrine effects, which represent targets for therapeutic studies.

Keywords: mitral valve; TGFβ; hypertrophic cardiomyopathy

1. Introduction

Mitral valve (MV) abnormalities occur commonly in hypertrophic cardiomyopathy (HCM) [1]. The most frequent and predominant changes include elongation of the anterior (AML) and/or posterior (PML) mitral leaflets and anterior displacement of the MV and papillary muscles within the left ventricular cavity [2]. These changes and their severity contribute to both the initiation and magnitude of systolic anterior motion (SAM) of the MV with variable dynamic left ventricular outflow tract (LVOT) obstruction and, consequently, mitral regurgitation (MR) due to MV deformation with inadequate leaflet coaptation [3–6]. The etiology of MV leaflet elongation in this setting is not well understood, but it has long been attributed to turbulence in the LVOT leading to repeated deformation and stretch of the MV [7]. Recent investigation with 3-D echocardiography demonstrated that individuals with HCM and LVOT obstruction have larger MV leaflets than those with HCM without LVOT obstruction, yet both groups had greater MV area than normal controls [8]. If LVOT turbulence were required for MV enlargement, then we would not expect MV enlargement in people without a significant LVOT gradient.

Several other factors have been recognized as contributing to increased MV length and thickness in other disorders. In a murine model of Marfan syndrome with MV prolapse, fibrillin-1 deficiency results in diminished binding of the latent form of TGFβ and localized increase in this growth factor, accompanied by increased Ki67-positive cells in the MV [9]. Antagonism of TGFβ leads to normalization of MV length and thickness in that model [9]. X-linked MVP is caused by missense mutations in *FLNA*, the gene encoding filamin A [10]. Developmental studies in filamin-A-deficient mice show perturbation of matrix remodeling in AV valves [11]. Chromosomal loci have been recognized to associate with non-syndromic familial MV prolapse with prolongation and thickening of the valve leaflets [12–14]. In contrast with some of these conditions, MV disease in HCM is typically fibrotic rather than myxomatous, yet overlap among these disorders provides rationale for the hypothesis that they share common pathophysiology.

Loss-of-function mutations in *MYBPC3*, encoding cardiac myosin binding protein C (cMyBP-C), are a common cause of HCM in people [15,16]. Mice with *Mybpc3* knockout (–/–) develop concentric ventricular hypertrophy with histopathological features of HCM [17]. Importantly, these mice do not have SAM or LVOT obstruction in the setting of diminished systolic LV function. Although there are no reports of humans with homozygous null *MYBPC3* mutations, there are reports of people with severe LVH due to compound heterozygous truncating mutations in this gene [18,19]. We reasoned that investigation of the MV in this model of cMyBP-C deficiency could help to understand the pathogenesis of structural MV abnormalities in HCM. We hypothesized that increased growth factor production in or near the MV leaflets would arise from the *Mybpc3* mutation, and that MV pathology would occur in these mice in the absence of LVOT turbulence.

2. Experimental Section

Mice: The murine studies conform to the ARRIVE guidelines, and the protocol was approved by the Paris Cardiovascular Research Center's Animal Care and Use Committee. Development of *Mybc3* (–/–) mice on a C57Bl/6 background strain was previously reported [17]. They were housed in a sterile facility at the Paris Cardiovascular Research Center using a standard diet.

Echocardiography: All echocardiograms were performed on adult mice aged 3–6 months, sedated with isofluorane using a VisualSonics Vevo 2100 imaging system and an MS400 (18–38 MHz) transducer (Fujifilm SonoSite, Inc.; Tokyo, Japan). The resolution for this device is 30 microns. The MV was imaged using a modified parasternal long axis view. Three separate measurements of the maximal diastolic length and thickness (at the mid-part of the leaflet) of AML and PML were obtained by a single observer blinded to the genotype of the mice on acquired cineloops using the zoom feature of the system, and a mean was calculated. Standard measures of the LV size, wall thickness, systolic LV function and left atrial anteroposterior dimension were included. We systematically searched for SAM using two-dimensional echocardiography and for LVOT flow acceleration using pulsed Doppler. Others have shown good correlation between this type of high frequency echocardiography and cardiac MRI in mice [20].

Micro-CT: Three consecutive mice of (–/–) and (+/+) genotype were chosen for high-resolution microCT imaging. MV annulus with intact leaflets and papillary muscle attachments were excised from mouse hearts after fixation in 10% buffered formalin. Cardiac muscle tissue was trimmed away from the annulus and chordal insertion sites prior to gross anatomical analysis and bright-field imaging. Leaflets were transferred to conical tubes containing 1% phosphotungstenic acid and imaged using Micro-CT as previously described [21]. Average leaflet thickness and volume and total leaflet area were measured using Microview (GE), an automated system that independently defines tissue boundaries, with a 25 μM^3 resolution.

Histology: Hearts were fixed in 10% buffered formalin, embedded in paraffin, and sectioned according to standard techniques [9]. Briefly, hearts were transected in the parasternal long axis to expose the MV and sectioned until MV leaflets were visible on unstained slides. Additional sections (10 μM thick, 4–6 sections) were mounted onto slides for additional analysis. To assess these MV leaflets for increased collagen, staining with modified Movat's techniques was performed in three mice of each +/+ and −/− genotypes. Immunostaining for periostin was performed using a rabbit polyclonal antibody (Abcam #ab14041) in three mice of each +/+ and −/− genotypes. To assess for additional markers of TGFβ signaling, immunostaining for phosphorylated Smad2 (pSmad2) was performed using a rabbit polyclonal antibody (Millipore #AB3849, Merck KGaA, Darmstadt, Germany) in three mice of each +/+ and −/− genotypes. Standard chromogens (Diaminobenzidine (DAB) or 3-Amino-9-Ethylcarbazole (AEC)) were used according to manufacturer's protocols (Vector Laboratories, Inc; Burlingame, CA; USA). All images were reviewed, and the amount of chromogen corresponding to target ligand was assessed by three blinded investigators. Relative quantification was determined by an arbitrary scale, ranging from (1) for no staining, to (5) for prominent staining; histology scores were averaged among the three observers. These investigations were used to support more quantitative methods of mRNA and protein analysis when differences were identified.

RNA analysis: In order to quantify differences observed with immunostaining, qRT-PCR expression assays were used to compare the mRNA expression of two genes that are induced by TGFβ: *Postn* encoding periostin and *Ctgf* encoding connective tissue growth factor (CTGF). The expression of these genes was compared in (+/+) and *Mybpc3* (−/−) MV, adjacent septum, and apex of the LV. For RNA extraction hearts were flushed with normal saline, and the MV was removed with a dissecting microscope, followed by immersion in Trizol (Invitrogen, Thermo Fisher Scientific, Waltham, MA, USA. Sections of adjacent (septum) and distant (apex) LV myocardium were also dissected and immersed in Trizol. RNA was extracted as previously reported [9]. Real-time PCR reactions were performed and analyzed using ABI PRISM 7900 (Applied Biosystems, Thermo Fisher Scientific, Waltham, MA, USA). Levels of mRNA for *Ctgf* and *Postn* were assessed in relation to expression of *Gapdh* using specific primer-probe from Applied Biosystems. Each experiment was performed in triplicate, blinded to MV imaging results, with three consecutive mice of each genotype at 6 months of age and with specimens from the same site in each genotype.

Protein analysis: Murine MV leaflets were dissected and snap frozen in lysis buffer. After homogenization, protein was quantified and equal amounts (4 μg) separated by gel electrophoresis as previously described [22]. The periostin primary antibody for Western analysis was generously provided by S. Hoffman, Medical University of South Carolina, Charleston, SC, USA. Periostin was normalized to β-actin to account for differences in protein loading.

Complementary human studies: Written informed consent was obtained from the individual who provided MV tissue. The study was conducted in accordance with the Declaration of Helsinki, and the protocol was approved by the Ethics Committee (CPP Ile de France VI, 25 June 2008) and Biomedicine Agency for genetic studies approval (12 December 2008). Movat's staining and immunohistochemical analyses were performed per standard protocols and as previously described (20). Proteins were extracted from excised MV leaflets of a 71-year-old patient with non-obstructive HCM due to

MYBPC3 mutation who underwent mitral valve surgery for chordal rupture and from normal control valves (n = 3, obtained from normal hearts that were not used for cardiac transplant) that had been previously processed, sectioned, and mounted. Valve sections were photographed and area measurements were used to equalize tissue amounts. Proteins were de-crosslinked and extracted using the Qproteome FFPE Tissue Extraction Kit according to manufacturer's recommendations (Qiagen, Hilden, Germany). Extracted protein lysate was mixed with appropriate amounts of 2 × SDS page loading dye and run on denaturing SDS-PAGE. Blots were probed with an α-Collagen-I antibody (1:1000, MD Biosciences GmbH, Zürich, Switzerland) and a secondary HRP-labeled goat-anti-rabbit antibody (Sigma-Aldrich, St. Louis, MO, USA) (1:7500). Bands were detected with Super Signal West Femto Substrate (Thermo Fisher Scientific, Waltham, MA, USA) and densitometric analyses were performed using Adobe Photoshop CS5. Analyses were performed in triplicate and results are graphically depicted.

Statistics: Statistical analysis for the MV comparisons used the SAS version 9.2 (statistical analysis system, Cary, NC, USA). MV leaflet length, LV end-diastolic volume and LV mass reached statistical criteria for normal distribution across groups, allowing the use of analysis of variance for comparisons. Comparisons of variables across groups were performed using analysis of variance without and with adjustment for LV mass and LV end-diastolic volume. A two-tailed p value <0.05 was considered as statistically significant. Pairwise comparisons were also analyzed using analysis of variance and p-value, adjusted for multiple testing (Tukey adjustment). Intra-observer and inter-observer variability of ultrasonic measurements was assessed blindly by linear regression analysis (R^2) using five separate measures in randomly chosen mice of the three genotypes ($N = 15$ for each). Results are provided with mean ± standard deviation, range.

3. Results and Discussion

3.1. Mybpc3 (−/−) Anterior Mitral Leaflet is Longer and Thicker than Wild-Type Anterior Mitral Leaflet by Echocardiographic Analysis

Data acquired by echocardiography are summarized in Table 1. The *Mybpc3* (−/−) mice had LV globular dilation with increased wall thickness and mass compared to both wild-type (+/+) and heterozygous (+/−) mice as previously reported [17]; neither SAM nor LVOT flow acceleration was present. The length of the anterior MV leaflet was greater in the (−/−) mice than in the (+/−) and (+/+) mice (1.92 ± 0.08 *vs.* 1.73 ± 0.07 *vs.* 1.73 ± 0.08 mm, respectively; $p < 0.0001$). After correction for LV mass, as well as for LV end-diastolic volume (EDV), or both, these differences remained highly significant ($p < 0.001$) (Figure 1, Table 1). The length of the posterior MV leaflet was similar in all three groups of mice. The aggregate MV leaflet thickness (AML + PML thickness) in (−/−) was greater than in (+/+) mice (0.23 ± 0.04 *vs.* 0.15 ± 0.02 mm, respectively; $p < 0.001$). Analysis of reproducibility of the echocardiographic measurements showed small intra-observer and inter-observer variability, with calculated R^2 of 0.88 and 0.90, respectively.

3.2. MicroCT Imaging Confirms the Results of Echocardiographic Imaging

The MV volume by microCT was greater in (−/−) mice than (+/+) mice (0.47 ± 0.06 *vs.* 0.15 ± 0.06 mm^3, respectively; $p = 0.018$). Similarly, the MV thickness in (−/−) mice was greater than in (+/+) mice (0.35 ± 0.02 *vs.* 0.12 ± 0.02 mm, respectively; $p = 0.002$). Total leaflet surface area was 7.35 ± 0.84 mm^2 in (+/+) mice *vs.* 3.68 ± 1.16 mm^2 in (+/+) mice ($p = 0.06$).

Table 1. Cardiac findings using high resolution echocardiography.

Parameter	+/+ N = 22	+/− N = 33	−/− N = 29	*p*
Length AML (mm)	1.72 ± 0.08 (1.64–1.94)	1.73 ± 0.07 (1.55–1.90)	1.92 ± 0.08 (1.80–2.09)	<0.001 *
Length PML (mm)	1.36 ± 0.07 (1.23–1.46)	1.33 ± 0.07 (1.20–1.45)	1.35 ± 0.07 (1.23–1.51)	NS *
Thickness AML + PML (mm)	0.15 ± 0.02 (0.11–0.18)	0.18 ± 0.04 (0.10–0.19)	0.23 ± 0.04 (0.14–0.29)	<0.001 *
LV Mass (mg)	80 ± 16 (55–109)	88 ± 7 (71–105)	129 ± 26 (99–173)	<0.0001
EF (%)	63 ± 5 (55–76)	62 ± 7 (52–80)	35 ± 7 (22–49)	<0.0001
ED Volume (mL)	67 ± 11 (43–88)	63 ± 11 (39–89)	118 ± 40 (42–175)	<0.0001

(*) indicates *p* values that are adjusted for LV mass and end-diastolic volume. Results are expressed as mean ± SD (range). All mice are age 3–6 months.

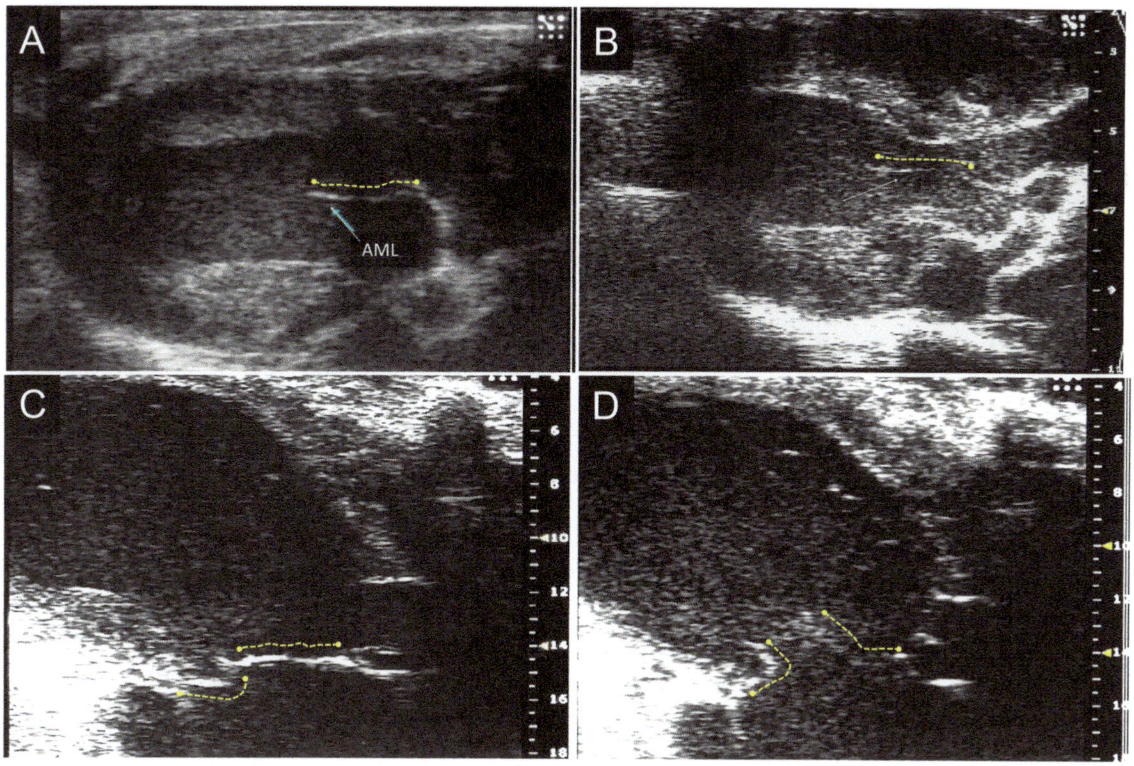

Figure 1. Imaging of the MV by high-resolution echocardiography. Representative echocardiographic images are shown from *Mybpc3* (−/−) (**A**,**C**,**D**) and (+/+); (**B**) mice; arrows show AML; Systolic (**C**) and diastolic (**D**) images are shown with AML and PML highlighted.

3.3. Mybpc3-*(−/−) Mitral Valve Leaflets Have Evidence of Increased TGFβ Signaling*

TGFβ is a growth factor that has been directly implicated in HCM pathogenesis, and its activity is assessed by downstream effects [23]. The *Mybpc3* (−/−) MV leaflets have increased nuclear pSmad2 immunostaining (Figure 2). Smad2 is a receptor-activated intracellular protein that becomes phosphorylated in response to TGFβ ligand interacting with the TGFβ receptor [24]. Upon phosphorylation, it combines with Smad4 and translocates to the nucleus. Nuclear immunostaining of pSmad2 is a commonly used marker of canonical TGFβ stimulation [25].

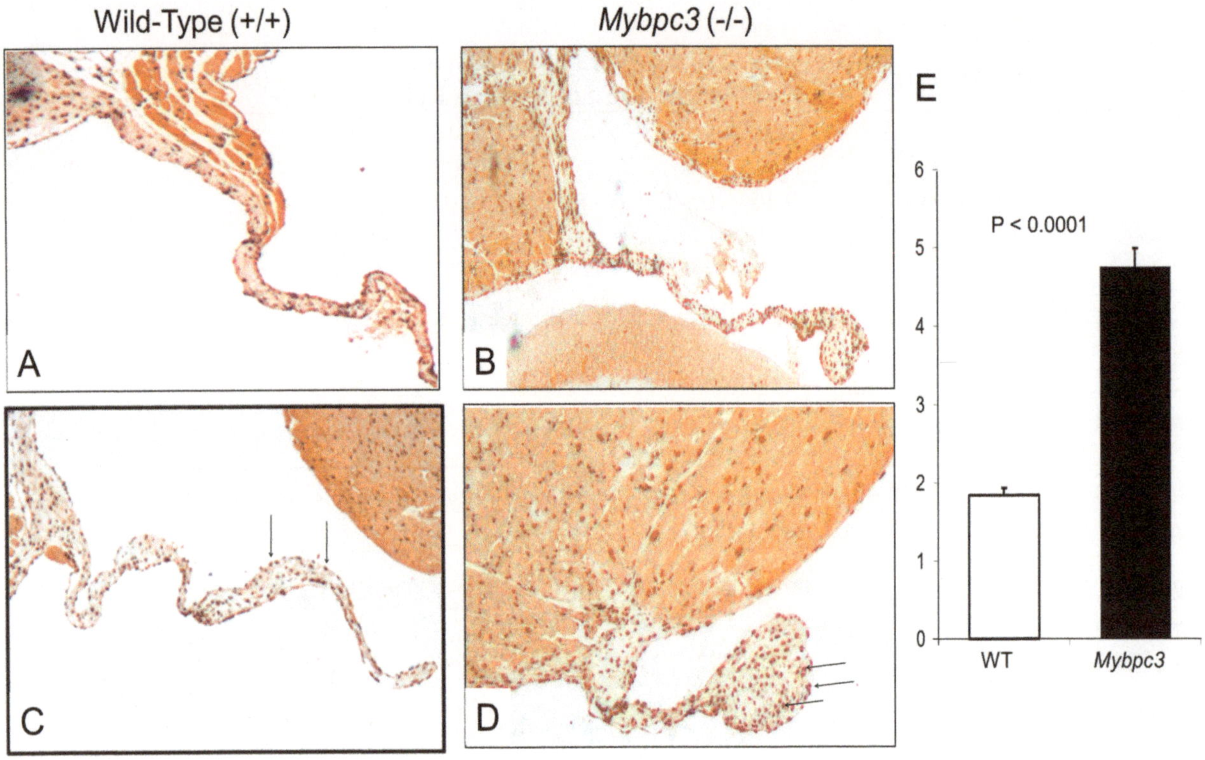

Figure 2. *Mybpc3* (−/−) MVs have increased nuclear pSmad2. Immunostaining for pSmad2 was performed using AEC as the chromogen (red) according to standard protocols (Vectorlabs). Representative 40× images are shown from (+/+) (**A**,**C**) and *Mybpc3* (−/−) (**B**,**D**) mice. Nuclear pSmad2 staining (arrows) is a marker for TGFβ activity. Relative quantification of immunostaining (**E**) was performed by blinded reviewers, using a scale from 1 (faint staining) to 5 (strong staining). Error bars show SEM.

Periostin is a secreted protein that is induced by TGFβ and regulates collagen production [22]. To investigate a downstream marker of TGFβ signaling, we analyzed periostin in both (−/−) and (+/+) mice. We reasoned that increased periostin could contribute to the MV phenotype in *Mybpc3* (−/−) mice. Indeed, immunostaining for periostin was markedly increased in the *Mybpc3* (−/−) mice compared to (+/+) mice (Figure 3). In order to quantify the increase in periostin in the *Mybpc3* (−/−) mouse MV and myocardium, we performed Western analyses (Figure 3). The ratio of periostin to β-actin in MV leaflets was greater in the (−/−) than in the (+/+) mice (3.40 ± 0.29 *vs.* 1.81 ± 0.50, respectively; p = 0.034). The ratio of periostin to β-actin in the myocardium was also greater in the (−/−) than the (+/+) mice (1.25 ± 0.01 *vs.* 0.92 ± 0.09, respectively; $p = 0.009$).

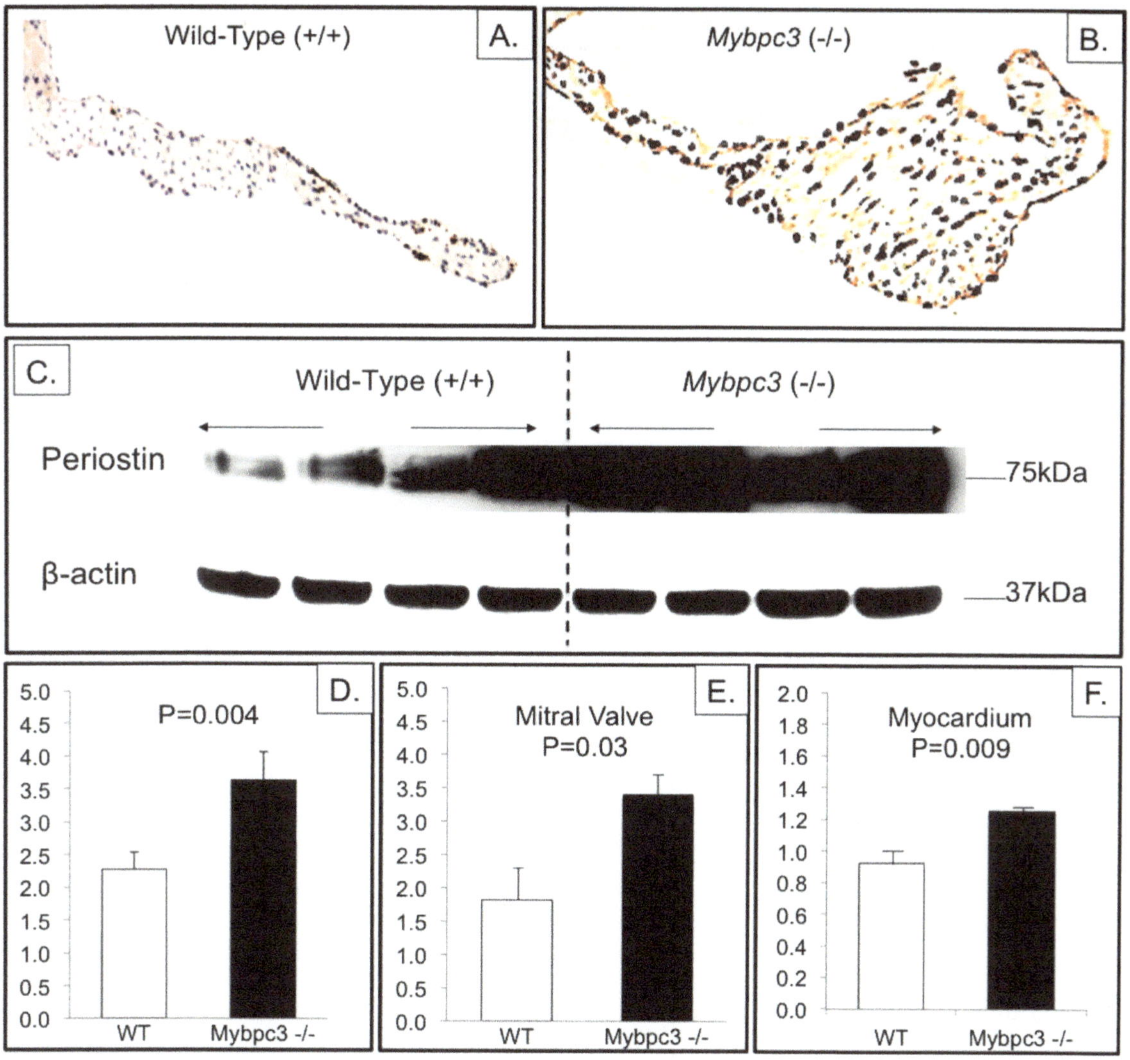

Figure 3. *Mybpc3* (−/−) MVs have increased periostin. Immunostaining for periostin was performed using DAB as the chromogen (brown). Representative low power (40×, **A**,**B**) images are shown from (+/+) (**A**) and *Mybpc3* (−/−) (**B**) mice. Increased periostin (brown) is evident in the *Mybpc3* (−/−) MV leaflets; (**C**) Western blot for quantification of periostin in MV leaflets comparing 4 (+/+) and 4 (−/−) leaflets, with use of β-actin to normalize for protein loading. Relative quantification of immunostaining (**D**) was performed by blinded reviewers using a scale from 1 (faint staining) to 5 (strong staining). Quantification of Western blots was performed by NIH ImageJ software, demonstrating increased periostin in both MV leaflets (**E**) and adjacent myocardium (**F**) in *Mybpc3* (−/−) mice compared to wild-type controls (+/+). Error bars show SEM.

Increased TGFβ activity stimulates production of collagen in MV leaflets in mice as shown using Movat's stains (Figure 4). The mouse MV leaflets in (−/−) mice have a greater abundance of collagen than in (+/+) mice, as determined by scoring for brown shading by blinded review of Movat's staining (Figure 4).

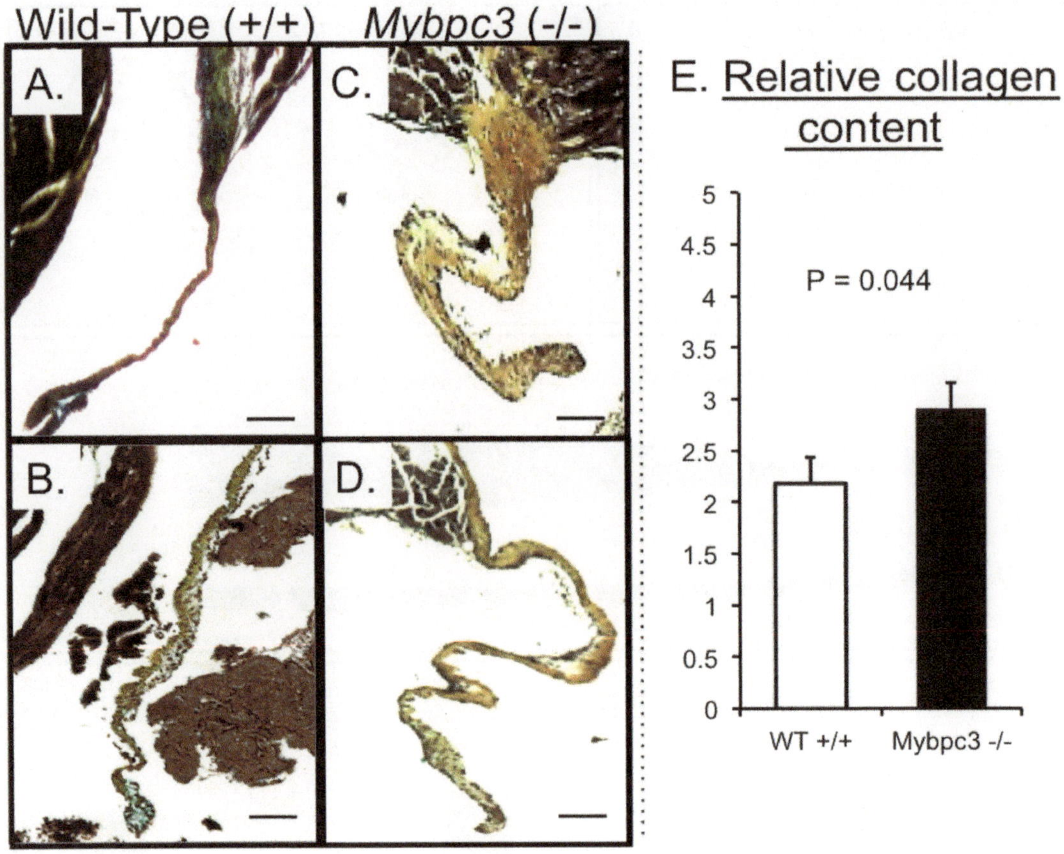

Figure 4. *Mybpc3* (−/−) MVs have more collagen. MVs were stained with modified Movat's (**A–D**). The *Mybpc3* (−/−) MV leaflets (**C,D**) show more collagen (yellow−brown in **C** and **D**) than the Wild-Type (+/+) MV leaflets (**A,B**). All size bars correspond to 100 μM. Relative quantification of collagen (**E**) on Movat's staining was performed by blinded reviewers, using a scale from 1 (blue valves without brown) to 5 (brown valves without blue). Error bars show SEM.

3.4. Quantitative PCR Analysis Confirms Increased Expression of TGFβ-Related Genes in Myocardium

Connective tissue growth factor is also produced in response to TGFβ, and increased expression of *Ctgf* mRNA has been demonstrated in another murine model with cardiac hypertrophy due to a sarcomere mutation [23]. Both the septum and apex from the *Mybpc3* (−/−) mice had markedly increased expression of *Ctgf* compared to (+/+) mice (4.2-fold increase for apex and 7.1-fold increase for septum, $p = 0.0008$ and 0.004 respectively) (Figure 5). The septum also had increased expression of *Postn* in the *Mybpc3* (−/−) compared to (+/+) mice (3.1-fold increase, $p = 0.01$), but there was similar expression of *Postn* at the apex ($p = 0.6$). The expression of genes encoding these two growth factors was similar when comparing RNA derived from the MV in the *Mybpc3* (−/−) and (+/+) mice ($p = 0.3$ for *Ctgf* and 0.5 for *Postn*) suggesting that the primary source for the increased protein present in MV leaflets is due to paracrine effects mediated by myocardial hypertrophy in adjacent myocardium.

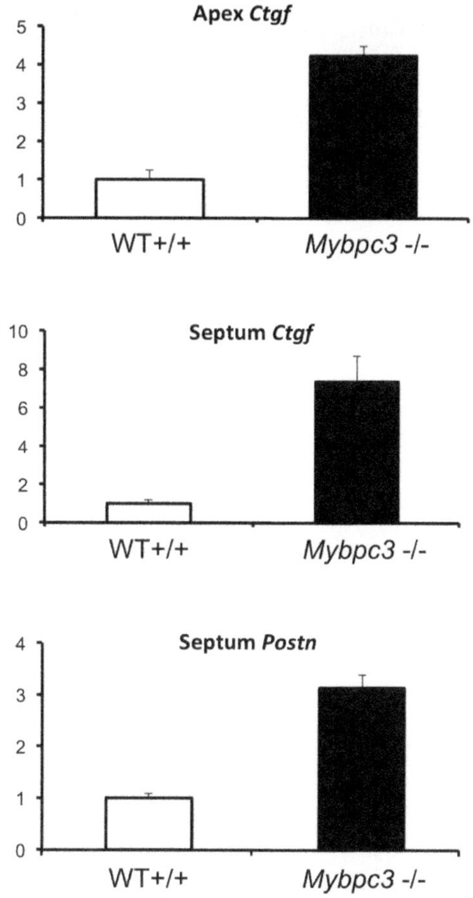

Figure 5. Increased expression of *Ctgf* and *Postn* in *Mybpc3* (−/−) hearts. The relative mRNA expression of *Ctgf*, encoding connective tissue growth factor, and *Postn*, encoding periostin, is shown with the wild-type (+/+) level set at 1.0. Bar graphs show the average relative gene quantification (N = 3 for each genotype and each tissue) with SEM.

3.5. MV Leaflets in Human Non-Obstructive Hypertrophic Cardiomyopathy (HCM) Exhibit Increase in Collagen along with Molecular Changes in TGFβ Signaling

These data were obtained to show that similar MV changes do in fact occur in the human HCM model with *MYBPC3* mutation, with histopathologic changes corresponding to the elongation described clinically by echo and anatomic pathology. It is unusual to obtain such a specimen, since these valves are only rarely excised. Therefore, only one MV specimen is available from an individual with HCM and *MYBPC3* mutation (p.Arg326Gln), which has previously been reported to cause HCM [26,27]. It was compared with normal human MVs obtained from unused normal cardiac transplant donor controls. Formalin-fixed, paraffin-embedded (FFPE) sections from an individual with *MYBPC3* mutation who underwent MV surgery were analyzed for TGFβ effectors. Immunofluorescence studies demonstrate an increase in the TGFβ-responsive extracellular matrix genes (collagen I, periostin, and hyaluronan), as well as an increase in both the TGFβ1 ligand and TGFβ1 signaling intermediate pSmad3 (Figure 6). Because TGFβ1 has previously been demonstrated as promoting a myofibroblastic phenotype during valve disease pathogenesis, we additionally examined the expression of α-smooth muscle actin (α-SMA). As shown in Figure 6, there was an increase in α-SMA expressing cells in the MV with *MYBPC3* mutation compared to controls. In order to quantify the increased level of type 1 collagen in *MYBPC3*-

mutant human MV leaflets, equal tissue volumes were analyzed by Western analysis. Proteins were de-crosslinked and isolated from deparaffinized FFPE MV tissue sections. Compared to control MV tissues, the HCM-associated MV leaflets had a >2-fold increase in collagen type I, αI (COL1A1) and a >-9-fold increase in collagen type I, α2 (COL1A2; p.0015 and .0002, respectively) (Figure 6). This demonstrates that similar MV abnormalities occurred in this person with HCM, although it is a single example. As such, it is not possible to draw broader conclusions from this individual.

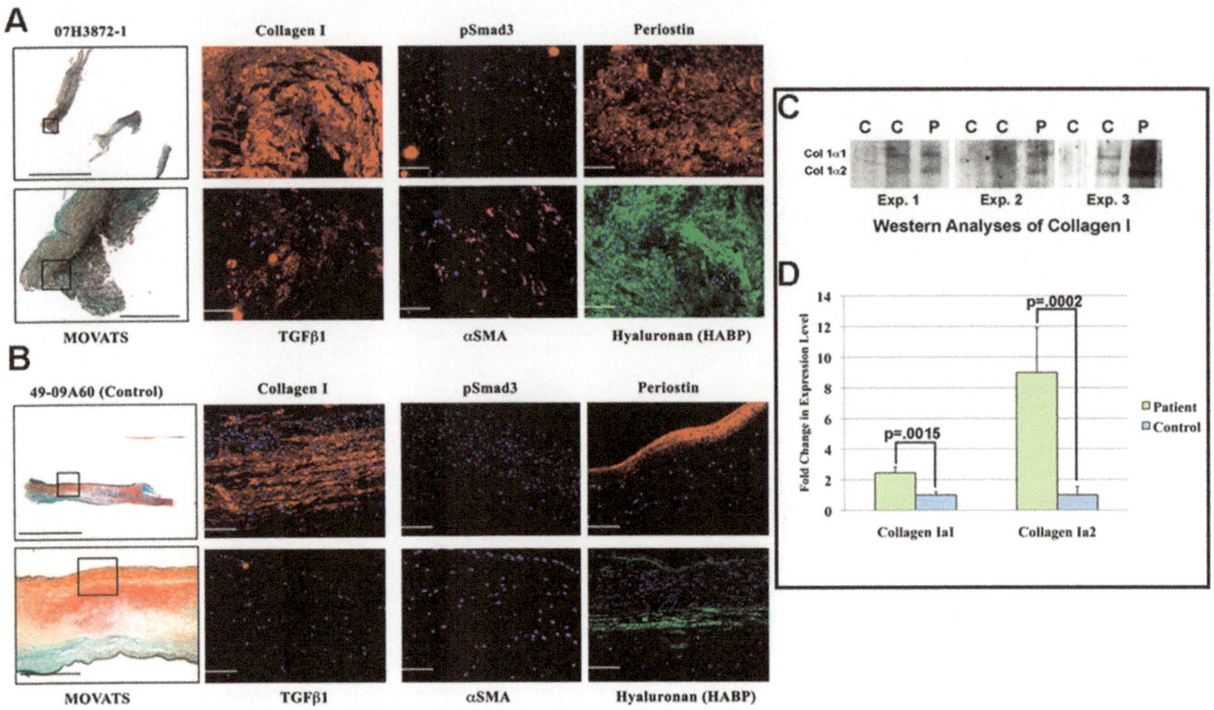

Figure 6. Comparison of excised MVs in an HCM patient with a *MYBPC3* mutation and in two normal hearts (controls, $n = 2$). Findings in the patient (**A**) and in a representative control (**B**) with histological (Movat's) and immunohistochemical stainings are shown. Boxed areas represent regions where protein stainings were captured. (**A**) The MV from the HCM patient exhibits a disruption of the normal stratified layers of the mitral leaflets with an increase in TGFβ downstream extracellular matrix proteins (collagen I, periostin, and hyaluronan). Higher levels of TGFβ1 were observed in the leaflets of the HCM valve as well as the TGFβ1 signaling intermediate, pSmad3. Moreover, α-SMA, a TGFβ-regulated gene and a marker of myofibroblast phenotype, was also increased in these leaflets. All proteins are depicted in red except hyaluronan, which is in green, while nuclei are blue; (**C**) Western analysis of excised proteins collected from the valve revealed a significant increase in both collagen 1α1 and collagen 1α2 in the HCM patient with *MYBPC3* mutation compared to the controls. Shown are each of the three Westerns performed on three different areas of the same human valve on the de-crosslinked proteins from human valve sections; they were compared against comparable areas in three separate controls (two controls are shown on the Westerns). Sample size was normalized based on similar tissue volumes used in the valve extraction procedure (see Experimental Section) (C = controls, P = patient); (**D**) Graphical depiction of fold-change in collagen expression ($N = 3$).

3.6. Discussion

Our results demonstrate that MV elongation and thickening occur in cMyBPC-null mice despite the absence of SAM or obstruction, and that the magnitude of excess tissue is independent of LV enlargement and hypertrophy. After adjustment for LV mass and size, high-resolution echocardiography shows a consistent 12% greater length in AML for the *Mybpc3* (−/−) mice, while the more detailed three-dimensional micro-CT measurements in a subset show 3-fold greater volume in the (−/−) as compared to (+/+) mice. Immunohistochemical analysis of the MV and adjacent LV myocardium in knock-out mice demonstrates increased collagen, which was also demonstrated in excised MV leaflets from an HCM patient with a *MYBPC3* mutation. Increased expression of growth factors in the LV myocardium of *Mybpc3* (−/−) strain of mice correlates with MV remodeling, which is consistent with the proposal that these growth factors contribute to its pathogenesis.

The mRNA expression of the genes encoding both periostin and CTGF was similar in the MV leaflets themselves, yet greater in the adjacent myocardium. The differences in periostin gene expression are greatest in the nearby myocardium, in contrast with the more homogeneously increased expression of CTGF. Within the MV leaflets, there is no significant difference in expression of these genes at this age (6 months), yet histological and quantitative protein (Western) analyses show increased periostin in the MV leaflets. This indicates a paracrine effect, wherein the origin of the increased protein is the adjacent myocardium, and its target is the nearby mitral valve.

Elongation of the MV leaflets commonly occurs in HCM [3,4]. A landmark study of MV abnormalities in HCM was published in 1992 [28]. In that report, the average leaflet area of the excised MV among a cohort of 94 patients with obstructive HCM was 12.9 ± 3.7 cm^2, as compared with a cohort of 45 normal controls wherein the MV leaflet area was $8.7 + 2.0$ cm^2; $p < 0.001$). Notably, the MV surface area in those with HCM widely varied, ranging from 6.3 to 23.0 cm^2, and 55 of the 94 (59%) had a MV surface area >95 percentile of the normal control MVs [28]. Another group found a wide spectrum of MV leaflet abnormalities among individuals undergoing surgical intervention for HCM with SAM, including degenerative, myxomatous, restrictive, and elongated AML as well as restrictive chordae and abnormal position of the papillary muscles [29]. This variability may reflect the intrinsic heterogeneity for the genetic causes in HCM, as well as the variability in other genetic and environmental factors that normally occur in patients. Our investigation utilized an inbred strain of mice in order to circumvent these factors.

The specificity of MV enlargement in HCM *vs.* other causes of LV hypertrophy was addressed in at least one prior pathological report in which sizes of excised MVs were compared among patients with aortic valve stenosis or regurgitation, with or without LV dilation, to MV size in HCM and controls [30]. In this study, compared to controls, MV size was similarly increased in HCM and in aortic stenosis patients with LV dilation, but remained unchanged when aortic stenosis occurred without LV dilation despite LVH.

There are many severe consequences of MV leaflet elongation in HCM [1,6,31]. First, elongation of the AML may result in displacement of a portion of the excess tissue interposed into the pathway of the LVOT at the beginning of systolic ejection, thereby facilitating SAM and obstruction and causing MR, the severity of which increases proportionally to the degree of mismatch between the AML and

PML length [32]; it also worsens left atrial enlargement and increases the risk for atrial fibrillation. Finally, obstruction increases the likelihood of death and progressive heart failure [33].

Although leaflet elongation in HCM has long been attributed to MV deformation with repeated stretch of the MV due to SAM, enlarged MV leaflets have also been reported in the absence of LVOT obstruction [8,28]. Two studies have recognized that healthy carriers of a gene mutation predisposing to HCM (without LVH) also have pathologic elongation of the AML [3,4]. This suggests that a process in the surrounding pre-hypertrophic LV exerts an early effect on the MV leaflets. Since the sarcomere proteins in which mutations typically occur in HCM are not abundant in the MV leaflets, it supports our hypothesis that increased expression of paracrine growth factors may arise in the surrounding myocardium where sarcomere proteins are abundant, with influence on the size of the adjacent MV. Our results in this murine model and in 1 person with HCM with a *MYBPC3* mutation confirm and extend this hypothesis, with recognition of specific alterations in the TGFβ pathway that contribute to both LVH and MV disease in this setting. While there may be a role for LVOT obstruction contributing to MV pathology, better models of HCM with and without obstruction are needed to address this issue.

Several lines of evidence emphasize the dynamic nature of MV disease in different contexts. MV area is increased by approximately 30% in people with inferior wall myocardial infarction and dilated cardiomyopathy compared to people with normal hearts [34]. A study in sheep that compared MV remodeling in response to inferior myocardial infarction with or without LV patch to prevent LV dilation showed that the increase in MV area correlates with LV dilation [35]. Thus, while it cannot be excluded that LV dilatation might have contributed to leaflet elongation in *Mybpc3*-mutant mice, the LV enlargement cannot solely explain the difference. Moreover, the MV leaflets do not appear tethered (Figure 1) or drawn down apically into the ventricular cavity with apically restricted closure and leaflet tenting, as sometimes occurs in dilated or ischemic cardiomyopathy [34,35]. Based on the absence of tethering or leaflet tenting, LV enlargement is unlikely to be the sole explanation for the leaflet enlargement. Our data suggest that increased growth factor signaling contributes to MV enlargement. It seems that increased MV area in dilated or ischemic cardiomyopathy is a limited process that is insufficient for preventing the occurrence of MR, while in HCM, greater proportional increases in MV size are observed, as shown here and in human studies.

Mice with a knock-in mutation in *Fbn1*, the gene encoding fibrillin-1, develop many systemic features of Marfan syndrome [9,36,37]. These mice similarly have pathological elongation and thickening of the MV leaflets [9,38]. Fibrillin-1 binds the inactive form of latent TGFβ, and its deficiency has been shown to result in increased activation and signaling of this pluripotent growth factor, including in the MV leaflets [9]. Therapies that modulate excessive TGFβ stimulation of MV leaflets have been shown to normalize the MV in *Fbn1*-mutant mice [9].

HCM is typically caused by dominant mutations in genes encoding elements of the cardiac sarcomere [39]. The process whereby sarcomere gene mutations result in HCM has been elegantly investigated over the past two decades. Recent work in this area has led to improved understanding of the role of a cascade of gene expression in non-myocyte cells within the LV that results in proliferation of non-myocyte cells and increased fibrosis [23]. Periostin contributes to this process, but *Postn*-null mice with an α-myosin heavy chain gene mutation and LVH are only partially normalized compared to those with normal periostin [23]. A critical role for TGFβ signaling in this process was demonstrated by gene expression analysis, immunostaining, and TGFβ-neutralizing therapies [23]. Our work extends these findings to the MV in HCM, providing both an explanation for MV disease in this disorder and an opportunity to investigate treatment for this with TGFβ-neutralizing therapies. Although this strain of mice does not have LVOT turbulence, it does have LVH due to a sarcomere gene mutation, and thus only partly recapitulates HCM.

One potential limitation in our analysis is the issue of blinding. Although the valve measures were made in a blinded fashion, with magnification to limit the ability of the interpreter to see the LV size and function, it is possible that bias could have entered into the analysis of echocardiograms. Thus, the microCT assessment was performed to independently assess MV size and thickness. Average leaflet thickness, volume, and total leaflet area were measured using an automated system that independently defines tissue boundaries with a 25 μM^3 resolution.

There are both benefits and limitations inherent in any investigation involving murine models of HCM [40–42]. In contrast with human HCM, this strain of mice with loss of cMyBP-C does not have LV hypercontractility, SAM, or LVOT obstruction. This model does mimic human disease by targeting the endogenous *Mybpc3* gene, rather than by transgenesis, although (in contrast with patients) hypertrophy is not substantial in the heterozygous mice. Thus, this mouse model is not a perfect model of human HCM, even if histopathological analysis of the LV in these (−/−) mice shows increased LV wall thickness compared to (+/+) mice at 3 months, with associated myofiber disarray and increased interstitial fibrosis, just as in people with HCM [17]. The myocardial walls also produce more CTGF and POSTN, as in other HCM mouse models [23]. Unfortunately, no HCM mouse model with LVOT obstruction is currently available, precluding any comparison between HCM mice with and without obstruction. In about 5% of people with HCM, two mutations (compound/digenic heterozygous or homozygous) are present, typically with a more severe phenotype [43]. There is at least one case published of a person with a homozygous p.Q76Ter nonsense mutation in *MYBPC3* predicted to produce no protein, and this parallels the *Mybpc3* knock-out mouse with a dilated, hypertrophied, and hypokinetic left ventricle and sudden death by 9 months of age [27]. LV enlargement and reduced contractility may be responsible for the increased markers of TGFβ activity, and this may further confound the analysis of MV leaflet length and thickness, despite controlling for these factors.

4. Conclusions

Mybpc3 (−/−) mice with LVH have longer and thicker MV leaflets compared to age-matched control (+/+) mice. Enlargement of the MV leaflets occurs in this model in the absence of SAM and LVOT obstruction. In this murine model of HCM, MV remodeling correlates with multiple markers of increased activity of TGFβ, a pleiotropic family of growth factors that is known to induce MV pathology in other settings, and that has been identified as a critical factor in the pathogenesis of HCM and pathologic MV leaflet elongation.

Acknowledgments

This work was funded by Fondation Leducq (07CVD04). The authors gratefully acknowledge and thank Elizabeth Huc for mouse colony maintenance, Núria Amat-Alarcon and Yan Chen for technical assistance, and members of the Leducq Mitral Network for scientific advice. Additional funding was provided by NIH-NHLBI: HL033756 (RRM and RAN) and NIH-NIGMS: GM103444-07 (RRM and

RAN). Some of this work was conducted in a facility constructed with support from the National Institutes of Health, Grant Number C06 RR018823 from the Extramural Research Facilities Program of the National Center for Research Resources.

Author Contributions

DPJ and AAH conceived and designed the experiments; DPJ, HN, RAN, JTB, KHK, QN, PB, EM, and AdV performed the experiments; DPJ, RAN, RAL, JTB, PB, M-CP, XJ, RM, LC, and AAH analyzed the data; NV and LC contributed critical reagents; DPJ and AAH wrote the first draft of this paper, and all authors reviewed and provided critical commentary.

Conflicts of Interest

The authors declare no conflict of interest.

References

1. Jiang, L.; Levine, R.A.; King, M.E.; Weyman, A.E. An integrated mechanism for systolic anterior motion of the mitral valve in hypertrophic cardiomyopathy based on echocardiographic observations. *Am. Heart J.* **1987**, *113*, 633–644.
2. Hagege, A.A.; Bruneval, P.; Levine, R.A.; Neamatalla, H.; Judge, D.P. The mitral valve in hypertrophic cardiomyopathy: Old *versus* new concepts. *J. Cardiovasc. Transl. Res.* **2011**, *4*, 757–766.
3. Hagege, A.A.; Dubourg, O.; Desnos, M.; Mirochnik, R.; Isnard, G.; Bonne, G.; Carrier, L.; Guicheney, P.; Bouhour, J.B.; Schwartz, K.; Komajda, M. Familial hypertrophic cardiomyopathy. Cardiac ultrasonic abnormalities in genetically affected subjects without echocardiographic evidence of left ventricular hypertrophy. *Eur. Heart J.* **1998**, *19*, 490–499.
4. Maron, M.S.; Olivotto, I.; Harrigan, C.; Appelbaum, E.; Gibson, C.M.; Lesser, J.R.; Haas, T.S.; Udelson, J.E.; Manning, W.J.; Maron, B.J. Mitral Valve Abnormalities Identified by Cardiovascular Magnetic Resonance Represent a Primary Phenotypic Expression of Hypertrophic Cardiomyopathy. *Circulation* **2011**, *124*, 40–47.
5. Schwammenthal, E.; Levine, R.A. Dynamic subaortic obstruction: A disease of the mitral valve suitable for surgical repair? *J. Am. Coll. Cardiol.* **1996**, *28*, 203–206.
6. Levine, R.A.; Vlahakes, G.J.; Lefebvre, X.; Guerrero, J.L.; Cape, E.G.; Yoganathan, A.P.; Weyman, A.E. Papillary muscle displacement causes systolic anterior motion of the mitral valve. Experimental validation and insights into the mechanism of subaortic obstruction. *Circulation* **1995**, *91*, 1189–1195.
7. Wigle, E.D.; Adelman, A.G.; Auger, P.; Marquis, Y. Mitral regurgitation in muscular subaortic stenosis. *Am. J. Cardiol.* **1969**, *24*, 698–706.
8. Kim, D.H.; Handschumacher, M.D.; Levine, R.A.; Choi, Y.S.; Kim, Y.J.; Yun, S.C.; Song, J.M.; Kang, D.H.; Song, J.K. *In vivo* measurement of mitral leaflet surface area and subvalvular geometry in patients with asymmetrical septal hypertrophy: Insights into the mechanism of outflow tract obstruction. *Circulation* **2010**, *122*, 1298–1307.

9. Ng, C.M.; Cheng, A.; Myers, L.A.; Martinez-Murillo, F.; Jie, C.; Bedja, D.; Gabrielson, K.L.; Hausladen, J.M.; Mecham, R.P.; Judge, D.P.; *et al.* TGF-β-dependent pathogenesis of mitral valve prolapse in a mouse model of Marfan syndrome. *J. Clin. Investig.* **2004**, *114*, 1586–1592.
10. Kyndt, F.; Gueffet, J.P.; Probst, V.; Jaafar, P.; Legendre, A.; le Bouffant, F.; Toquet, C.; Roy, E.; McGregor, L.; Lynch, S.A.; *et al.* Mutations in the Gene Encoding Filamin A as a Cause for Familial Cardiac Valvular Dystrophy. *Circulation* **2007**, *115*, 40–49.
11. Sauls, K.; de Vlaming, A.; Harris, B.S.; Williams, K.; Wessels, A.; Levine, R.A.; Slaugenhaupt, S.A.; Goodwin, R.L.; Pavone, L.; Merot, J.; *et al.* Developmental Basis for Filamin-A Associated Myxomatous Mitral Valve Disease. *Cardiovasc. Res.* **2012**, *96*, 109–119.
12. Disse, S.; Abergel, E.; Berrebi, A.; Houot, A.M.; le Heuzey, J.Y.; Diebold, B.; Guize, L.; Carpentier, A.; Corvol, P.; Jeunemaitre, X. Mapping of a first locus for autosomal dominant myxomatous mitral-valve prolapse to chromosome 16p11.2–p12.1. *Am. J. Hum. Genet.* **1999**, *65*, 1242–1251.
13. Freed, L.A.; Acierno, J.S., Jr.; Dai, D.; Leyne, M.; Marshall, J.E.; Nesta, F.; Levine, R.A.; Slaugenhaupt, S.A. A locus for autosomal dominant mitral valve prolapse on chromosome 11p15.4. *Am. J. Hum. Genet.* **2003**, *72*, 1551–1559.
14. Nesta, F.; Leyne, M.; Yosefy, C.; Simpson, C.; Dai, D.; Marshall, J.E.; Hung, J.; Slaugenhaupt, S.A.; Levine, R.A. New locus for autosomal dominant mitral valve prolapse on chromosome 13: Clinical insights from genetic studies. *Circulation* **2005**, *112*, 2022–2030.
15. Millat, G.; Bouvagnet, P.; Chevalier, P.; Dauphin, C.; Jouk, P.S.; da Costa, A.; Prieur, F.; Bresson, J.L.; Faivre, L.; Eicher, J.C.; *et al.* Prevalence and spectrum of mutations in a cohort of 192 unrelated patients with hypertrophic cardiomyopathy. *Eur J. Med. Genet.* **2010**, *53*, 261–267.
16. Watkins, H.; Conner, D.; Thierfelder, L.; Jarcho, J.A.; MacRae, C.; McKenna, W.J.; Maron, B.J.; Seidman, J.G.; Seidman, C.E. Mutations in the cardiac myosin binding protein-C gene on chromosome 11 cause familial hypertrophic cardiomyopathy. *Nat. Genet.* **1995**, *11*, 434–437.
17. Carrier, L.; Knoll, R.; Vignier, N.; Keller, D.I.; Bausero, P.; Prudhon, B.; Isnard, R.; Ambroisine, M.L.; Fiszman, M.; Ross, J., Jr.; *et al.* Asymmetric septal hypertrophy in heterozygous cMyBP-C null mice. *Cardiovasc. Res.* **2004**, *63*, 293–304.
18. Lekanne Deprez, R.H.; Muurling-Vlietman, J.J.; Hruda, J.; Baars, M.J.H.; Wijnaendts, L.C.D.; Stolte-Dijkstra, I.; Alders, M.; van Hagen, J.M. Two cases of severe neonatal hypertrophic cardiomyopathy caused by compound heterozygous mutations in the MYBPC3 gene. *J. Med. Genet.* **2006**, *43*, 829–832.
19. Xin, B.; Puffenberger, E.; Tumbush, J.; Bockoven, J.R.; Wang, H. Homozygosity for a novel splice site mutation in the cardiac myosin-binding protein C gene causes severe neonatal hypertrophic cardiomyopathy. *Am. J. Med. Genet. A* **2007,** *143A*, 2662–2667.
20. Bhan, A.; Sirker, A.; Zhang, J.; Protti, A.; Catibog, N.; Driver, W.; Botnar, R.; Monaghan, M.J.; Shah, A.M. High-frequency speckle tracking echocardiography in the assessment of left ventricular function and remodeling after murine myocardial infarction. *Am. J. Physiol. Heart Circ. Physiol.* **2014**, *306*, H1371–H1383.
21. Henning, A.L.; Jiang, M.X.; Yalcin, H.C.; Butcher, J.T. Quantitative three-dimensional imaging of live avian embryonic morphogenesis via micro-computed tomography. *Dev. Dyn.* **2011**, *240*, 1949–1957.

22. Norris, R.A.; Potts, J.D.; Yost, M.J.; Junor, L.; Brooks, T.; Tan, H.; Hoffman, S.; Hart, M.M.; Kern, M.J.; Damon, B.; *et al.* Periostin promotes a fibroblastic lineage pathway in atrioventricular valve progenitor cells. *Dev. Dyn.* **2009**, *238*, 1052–1063.
23. Teekakirikul, P.; Eminaga, S.; Toka, O.; Alcalai, R.; Wang, L.; Wakimoto, H.; Nayor, M.; Konno, T.; Gorham, J.M.; Wolf, C.M.; *et al.* Cardiac fibrosis in mice with hypertrophic cardiomyopathy is mediated by non-myocyte proliferation and requires TGF-β. *J. Clin. Investig.* **2010**, *120*, 3520–3529.
24. Massague, J.; Seoane, J.; Wotton, D. Smad transcription factors. *Genes Dev.* **2005**, *19*, 2783–2810.
25. Habashi, J.P.; Judge, D.P.; Holm, T.M.; Cohn, R.D.; Loeys, B.L.; Cooper, T.K.; Myers, L.; Klein, E.C.; Liu, G.; Calvi, C.; *et al.* Losartan, an AT1 Antagonist, Prevents Aortic Aneurysm in a Mouse Model of Marfan Syndrome. *Science* **2006**, *312*, 117–121.
26. Morner, S.; Richard, P.; Kazzam, E.; Hellman, U.; Hainque, B.; Schwartz, K.; Waldenstrom, A. Identification of the genotypes causing hypertrophic cardiomyopathy in northern Sweden. *J. Mol. Cell. Cardiol.* **2003**, *35*, 841–849.
27. Richard, P.; Charron, P.; Carrier, L.; Ledeuil, C.; Cheav, T.; Pichereau, C.; Benaiche, A.; Isnard, R.; Dubourg, O.; Burban, M.; *et al.* Hypertrophic cardiomyopathy: Distribution of disease genes, spectrum of mutations, and implications for a molecular diagnosis strategy. *Circulation* **2003**, *107*, 2227–2232.
28. Klues, H.G.; Maron, B.J.; Dollar, A.L.; Roberts, W.C. Diversity of structural mitral valve alterations in hypertrophic cardiomyopathy. *Circulation* **1992**, *85*, 1651–1660.
29. Kaple, R.K.; Murphy, R.T.; DiPaola, L.M.; Houghtaling, P.L.; Lever, H.M.; Lytle, B.W.; Blackstone, E.H.; Smedira, N.G. Mitral valve abnormalities in hypertrophic cardiomyopathy: Echocardiographic features and surgical outcomes. *Ann. Thorac. Surg.* **2008**, *85*, 1527–1535.
30. Mautner, S.L.; Klues, H.G.; Mautner, G.C.; Proschan, M.A.; Roberts, W.C.; Maron, B.J. Comparison of mitral valve dimensions in adults with valvular aortic stenosis, pure aortic regurgitation and hypertrophic cardiomyopathy. *Am. J. Cardiol* **1993**, *71*, 949–953.
31. Shah, P.M.; Taylor, R.D.; Wong, M. Abnormal mitral valve coaptation in hypertrophic obstructive cardiomyopathy: Proposed role in systolic anterior motion of mitral valve. *Am. J. Cardiol.* **1981**, *48*, 258–262.
32. Schwammenthal, E.; Nakatani, S.; He, S.; Hopmeyer, J.; Sagie, A.; Weyman, A.E.; Lever, H.M.; Yoganathan, A.P.; Thomas, J.D.; Levine, R.A. Mechanism of Mitral Regurgitation in Hypertrophic Cardiomyopathy: Mismatch of Posterior to Anterior Leaflet Length and Mobility. *Circulation* **1998**, *98*, 856–865.
33. Petrone, R.K.; Klues, H.G.; Panza, J.A.; Peterson, E.E.; Maron, B.J. Coexistence of mitral valve prolapse in a consecutive group of 528 patients with hypertrophic cardiomyopathy assessed with echocardiography. *J. Am. Coll. Cardiol.* **1992**, *20*, 55–61.
34. Chaput, M.; Handschumacher, M.D.; Tournoux, F.; Hua, L.; Guerrero, J.L.; Vlahakes, G.J.; Levine, R.A. Mitral leaflet adaptation to ventricular remodeling: Occurrence and adequacy in patients with functional mitral regurgitation. *Circulation* **2008**, *118*, 845–852.
35. Messas, E.; Bel, A.; Szymanski, C.; Cohen, I.; Touchot, B.; Handschumacher, M.D.; Desnos, M.; Carpentier, A.; Menasche, P.; Hagege, A.A.; *et al.* Relief of mitral leaflet tethering following chronic myocardial infarction by chordal cutting diminishes left ventricular remodeling. *Circ. Cardiovasc. Imaging* **2009**, *3*, 679–686.

36. Judge, D.P.; Biery, N.J.; Keene, D.R.; Geubtner, J.; Myers, L.; Huso, D.L.; Sakai, L.Y.; Dietz, H.C. Evidence for a critical contribution of haploinsufficiency in the complex pathogenesis of Marfan syndrome. *J. Clin. Investig.* **2004**, *114*, 172–181.
37. Judge, D.P.; Rouf, R.; Habashi, J.; Dietz, H.C. Mitral valve disease in Marfan syndrome and related disorders. *J. Cardiovasc. Transl. Res.* **2011**, *4*, 741–747.
38. Gould, R.A.; Sinha, R.; Aziz, H.; Rouf, R.; Dietz, H.C., 3rd; Judge, D.P.; Butcher, J. Multi-scale biomechanical remodeling in aging and genetic mutant murine mitral valve leaflets: Insights into Marfan syndrome. *PLoS One* **2012**, *7*, e44639.
39. Seidman, J.G.; Seidman, C. The Genetic Basis for Cardiomyopathy: From Mutation Identification to Mechanistic Paradigms. *Cell* **2001**, *104*, 557–567.
40. Harris, S.P.; Lyons, R.G.; Bezold, K.L. In the Thick of It. *Circ. Res.* **2011**, *108*, 751–764.
41. Shephard, R.; Semsarian, C. Role of animal models in HCM research. *J. Cardiovasc. Transl. Res.* **2009**, *2*, 471–482.
42. McConnell, B.K.; Jones, K.A.; Fatkin, D.; Arroyo, L.H.; Lee, R.T.; Aristizabal, O.; Turnbull, D.H.; Georgakopoulos, D.; Kass, D.; Bond, M.; *et al.* Dilated cardiomyopathy in homozygous myosin-binding protein-C mutant mice. *J. Clin. Investig.* **1999**, *104*, 1235–1244.
43. Judge, D.P.; Johnson, N.M. Genetic evaluation of familial cardiomyopathy. *J. Cardiovasc. Transl. Res.* **2008**, *1*, 144–154.

3

Rationale for the Cytogenomics of Cardiovascular Malformations Consortium: A Phenotype Intensive Registry Based Approach

Robert B. Hinton [1], Kim L. McBride [2], Steven B. Bleyl [3], Neil E. Bowles [3], William L. Border [4], Vidu Garg [2], Teresa A. Smolarek [1], Seema R. Lalani [5] and Stephanie M. Ware [6,*]

[1] Divisions of Cardiology and Genetics, Cincinnati Children's Hospital Medical Center, Cincinnati, OH 45229, USA; E-Mails: bingrbh@icloud.com (R.B.H.); teresa.smolarek@cchmc.org (T.A.S.)

[2] Center for Cardiovascular and Pulmonary Research and Heart Center, Nationwide Children's Hospital and Department of Pediatrics, Ohio State University, Columbus, OH 43205, USA; E-Mails: kim.mcbride@nationwidechildrens.org (K.L.M.); vidu.garg@nationwidechildrens.org (V.G.)

[3] Division of Pediatric Cardiology, University of Utah School of Medicine, Salt Lake City, UT 84132, USA; E-Mails: steven.bleyl@utah.edu (S.B.B.); neil.bowles@hsc.utah.edu (N.E.B.)

[4] Division of Cardiology, Children's Healthcare of Atlanta, Atlanta, GA 30322, USA; E-Mail: borderw@kidsheart.com

[5] Department of Molecular and Human Genetics, Baylor College of Medicine, Houston, TX 77030, USA; E-Mail: seemal@bcm.edu

[6] Departments of Pediatrics and Medical and Molecular Genetics, Indiana University School of Medicine, Indianapolis, IN 46202, USA

* Author to whom correspondence should be addressed; E-Mail: stware@iu.edu

Academic Editors: Cheryl L. Maslen and Russell Norris

Abstract: Cardiovascular malformations (CVMs) are the most common birth defect, occurring in 1%–5% of all live births. Although the genetic contribution to CVMs is well recognized, the genetic causes of human CVMs are identified infrequently. In addition, a failure of systematic deep phenotyping of CVMs, resulting from the complexity and heterogeneity of malformations, has obscured genotype-phenotype correlations and contributed to a lack of understanding of disease mechanisms. To address these knowledge gaps, we have developed the Cytogenomics of Cardiovascular Malformations (CCVM) Consortium, a multi-site alliance of geneticists and cardiologists, contributing to a database registry of submicroscopic genetic copy number variants (CNVs) based on clinical chromosome microarray testing in individuals with CVMs using detailed classification schemes. Cardiac classification is performed using a modification to the National Birth Defects Prevention Study approach, and non-cardiac diagnoses are captured through ICD-9 and ICD-10 codes. By combining a comprehensive approach to clinically relevant genetic analyses with precise phenotyping, the Consortium goal is to identify novel genomic regions that cause or increase susceptibility to CVMs and to correlate the findings with clinical phenotype. This registry will provide critical insights into genetic architecture, facilitate genotype-phenotype correlations, and provide a valuable resource for the medical community.

Keywords: genetics; genomics; pediatrics; cardiovascular malformation; registry; chromosome microarray; copy number variation

1. Introduction

Chromosomal abnormalities account for 12%–14% of all live born cases and 20%–33% of fetal cases of congenital cardiovascular malformations (CVMs), indicating that the proper genetic control of cardiac development is essential for normal anatomic structure [1–4]. The complex development of the heart suggests the involvement of numerous genes in normal cardiac morphogenesis and, hence, numerous chromosomal loci [5]. In addition, syndromic CVMs can be quite difficult to distinguish from isolated CVMs, especially in early childhood [6,7]. Since early diagnosis of any genetic condition can inform clinicians in how best to optimize medical management, developmental intervention, and therapy, it becomes even more critical to more precisely delineate etiology. Additional benefits of a precise diagnosis include determination of prognosis and more accurate counseling about recurrence risk [8].

CVMs in humans commonly display incomplete penetrance and variable expressivity, with extensive allelic heterogeneity. This complex inheritance suggests a central contribution of as yet unidentified genetic modifiers. The high frequency of CVMs and their evident heterogeneity poses substantial problems in understanding the genetic causes underlying these common birth defects. However, by grouping CVMs that are mechanistically related, such as left ventricular outflow tract obstructive defects (LVOTO), heritability patterns can be identified [9–14]. These analyses have demonstrated that mild CVMs such as bicuspid aortic valve (BAV) may represent a *forme fruste* of severe CVMs, e.g., hypoplastic left heart syndrome (HLHS). Genetically mediated cardiac diseases that may not be present or ascertained at birth, e.g., BAV (present in ~2% of the population) or aortic dilation, are much more common than previously thought. When considering the etiology of CVMs, as opposed to the proportion of CVM cases that manifest as disease at birth, the incidence increases to approximately 5%.

Increasingly sophisticated genetic analyses, including chromosome microarray analysis (CMA) and next generation sequencing, are improving the ability to identify genetic causation and susceptibility of CVMs. CMA can also be used to analyze regions of homozygosity, which may unmask an autosomal recessive disorder. In addition, abnormalities in the parent of origin or imprinted chromosomal material (e.g., uniparental disomy) can contribute to CVMs and are detectable by current tests for copy number abnormalities [15,16]. CMA is standard of care testing for patients with developmental disability or multiple congenital anomalies and is considered first line testing for many patients with CVMs [17]. Copy number variation (CNV) refers to genetic deletions or duplications that are not identifiable by traditional chromosome analysis. These alterations may result from recombination within the genome, typically as a result of instability of regional genetic architecture, and vary in size. CNVs are more common than single nucleotide variants, and therefore generate important variation in the genome. CNVs are common, comprising approximately 12% of the genome of an individual and typically have no phenotypic consequence. However, CNVs containing dosage sensitive gene(s) result in phenotypic abnormalities due to alterations in gene expression, suggesting CNVs may represent major genetic modifiers in addition to their role in disease causation. The mechanisms of CNVs in disease have been the subject of recent reviews [18–21].

CNVs containing dosage sensitive genes are a well-described cause of genomic disorders associated with CVMs such as 22q11.2 deletion syndrome and Williams-Beuren syndrome, where *TBX1* and *ELN*, respectively, are critical dosage sensitive genes involved in the pathogenesis of these syndromes. These recurrent CNVs are associated with highly penetrant CVMs when haploinsufficient. More recent studies support a role for rare recurrent CNVs in CVMs with extracardiac malformations, as well as isolated CVMs [22,23]. It is estimated that CNVs contribute to 3%–25% of CVMs associated with extracardiac abnormalities and 3%–10% of isolated CVMs reviewed in [24,25] and this may be a significant underestimate given the current lack of understanding surrounding the contribution of genetic modifiers to the genetic basis of CVM.

Classification approaches for CVMs continue to present significant challenges for both clinicians and researchers. *The Atlas of Congenital Cardiac Disease*, based on Maude Abbott's systematic catalogue of CVM gross pathology published in 1908 is the first classification system for clinical pediatric cardiology [26]. Subsequently, beginning in earnest in the 1950s, the rapid evolution of surgical intervention for CVMs defined a detailed clinical taxonomy that was based on anatomy and physiology [27]. Organizing malformations requires consideration of cause, and only recently, in the context of significant strides in our understanding of the genetic basis underlying CVMs, have there been efforts to reconcile etiologic factors in a clinically meaningful manner and integrate this information into the existing classification scheme [8,28]. As our understanding of cardiac morphogenesis improved, hypothetical classification paradigms were developed that took into account the developmental relationships of lesions (in addition to the anatomic relationships previously described) to increase confidence in grouping [29]. As the genetic basis of CVMs has emerged, it has become clear that this knowledge will challenge our clinical taxonomy in fundamental ways. The National Birth Defects Prevention Study (NBDPS) developed an exhaustive taxonomy that organizes CVMs in multiple ways, including the most specific definition of a single defect (the "splitting" approach) and the broadest groupings (the "clumping" approach), as well as intermediate levels that allow flexibility with the analysis of common associations [30]. A classification system that incorporates etiologic factors as well as careful clinical phenotyping is necessary for clinical and research advances alike, including the large scale multi-site efforts required to address the relatively small frequency of CVMs per center.

A goal of the registry is to collect and annotate cytogenetic and phenotypic findings in patients with CVMs in a comprehensive and standardized manner to promote an understanding of the genetic basis of cardiac disease. A lack of systematic deep phenotyping of CVMs, resulting from the complexity and heterogeneity of malformations, has obscured genotype-phenotype correlations and contributed to a lack of understanding of disease mechanisms. Defining critical genes within CNVs, establishing rare recurrent CNVs associated with CVMs, and defining cardiac phenotypes of genomic disorders are all important objectives of this Registry. The high frequency of CVMs, large number of genes playing a role in normal cardiac development, and incomplete penetrance of phenotypes suggests that large numbers of cases will be required to identify causes and determine associations and susceptibility factors. Given the established phenotypic variability associated with genetic causes of CVMs, it is necessary to use a detailed and etiology-centric classification system to leverage the information learned from these associations. The CCVM Registry is a cost-effective resource to identify novel loci associated with isolated or syndromic CVMs, establish genotype-phenotype correlations, and facilitate discovery of new candidate genes for normal and abnormal cardiac development.

2. Experimental Section

2.1. Registry Organization

The CCVM Consortium is a collaborative group of 6 pediatric clinical centers, with different areas of expertise but common interests and broad experience in the genetics of CVMs, cytogenetics, pediatric cardiology, including specifically echocardiography, clinical genetics, and database/registry/biobank expertise.

The Investigator Group encompasses clinical expertise in cardiology (Border, Garg, Hinton, with specialized imaging expertise by Border, Hinton), clinical genetics (Bleyl, Lalani, McBride, Ware), and cytogenetics (Lalani, Smolarek,); research expertise in human genetics (Bleyl, Bowles, Garg, Hinton, Lalani, McBride, Ware), cardiac development (Bleyl, Garg, Hinton, Ware), clinical research (Border, McBride); and database/registry/biobank experience (Bleyl, Bowles, Hinton, McBride, Ware).

2.2. Study Population and Study Design

This is a cohort study of abnormal CMA cases in patients for whom echocardiography has been performed. To be eligible for the study, a patient is required to have had an abnormal CMA result, defined as a result interpreted to be clinically significant, disease causing, or of unknown clinical significance. Patients with no CMA results or normal testing are excluded. Of note, an iterative search process is implemented such that patients with abnormal CMA in whom no echocardiogram has been performed will remain potentially eligible, thus capturing patients with later diagnoses. Patients with isolated abnormalities in cardiac rhythm will be excluded from this study. The Institutional Review Boards of all participating study sites have approved the Registry and data use agreements have been executed to allow sharing of limited datasets.

2.3. Cytogenetic Data Elements

As certified clinical diagnostic laboratories, cytogenetics laboratories at the 6 sites have standardized requirements for processing and tracking patient samples as well as analyzing, interpreting, and recording analyses. Cytogenetic variables from each site have been standardized for collection_(Table 1). Each patient sample is assigned a case number with a unique identifier, and the cytogenetic laboratory maintains a large database of case numbers, results, and clinical interpretation. A DNA repository of samples is maintained long term for auditing and regulatory compliance. Due to the high standards for regulatory compliance and clinical interpretation inherent in the operation of a clinical diagnostic laboratory, the analyses represent a very well validated dataset. CMA frequently uncovers novel submicroscopic abnormalities [23]. In some cases, results are confirmed by a second method, most often fluorescence in situ hybridization. In addition, in cases of uncertain significance, parental samples are obtained when available to determine whether the submicroscopic gain or loss is *de novo*, to aid interpretation of pathogenicity. Literature and database searches are also performed for better interpretation of the data. CMA analytic tools are routinely used for interpretation of novel variants. These interpretation results are maintained in the Registry. Table 1 shows variables collected with example results shown for 22q11.2 deletion syndrome.

Table 1. Cytogenetic Data Elements.

Variable	Example
Platform	SNP
Chromosome	22
Cytolocation	22q11.21
Position Beginning	17,074,487
Position End	19,806,645
Version	HG18
CNV Value	1
Gain/Loss	Loss
Gene	USP18, DGCR6, PRODH, DGCR2, DGCR14, TSSK2, GSC2, SLC25A1, CLTCL1, HIRA, MRPL40, UFD1L, CDC45L, CLDN5, SEPT5, GP1BB, TBX1, GNB1L, TXNRD2, COMT, ARVCF, DGCR8, TRMT2A, RANBP1, ZDHHC8, RTN4R, DGCR6L, GGTLC3, RIMBP3, ZNF74, SCARF2, MED15, PI4KA, SERPIND1, SNAP29, CRKL, LZTR1, THAP7, P2RX6, SLC7A4, BCRL2
Inheritance	*De novo*
Size	2732158 bp
Probes	N/A
Number of Probes	1,140,419
Analysis	arr 22q11.21(17,074,487 − 19,806,645) × 1
Result	Consistent with a single copy loss of genomic segment or heterozygous deletion of approximately 2.73 Mb on chromosome 22q11.21. This finding confirms the concurrent FISH analysis, which showed a 22q11.2 deletion associated with DiGeorge syndrome. The deleted 22q11.21 region overlaps with the region associated with the 22q11.2 deletion syndrome (DiGeorge syndrome) and contains several disease genes including the TBX1 gene known to cause clinical phenotypes seen in patients with the syndrome. The deleted region is proximal to the SMARCB1 locus and no deletion of the SMARCB1 gene was detected in this assay.

2.4. Detailed Cardiac and Extra-Cardiac Phenotyping

Comprehensive segmental anatomy is collected from echocardiograms performed for clinical care at each site. All primary echocardiogram data is evaluated directly at each site and classified to ensure exceptionally accurate phenotyping, which is an absolutely essential prerequisite for meaningful analysis and interpretation of genetic data. Non-cardiac medical diagnoses (e.g., dysmorphic features, developmental delay, neurologic findings) are recorded in the composite database using ICD-9 and now ICD-10 coding. Criteria established by the National Birth Defects Prevention Study (NBDPS) are being used to collect extensive phenotype information regarding the CVMs [30]. These criteria have been adapted to optimize capture of all cardiac defects that may be attributed to genetic causes, using the term "malformation" broadly with the assumption that the vast majority of cases of pediatric heart disease has a genetic basis (Table 2). Adaptations include the addition of other forms of pediatric heart disease, including rare developmental aberrations that were not included in the NBDPS scheme, such as arteriopathy, coronary artery abnormalities, and latent cardiovascular disease that is not present at birth but has been associated with genomic abnormalities, such as cardiomyopathy and aortopathy, all lesions that might now be considered 'malformations' in a genetic and pathogenesis sense if not strictly pathologic. Importantly, functional deficits of unclear significance are captured in addition to structural defects, e.g., left ventricular systolic dysfunction. In addition, subclinical CVMs are included, such as BAV. In light of added items, new associations are added. Finally, persistent fetal communications that may represent malformation are tracked when present beyond the first year of life, e.g., patent ductus arteriosus. In addition, there is a free text field allowing capture of additional items that are not systematically screened for but may be considered subclinical and abnormal, for example isolated left superior vena cava. As specified by the original NBDPS, each case was assigned a classification based on three axes: cardiac phenotype, cardiac complexity, and the presence and type of extracardiac malformations [30]. The CCVM modified classification scheme is shown in the case report form in Supplemental Table S1.

Table 2. Basic Tenets of National Birth Defect Prevention Study (NBDPS) Classification and Cytogenomics of Cardiovasscular Malformations (CCVM) Consortium Modifications.

The NBDPS describes each patient's cardiovascular malformation (CVM) as a specific lesion and groups the lesion in fine, intermediate and coarse levels of detail to increase precision and allow flexibility in analyses [28]
The NBDPS describes complexity of CVM and patterns of associated anomalies
The CCVM Registry includes latent types of pediatric heart disease that have an established genetic etiology, including cardiomyopathy and aortopathy
The CCVM Registry includes vasculopathies and coronary artery abnormalities
The CCVM Registry includes subclinical CVMs, such as bicuspid aortic valve
The CCVM Registry includes persistent fetal connections when present beyond one year of life, such as patent ductus arteriosus
The CCVM Registry includes functional deficits that may identify emerging defects, such as left ventricular systolic dysfunction

All echocardiographic reports are reviewed at a single center (IU) and CVM phenotype designation is made at that time. Due to differences in reporting across study sites, regular conference calls address designation choices and studies of uncertain classification. A cardiologist will over-read 10% of studies, excluding straightforward lesions (e.g., isolated septal defects), and the central study site will address discrepancies.

2.5. Data and Information Management

Using Good Clinical Data Management principles and processes, as well as institutionally sanctioned standard operating procedures, the DCC ensures that data are valid, reliable and accurate leading to reproducible results. Demographic and cardiac indications/echocardiography results are recorded onto paper case report forms (CRFs) and sent to IU DCC for entry into a REDCap (Research Electronic Data Capture) database. Cytogenetic data are de-identified and transferred securely. The DCC is responsible for maintaining the existing database system, importing external data, programming data quality checks, query resolution, generation of reports, data exports and preparation for analysis. A detailed data management plan is be maintained to document all processes. A data use agreement outlines the proper use of the data and publication plans.

The study complies with all Federal and local privacy laws and regulations, including the Department of Health and Human Services (HHS) Protection of Human Subjects Regulations (45 CFR part 46 and 21 CFR parts 50) and The Health Insurance Portability and Accountability Act (HIPAA) Privacy Rule. Phenotypic information is linked to the cytogenetic information and a unique identifier number will be assigned within the composite database. REDCap provides a secure, web-based application that is flexible and provides (1) an intuitive interface for data entry and real time validation rules at the time of entry; (2) HIPAA-compliant and 21 CFR Part 11-ready audit trails for tracking page views, data manipulation and export procedures; (3) record locking and electronic signature functions; (4) fine grained control of user rights to view/manipulate data; (5) a report builder for reporting, monitoring and querying patient records; and (6) automated export procedures for seamless data downloads [31].

3. Results and Discussion

3.1. Study Population Enrollment

The cohort is geographically, racially, and ethnically diverse which represents a strength for genetic studies. Current and projected enrollment is shown in Table 3. The Utah site is predicted to have fewer cases, but a higher proportion will be linked in large non-syndromic CVM families, due to the availability of extended family data from the Utah Population Database, a computerized data warehouse with an extensive set of genealogy data (~12 million records) linked to medical information.

Table 3. Current and Projected Enrollment.

Site	Current Cases	Yr1	Yr2	Yr3	
BCM	305	75	85	85	
CCHMC	174	55	60	60	
Nationwide	76	55	60	60	
Emory/CHOA	67	30	35	40	
Utah	N/A	15	20	20	
Totals	622	230	260	265	1377

3.2. Genetic Descriptors

As part of the Registry, we expect to capture known genetic syndromic diagnoses that are commonly associated with CVMs such as 22q11.2 deletion syndrome and its reciprocal duplication, 22q11.2 duplication syndrome, and Williams-Beuren syndrome and its reciprocal duplication, 7q11.23 duplication syndrome. In addition, trisomy 21 may be detected by CMA in infants in whom a diagnosis of Down syndrome was not suspected and CMA was performed. In order to determine the degree to which these common diagnoses made by CMA contribute to the registry, we performed manual review of the initial 291 records. The results are shown in Table 4. These data demonstrate that these well-described genetic syndromes do not comprise a majority of results for subjects with CVMs and abnormal CMA findings within the Registry. Epidemiologic data from the Baltimore Washington Infant Study indicated that approximately 76% of cases of CVMs were isolated, 12% resulted from aneuploidies such as trisomy 13, 18, 21, and Turner syndrome, and 12% encompassed Mendelian disorders, clinical syndromes, genomic disorders, or other complex phenotypes suggestive of genetic syndromic conditions. Because we anticipate that the majority of patients with aneuploidies will not be diagnosed using CMA, the prevalence of the most common genetic syndromic conditions associated with CVMs in the Registry appears to approximate epidemiologic estimates.

3.3. Cardiac Phenotyping

A subset of the current cases identified as having CMA abnormalities have undergone cardiac classification. The results are shown in Figure 1, which shows the highest level subgrouping of CVMs. As expected, septal defects are the most common. The conotruncal and LVOTO categories are the next most common groups of defects, with approximately equivalent numbers. Heterotaxy CVM numbers are slightly higher than might be expected, perhaps reflecting the high prevalence of heterotaxy in Texas and the overrepresentation of cases from that region in the current Registry. Importantly, aortopathy, arteriopathy, and cardiomyopathy, all defects not captured by the NBDPS, are well represented in this cohort of patients with CMA abnormalities.

Table 4. Prevalence of Common Genetic Syndromes with CVM in Registry Database.

Genetic Syndrome	N in Registry [1]	% of Registry Cases
22q11.2 deletion syndrome (DiGeorge, Velocardiofacial syndrome)	19	6.5%
22q11.2 duplication syndrome	3	1.0%
Williams-Beuren syndrome (7q11.23 deletion)	12	4.1%
7q11.23 duplication syndrome	3	1.0%
Trisomy 21	1	0.3%
Total	38	13.0%

[1] Based on review of 291 cases.

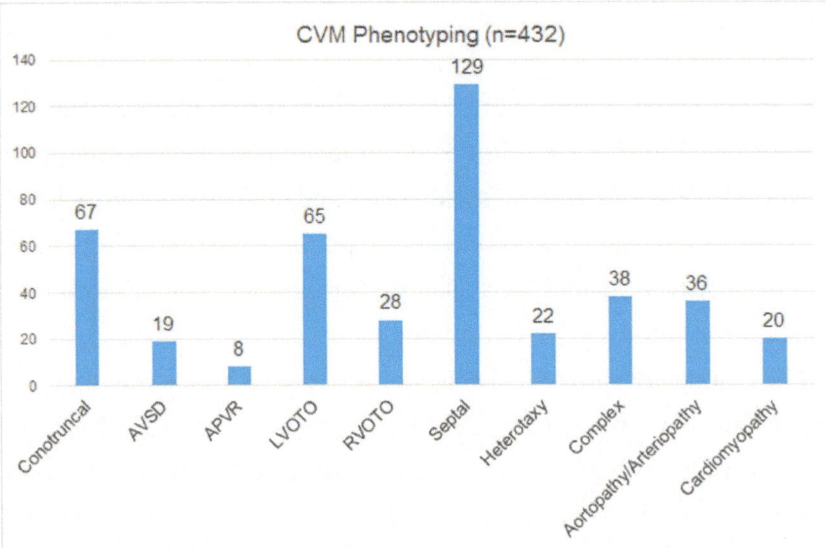

Figure 1. Cardiac classification groups for CCVM registry. AVSD (atrioventricular septal defects); APVR (anomalous pulmonary venous return); LVOTO (left ventricular outflow tract obstruction); RVOTO (right ventricular outflow tract obstruction).

As the clinical genetic testing paradigms for CVMs evolve, we expect to capture increasing numbers of isolated CVM subjects. It has been shown in a cohort of infants with CVMs that fewer patients were undergoing genetic testing than would be predicted to have syndromic disease based on epidemiologic data [10,32]. In addition, many patients who do undergo genetic testing have multiple, redundant tests resulting in cost inefficiencies [33,34]. While a conventional tiered approach to genetic testing is important, these studies have identified circumstances when broader testing may be indicated. Four of the six sites involved with the Registry have implemented institution-specific approach to infants with cyanotic CVMs, with standardized approaches for genetic testing and/or cardiovascular genetics consultation, increasing the comprehensive evaluation of infants with CVMs. Recent studies showing the diagnostic yield of CMA in isolated CVM cases provides rationale for clinical testing [24,35,36]. The CCVM Registry may provide a repository to determine the yield of testing within certain classes of CVMs, thereby providing an improved ability to implement genetic testing appropriately.

3.4. Proof of Principle: Anticipated Outcomes

3.4.1. Delineation of Cardiac Features for Well Characterized Genomic Disorders

Because CVMs are the most common birth defects, many well-characterized genomic disorders have CVMs associated as part of the phenotype. In many cases, careful description of the CVMs associated with these disorders has been lacking, and for some genetic syndromes, no specific information exists about the type of heart defects identified. An anticipated and important function of the CCVM Registry will be to provide deep phenotyping of CVMs for a number of recurrent genomic disorders that have not been carefully studied. For example, we recently published a case series of eight patients with 7q11.23 duplication and aortopathy [37]. The 7q11.23 microduplication syndrome is a genomic disorder with an emerging clinical phenotype including dysmorphic features, hypotonia, developmental delay with prominent speech delay, and autistic features. CVMs, most commonly patent ductus arteriosus, have been reported in a subset of cases. We identified a series of eight pediatric patients and one adult with 7q11.23 microduplication syndrome, all of whom had aortic dilation, the opposite vascular phenotype of the typical supravalvar aortic stenosis found in Williams-Beuren syndrome. The ascending aorta was most commonly involved, while dilation was less frequently identified at the aortic root and sinotubular junction. Inclusion and systematic evaluation of aorta dimensions, as part of the comprehensive phenotyping approach, allowed the identification of these patients. These initial patients were ascertained at a single institution, and CCVM Registry participation allowed the identification of additional subjects. The incidence of 7q11.23 duplication syndrome is estimated at 1/13,000 to 1/20,000 births and therefore no single institution would be expected to have a large cohort of patients. This example indicates that the CCVM Registry is an important resource for better defining cardiac features in genetic syndromes that are still being characterized or for which cardiac features are less common. Importantly, in this example the findings led to a management recommendation for cardiovascular surveillance in patients with 7q11.23 microduplication syndrome.

3.4.2. Identification of Novel Loci that Confer CVM Susceptibility

The widespread use of CMA for diagnosis in patients with developmental disability or congenital anomalies has led to the identification of many new genomic disorders as well as CNVs of uncertain clinical significance. There are a large number of genes predicted to impact cardiac development and therefore we have hypothesized that some submicroscopic deletions or duplications associated with CVMs may be quite rare. Rare, recurrent CNVs associated with CVMs are important to identify because they allow further delineation of the clinical spectrum of disease, allow refinement of the critical region for specific phenotypic features, and provide a mechanism to identify novel candidate genes for CVMs. Recently, Lalani *et al*., undertook a large study of rare, recurrent CNVs associated with CVMs in patients with abnormal CMA findings and extracardiac anomalies [22] and identified 16 unique CNVs, 12 of which were novel loci, including 16q24.3 loss and 2q31.3–q32.1 loss. In addition, the study narrowed critical intervals in three well-recognized genomic disorders with CVMs.

3.4.3. Identification of Novel Genes Causing CVMs

Coarctation of the aorta (CoA) and HLHS, both LVOTO defects, have been reported in rare individuals with large terminal deletions of chromosome 15q26. However, no single gene important for left ventricular outflow tract development has been identified in this region. Clinical CMA testing through the Kleberg Laboratory at Baylor College of Medicine identified two half-siblings with CoA with a 2.2 Mb deletion on 15q26.2, inherited from their mother, who was mosaic for this deletion. This interval contains a single gene, *MCTP2* (multiple C2-domains with two transmembrane regions 2). The CCVM Registry can be used to further investigate candidate genes identified in novel CNVs and/or to further narrow critical regions for loci previously associated with CVMs. These candidate genes can be further investigated using genetic and developmental approaches. In the case of *MCTP2*, gene-specific array screening in 146 individuals with non-syndromic LVOTO defects identified another individual with a *de novo* 41 kb intragenic duplication within *MCTP2*, predicted to result in premature truncation, p.F697X [38]. Alteration of *Mctp2* gene expression in *Xenopus laevis* embryos by morpholino knockdown and mRNA overexpresssion resulted in failure of proper outflow tract development, confirming the functional importance of this dosage sensitive gene for cardiogenesis and illustrating the importance of precise phenotyping. Our results identify *MCTP2* as a novel genetic cause of CoA and related cardiac malformations.

In addition, we identified a patient with unbalanced atrioventricular septal defect (AVSD) and hypoplastic left ventricle who harbored an ~0.3 Mb deletion on chromosome 3p14.1 [39]. The deletion encompassed the first four exons of *FOXP1*, a gene critical for normal heart development that represses cardiomyocyte proliferation and expression of Nkx2.5. Identification of this candidate gene led to sequence based approaches within patients with CVMs to determine whether single nucleotide variants in *FOXP1* cause or increase susceptibility to CVMs. It should be noted that the CCVM Registry only captures patients with abnormal CMA, and thus no sequence-based interrogation has been performed. Sequencing *FOXP1* in 82 patients with AVSD or HLHS led to the identification of two patients with a variant that showed abnormal transactivation in functional assays as well as alterations in cardiomyoblast proliferation, suggesting that haploinsufficiency of *FOXP1* is associated with human CVMs.

3.5. Approaches for Genetic Identification of CVMs

There is a clear need presently for combining clinical genetic testing with deep phenotyping, and this need requires flexibility on both the genotype and phenotype spectrums due to substantial heterogeneity. In addition to careful cardiac phenotyping, there is a growing appreciation that extra-cardiac organ systems should be considered in all cases of CVMs, and there is a growing appreciation of central nervous system abnormalities that significantly impact both a patient's medical status and his or her quality of life. A strength of this Registry is the careful cardiac phenotyping combined with the systematic collection of extracardiac findings, bolstering analyses focusing on the genetic underpinnings of these specific findings and associations. For example, we recently reported twins with progressive aortopathy, recurrent dissections and an *ACTA2* mutation [40]. Interestingly, in addition to illustrating the potential for genotype-phenotype correlations that directly impact clinical care, this example also illustrates the potential use of non-cardiac findings to direct cardiac care. These twins were diagnosed with mydriasis years prior to their aortopathy being recognized, and because mydriasis is a manifestation of smooth muscle dysfunction this might prompt a heightened index of suspicion for aortopathy and therefore surveillance. These types of associations challenge previous system based models of disease and allow paradigms whereby genetic information is integrated into clinical practice. A limitation of the Registry is that it is currently focused only on CNVs as a mechanism for CVM causation and susceptibility. In its present form, it does not incorporate sequence based approaches to genetic diagnosis, and this is a clear need for future iterations.

Patients with CVMs are managed clinically by pediatric cardiologists and pediatric cardiothoracic surgeons primarily, but several types of specialists are now routinely involved in the delivery of comprehensive care, importantly including increasing numbers of health care providers with specific expertise in cardiovascular genetics such as geneticists and genetic counselors [41,42]. Distinct nomenclature systems have been developed in both disciplines. For example, surgical paradigms of CVM have been systematically archived by the Society of Thoracic Surgeons (STS) by lesion [43] using an extreme reductionist approach to classification. The Pediatric Heart Network is a multi-site network that conducts clinical trials, and uses project specific phenotyping, but is charged with partnering with the Pediatric Cardiovascular Genomic Consortium, a rapidly growing registry of CVM patients and biorepository of DNA that uses a variation of the Fyler classification scheme based on anatomy and physiology [44,45]. The CCVM Registry presented in this manuscript uses an inclusive approach to an etiology centric classification scheme. When considering cause, it is important to group lesions appropriately and avoid misclassification that may confound interpretation. Importantly, these approaches to phenotypic details are different, potentially confounding analyses. A central need in the field is for consensus regarding careful phenotyping, and this will be made more challenging by the emerging molecular taxonomy. Because the genetic basis of CVMs, and more broadly pediatric heart disease, is characterized by both phenotypic and genetic heterogeneity, with an anticipated central role for common major modifiers, a defined genetic understanding of CVMs will greatly inform complete phenotyping, potentially impacting diagnosis, prognosis and treatment decisions, as well as counseling for families. Therefore, it is crucial that the larger CVM community reconcile different approaches to careful phenotyping to fully leverage the potential of current large registries.

Molecular taxonomies, defined by human genetics, are going to impact established clinical taxonomies and change approaches to care, resulting in the increased use of preventive and proactive strategies. The definition of a syndrome is less straightforward than in previous years, as single gene defects may result in apparently isolated CVMs in some individuals, and CVMs with extracardiac findings in others. Therefore, one specific opportunity lies in the ability to delineate both genetic modifiers and phenotypic variability, e.g., the same gene mutation resulting in varying CVMs in a given family or within a known syndrome [46,47]. Given the analytic challenges involved, recent recommendations from the American Heart Association state that Centers with Cardiovascular Genetics Centers should direct testing and interpretation and participate in subsequent management decisions, especially as exome testing becomes more common [48]. The most effective approaches for delivering cardiovascular genetics services have not been completely defined, and the composition of clinics and expertise can vary [49]. Coordinated and uniform practices in cardiovascular genetics will be increasingly important as the causes of heritable CVMs are identified, risk variants are defined, and personalized medicine efforts become mainstream [49]. To further these efforts, it is imperative that the field reconcile different ways of approaching both genetic and phenotypic schemes. The success of the Children's Oncology Group has been attributed in large part to overcoming these very challenges. In addition, they have been successful at reconciling registries and compliance issues between study sites and using collective biospecimens [50,51] and may serve as an ideal model for pediatric heart disease. Ultimately, consensus on phenotyping between centers is necessary for national and international network, consortium and registry research efforts to fully realize their potential and truly impact patient care.

4. Conclusions

Identification of the genetic causes of CVMs has been challenging. Although the developmental basis for many cardiac defects has been investigated in model organisms, identification of genetic causes in human CVMs has been less successful. The current experimental framework for studying CVMs is clearly deficient. The attempt to translate bench (animal models) to bedside (identification of human mutations) has not been straightforward. This has led to the paradigm that CVMs are too heterogeneous and multifactorial in origin to genetically characterize except in rare familial cases, resulting in stagnation of clinical and translational investigation and diagnostic test development. The development of the CCVM Consortium is an important step toward achieving the goal of identifying the genetic basis of CVMs. Using innovative technology, clinical expertise, and clinical diagnostic laboratory expertise, this alliance will determine the importance of structural genome variation in CVMs and enable the identification of novel loci, delineation of genetic syndromes, and genotype-phenotype analyses. In turn, this will facilitate the development of disease specific therapy, accurate diagnostic algorithms, effective management, and assignment of precise recurrence risk.

Acknowledgments

This project is supported by a March of Dimes Foundation grant 6-FY13-167 (S.M.W.).

Author Contributions

RBH, SRL, and SMW designed the research. RBH, KLM, SBB, NEB, WLB, VG, TAS, SRL, and SMW reviewed the data collection elements and analyzed the data. RBH and SMW wrote the paper. RBH, KLM, SBB, NEB, WLB, VG, TAS, SRL, and SMW read and approved the final manuscript.

Conflicts of Interest

The authors declare no conflict of interest.

References

1. Gillum, R.F. Epidemiology of congenital heart disease in the united states. *Am. Heart J.* **1994**, *127*, 919–927.
2. Chaoui, R.; Korner, H.; Bommer, C.; Goldner, B.; Bierlich, A.; Bollmann, R. Prenatal diagnosis of heart defects and associated chromosomal aberrations. *Ultraschall Med.* **1999**, *20*, 177–184.
3. Tennstedt, C.; Chaoui, R.; Korner, H.; Dietel, M. Spectrum of congenital heart defects and extracardiac malformations associated with chromosomal abnormalities: Results of a seven year necropsy study. *Heart (Br. Card. Soc.)* **1999**, *82*, 34–39.
4. Ferencz, C.; Boughman, J.A.; Neill, C.A.; Brenner, J.I.; Perry, L.W. Congenital cardiovascular malformations: Questions on inheritance. Baltimore-Washington Infant Study Group. *J. Am. Coll. Cardiol.* **1989**, *14*, 756–763.
5. Bruneau, B.G. The developmental genetics of congenital heart disease. *Nature* **2008**, *451*, 943–948.
6. Erdogan, F.; Larsen, L.A.; Zhang, L.; Tumer, Z.; Tommerup, N.; Chen, W.; Jacobsen, J.R.; Schubert, M.; Jurkatis, J.; Tzschach, A.; *et al.* High frequency of submicroscopic genomic aberrations detected by tiling path array comparative genome hybridisation in patients with isolated congenital heart disease. *J. Med. Genet.* **2008**, *45*, 704–709.

7. Lu, X.Y.; Phung, M.T.; Shaw, C.A.; Pham, K.; Neil, S.E.; Patel, A.; Sahoo, T.; Bacino, C.A.; Stankiewicz, P.; Kang, S.H.; *et al.* Genomic imbalances in neonates with birth defects: High detection rates by using chromosomal microarray analysis. *Pediatrics* **2008**, *122*, 1310–1318.
8. Pierpont, M.E.; Basson, C.T.; Benson, D.W., Jr.; Gelb, B.D.; Giglia, T.M.; Goldmuntz, E.; McGee, G.; Sable, C.A.; Srivastava, D.; Webb, C.L. Genetic basis for congenital heart defects: Current knowledge. A scientific statement from the American Heart Association congenital cardiac defects committee, Council on Cardiovascular Disease in the Young. *Circulation* **2007**, *115*, 3015–3038.
9. Øyen, N.; Poulsen, G.; Wohlfahrt, J.; Boyd, H.A.; Jensen, P.K.; Melbye, M. Recurrence of discordant congenital heart defects in families. *Circ. Cardiovasc. Genet.* **2010**, *3*, 122–128.
10. Øyen, N.; Poulsen, G.; Boyd, H.A.; Wohlfahrt, J.; Jensen, P.K.; Melbye, M. Recurrence of congenital heart defects in families. *Circulation* **2009**, *120*, 295–301.
11. Hinton, R.B.; Martin, L.J.; Rame-Gowda, S.; Tabangin, M.E.; Cripe, L.H.; Benson, D.W. Hypoplastic left heart syndrome is heritable. *J. Am. Coll. Cardiol.* **2007**, *50*, 1590–1595.
12. Hinton, R.B.; Martin, L.J.; Rame-Gowda, S.; Tabangin, M.E.; Cripe, L.H.; Benson, D.W. Hypoplastic left heart syndrome links to chromosomes 10q and 6q and is genetically related to bicuspid aortic valve. *J. Am. Coll. Cardiol.* **2009**, *53*, 1065–1071.
13. McBride, K.L.; Pignatelli, R.; Lewin, M.; Ho, T.; Fernbach, S.; Menesses, A.; Lam, W.; Leal, S.M.; Kaplan, N.; Schliekelman, P.; *et al.* Inheritance analysis of congenital left ventricular outflow tract obstruction malformations: Segregation, multiplex relative risk, and heritability. *Am. J. Med. Genet A* **2005**, *134A*, 180–186.
14. McBride, K.L.; Zender, G.A.; Fitzgerald-Butt, S.M.; Koehler, D.; Menesses-Diaz, A.; Fernbach, S.; Lee, K.; Towbin, J.A.; Leal, S.; Belmont, J.W. Linkage analysis of left ventricular outflow tract malformations (aortic valve stenosis, coarctation of the aorta, and hypoplastic left heart syndrome). *Eur. J. Hum. Genet.* **2009**, *17*, 811–819.
15. Pires, R.; Pires, L.M.; Vaz, S.O.; Maciel, P.; Anjos, R.; Moniz, R.; Branco, C.C.; Cabral, R.; Carreira, I.M.; Mota-Vieira, L. Screening of copy number variants in the 22q11.2 region of congenital heart disease patients from the São Miguel Island, Azores, revealed the second patient with a triplication. *BMC Genet* **2014**, *15*, 115, doi:10.1186/s12863-014-0115-6.
16. Sahoo, T.; Wang, J.C.; Elnaggar, M.M.; Sanchez-Lara, P.; Ross, L.P.; Mahon, L.W.; Hafezi, K.; Deming, A.; Hinman, L.; Bruno, Y.; *et al.* Concurrent triplication and uniparental isodisomy: Evidence for microhomology-mediated break-induced replication model for genomic rearrangements. *Eur. J. Hum. Genet* **2015**, *23*, 61–66.
17. Miller, D.T.; Adam, M.P.; Aradhya, S.; Biesecker, L.G.; Brothman, A.R.; Carter, N.P.; Church, D.M.; Crolla, J.A.; Eichler, E.E.; Epstein, C.J.; *et al.* Consensus statement: Chromosomal microarray is a first-tier clinical diagnostic test for individuals with developmental disabilities or congenital anomalies. *Am. J. Hum. Genet* **2010**, *86*, 749–764.
18. Stankiewicz, P.; Lupski, J.R. Structural variation in the human genome and its role in disease. *Annu. Rev. Med.* **2010**, *61*, 437–455.
19. Riccardi, V.M.; Lupski, J.R. Duplications, deletions, and single-nucleotide variations: The complexity of genetic arithmetic. *Genet Med.* **2013**, *15*, 172–173.
20. Zhang, F.; Carvalho, C.M.B.; Lupski, J.R. Complex human chromosomal and genomic rearrangements. *Trends Genet* **2009**, *25*, 298–307.

21. Zhang, F.; Gu, W.; Hurles, M.E.; Lupski, J.R. Copy number variation in human health, disease, and evolution. *Annu. Rev. Genomics Hum. Genet* **2009**, *10*, 451–481.
22. Lalani, S.R.; Shaw, C.; Wang, X.; Patel, A.; Patterson, L.W.; Kolodziejska, K.; Szafranski, P.; Ou, Z.; Tian, Q.; Kang, S.H.; *et al.* Rare DNA copy number variants in cardiovascular malformations with extracardiac abnormalities. *Hum. Mol. Genet* **2013**, *22*, 4339–4348.
23. Shaffer, L.G.; Bejjani, B.A.; Torchia, B.; Kirkpatrick, S.; Coppinger, J.; Ballif, B.C. The identification of microdeletion syndromes and other chromosome abnormalities: Cytogenetic methods of the past, new technologies for the future. *Am. J. Med. Genet C Semin. Med. Genet* **2007**, *145C*, 335–345.
24. Lander, J.; Ware, S.M. Copy Number Variation in Congenital Heart Defects. *Curr. Genet Med. Rep.* **2014**, *2*, 168–178.
25. Cowan, J.; Ware, S.M. Genetics and Genetic Testing in Congenital Heart Disease. *Clin. Perinatol.* **2015**, in press.
26. Abbott, M.E. Statistics of Congenital Cardiac Disease: 400 Cases Analyzed. *J. Med. Res.* **1908**, *19*, 77–81.
27. Fyler, D.C.; Rudolph, A.M.; Wittenborg, M.H.; Nadas, A.S. Ventricular septal defect in infants and children; a correlation of clinical, physiologic, and autopsy data. *Circulation* **1958**, *18*, 833–851.
28. Jenkins, K.J.; Correa, A.; Feinstein, J.A.; Botto, L.; Britt, A.E.; Daniels, S.R.; Elixson, M.; Warnes, C.A.; Webb, C.L. American Heart Association Council on Cardiovascular Disease in the Young. Noninherited risk factors and congenital cardiovascular defects: Current knowledge: A scientific statement from the American Heart Association Council on Cardiovascular Disease in the Young: Endorsed by the American Academy of Pediatrics. *Circulation* **2007**, *115*, 2995–3014.
29. Clark, E.B. Pathogenetic mechanisms of congenital cardiovascular malformations revisited. *Semin. Perinatol.* **1996**, *20*, 465–472.
30. Botto, L.D.; Lin, A.E.; Riehle-Colarusso, T.; Malik, S.; Correa, A. National Birth Defects Prevention Study. Seeking causes: Classifying and evaluating congenital heart defects in etiologic studies. *Birth Defects Res. A Clin. Mol. Teratol.* **2007**, *79*, 714–727.
31. Harris, P.A.; Taylor, R.; Thielke, R.; Payne, J.; Gnzalez, N.; Conde, J.G. Research electronic data capture (REDCap)—A metadata-driven methodology and workflow process for providing translational research informatics support. *J. Biomed. Inform.* **2009**, *42*, 377–381.
32. Ferencz, C.; Rubin, J.; Loffredo, C.; Wilson, P. Genetic and environmental risk factors of major cardiovascular malformations: The Baltimore-Washington Infant Study 1981–1989. In *Perspectives in Pediatric Cardiology*; Futura Publishing: Armonk, NY, USA, 1997; Volume 5, pp. 1–189.
33. Connor, J.A.; Hinton, R.B.; Miller, E.M.; Sund, K.L.; Ruschman, J.G.; Ware, S.M. Genetic testing practices in infants with congenital heart disease. *Congenit. Heart Dis.* **2014**, *9*, 158–167.
34. Geddes, G.C.; Butterly, M.; Sajan, I. FISH for 22q11.2 Deletion Not Cost-Effective for Infants with Congenital Heart Disease with Microarray. *Pediatr. Cardiol.* **2015**, *36*, 531–536.
35. Carey, A.S.; Liang, L.; Edwards, J.; Brandt, T.; Mei, H.; Sharp, A.J.; Hsu, D.T.; Newburger, J.W.; Ohye, R.G.; Chung, W.K.; *et al.* Effect of copy number variants on outcomes for infants with single ventricle heart defects. *Circ. Cardiovasc. Genet.* **2013**, *6*, 444–451.

36. Greenway, S.C.; Pereira, A.C.; Lin, J.C.; DePalma, S.R.; Israel, S.J.; Mesquita, S.M.; Ergul, E.; Conta, J.H.; Korn, J.M.; McCarroll, S.A.; *et al.* De novo copy number variants identify new genes and loci in isolated sporadic tetralogy of Fallot. *Nat. Genet.* **2009**, *41*, 931–935.
37. Parrott, A.; James, J.; Goldenberg, P.; Hinton, R.B.; Miller, E.; Shikany, A.; Aylsworth, A.S.; Kaiser-Rogers, K.; Ferns, S.J.; Lalani, S.R.; *et al.* Aortopathy in the 7q11.23 microduplication syndrome. *Am. J. Med. Genet A* **2015**, *167A*, 363–370.
38. Lalani, S.R.; Ware, S.M.; Wang, X.; Zapata, G.; Tian, Q.; Franco, L.M.; Jiang, Z.; Bucasas, K.; Scott, D.A.; Campeau, P.M.; *et al.* MCTP2 is a dosage-sensitive gene required for cardiac outflow tract development. *Hum. Mol. Genet* **2013**, *22*, 4339–4348.
39. Chang, S.W.; Mislankar, M.; Misra, C.; Huang, N.; Dajusta, D.G.; Harrison, S.M.; McBride, K.L.; Baker, L.A.; Garg, V. Genetic abnormalities in FOXP1 are associated with congenital heart defects. *Hum. Mutat* **2013**, *34*, 1226–1230.
40. Ware, S.M.; Shikany, A.; Landis, B.J.; James, J.F.; Hinton, R.B. Twins with progressive thoracic aortic aneurysm, recurrent dissection and ACTA2 mutation. *Pediatrics* **2014**, *134*, e1218–e1223.
41. Parrott, A.; Ware, S.M. The Role of the Geneticist and Genetic Counselor in an ACHD Clinic. *Prog. Pediatr. Cardiol.* **2012**, *34*, 15–20.
42. Somers, A.E.; Ware, S.M.; Collins, K.; Jefferies, J.L.; He, H.; Miller, E.M. Provision of cardiovascular genetic counseling services: Current practice and future directions. *J. Genet Couns.* **2014**, *23*, 976–983.
43. Jacobs, J.P.; Mavroudis, C.; Jacobs, M.L.; Lacour-Gayet, F.G.; Tchervenkov, C.I.; William Gaynor, J.; Clarke, D.R.; Spray, T.L.; Maruszewski, B.; Stellin, G.; *et al.* Lessons learned from the data analysis of the second harvest (1998–2001) of the Society of Thoracic Surgeons (STS) Congenital Heart Surgery Database. *Eur. J. Cardiothorac. Surg.* **2004**, *26*, 18–37.
44. Zaidi, S.; Choi, M.; Wakimoto, H.; Ma, L.; Jiang, J.; Overton, J.D.; Romano-Adesman, A.; Bjornson, R.D.; Breitbart, R.E.; Brown, K.K.; *et al.* De novo mutations in histone-modifying genes in congenital heart disease. *Nature* **2013**, *498*, 220–223.
45. Pediatric Cardiac Genomics Consortium; Gelb, B.; Brueckner, M.; Chung, W.; Goldmuntz, E.; Kaltman, J.; Kaski, J.P.; Kim, R.; Kline, J.; Mercer-Rosa, L.; Porter, G.; *et al.* The Congenital Heart Disease Genetic Network Study: Rationale, design, and early results. *Circ. Res.* **2013**, *112*, 698–706.
46. McBride, K.L.; Ware, S.M. Modifying Mendel: Approaches for identification of susceptibility alleles for human cardiovascular malformations. *Circ. Cardiovasc. Genet* **2012**, *5*, 274–276.
47. Arrington, C.B.; Bleyl, S.B.; Matsunami, N.; Bonnell, G.D.; Otterud, B.E.; Nielsen, D.C.; Stevens, J.; Levy, S.; Leppert, M.F.; Bowles, N.E. Exome analysis of a family with pleiotropic congenital heart disease. *Circ. Cardiovasc. Genet* **2012**, *5*, 175–182.
48. Ashley, E.A.; Hershberger, R.E.; Caleshu, C.; Ellinor, P.T.; Garcia, J.G.; Herrington, D.M.; Ho, C.Y.; Johnson, J.A.; Kittner, S.J.; Macrae, C.A.; *et al.* American Heart Association Advocacy Coordinating Committee. Genetics and cardiovascular disease: A policy statement from the American Heart Association. *Circulation* **2012**, *126*, 142–157.
49. Lin, A.E.; Salbert, B.A.; Belmont, J.; Smoot, L. Total is more than the sum of the parts: Phenotyping the heart in cardiovascular genetics clinics. *Am. J. Med. Genet A* **2004**, *131*, 111–114.

50. Teot, L.A.; Sposto, R.; Khayat, A.; Qualman, S.; Reaman, G.; Parham, D.; Children's Oncology Group. The problems and promise of central pathology review: Development of a standardized procedure for the Children's Oncology Group. *Pediatr. Dev. Pathol.* **2007**, *10*, 199–207.
51. Malempati, S.; Hawkins, D.S. Rhabdomyosarcoma: Review of the Children's Oncology Group (COG) Soft-Tissue Sarcoma Committee experience and rationale for current COG studies. *Pediatr. Blood Cancer* **2012**, *59*, 5–10.

4

N-acetylglucosamine-1-Phosphate Transferase Suppresses Lysosomal Hydrolases in Dysfunctional Osteoclasts: A Potential Mechanism for Vascular Calcification

Yang Lei, Masaya Iwashita, Jung Choi, Masanori Aikawa and Elena Aikawa *

Center for Interdisciplinary Cardiovascular Sciences, Division of Cardiovascular Medicine, Brigham and Women's Hospital, Harvard Medical School, Boston, MA 02115, USA; E-Mails: ylei3@partners.org (Y.L.); miwashita@partners.org (M.I.); jchoi22@partners.org (J.C.); maikawa@rics.bwh.harvard.edu (M.A.)

* Author to whom correspondence should be addressed; E-Mail: eaikawa@partners.org

Academic Editors: Cheryl L. Maslen and Russell Norris

Abstract: In addition to increased differentiation of vascular smooth muscle cells into osteoblast-like phenotypes, the limited accumulation of osteoclasts in atherosclerotic plaques or their dysfunction may participate in potential mechanisms for vascular calcification. *N*-acetylglucosamine-1-phosphate transferase containing alpha and beta subunits (GNPTAB) is a transmembrane enzyme complex that mediates the vesicular transport of lysosomal hydrolases. GNPTAB may also regulate the biogenesis of lysosomal hydrolases from bone-marrow derived osteoclasts. In this study, the areas surrounding calcification in human atherosclerotic plaques contained high levels of GNPTAB and low levels of lysosomal hydrolases such as cathepsin K (CTSK) and tartrate-resistant acid phosphatase (TRAP), as demonstrated by immunohistochemistry and laser-capture microdissection-assisted mRNA expression analysis. We therefore hypothesized that GNPTAB secretion may suppress the release of CTSK and TRAP by vascular osteoclast-like cells, thus causing their dysfunction and reducing the resorption of calcification. We used human primary macrophages derived from peripheral blood mononuclear cells, an established osteoclast differentiation model. GNPTAB siRNA silencing accelerated the formation of functional osteoclasts as detected by increased secretion of CTSK and TRAP and increased their bone resorption activity as gauged by resorption pits assay. We concluded that high levels of GNPTAB inhibit secretion of lysosomal hydrolases in dysfunctional osteoclasts, thereby affecting their resorption potential in cardiovascular calcification.

Keywords: GNPTAB; vascular calcification; osteoclast; lysosomal hydrolases

1. Introduction

Previous studies have proposed several mechanisms for vascular calcification, including osteoblastic differentiation of smooth muscle cells (SMCs) [1–3], limited accumulation of osteoclasts and their dysfunction [4–7], loss of endogenous inhibitors of mineralization [8,9], cell death [10], and thermodynamic mechanisms via elevated calcium and phosphate levels [11]. Similarly, bone mineralization involves multiple mechanisms [12]. Bone homeostasis depends on the balance between bone formation by osteoblasts and bone resorption by osteoclasts [13]. Osteoclasts originated from hematopoietic progenitors of the monocyte/macrophage lineage differentiate into functional osteoclasts and resorb mineralized tissues [14]. To solubilize the mineral component of bone, osteoclasts secrete various enzymes such as tartrate-resistant acid phosphatase (TRAP) [15], cathepsin K (CTSK) [16], and carbonic anhydrase II [17]. TRAP, an osteoclast differentiation marker, regulates bone mineral matrix resorption [15]; CTSK cleaves collagen [16]; and carbonic anhydrase II facilitates proton production and thus maintains acidification of the resorption lacuna [17,18].

While the sources of osteoclasts and osteoblasts in vasculature and bone could be different, vascular calcification and bone mineralization share similar mechanisms, including the maintenance of a balance between bone forming osteoblasts and bone resorbing osteoclasts. Pluripotent cells exist in arteries, and studies showed that peripheral mononuclear phagocytic cells can differentiate into osteoclast-like cells with receptor activator of nuclear factor-κB ligand (RANKL) and macrophage colony-stimulating factor (MCSF) signaling [19]. Net calcium deposition in calcified atherosclerotic plaques occurs due to imbalance between the functional activity of osteoclast-like cells and osteoblast-like cells in vascular system [20,21].

N-acetylglucosamine-1-phosphate transferase, alpha and beta subunits (GNPTAB), is a transmembrane enzyme complex which catalyzes the formation of the mannose-6-phosphate (M6P) recognition on high mannose type oligosaccharides in lysosomal hydrolases. The M6P pathway regulates most lysosomal hydrolases, which are synthesized in the endoplasmic reticulum. The modified lysosomal hydrolases are then packaged into clathrin-coated transport vesicles for delivery to endosomes and lysosomes [22,23]. GNPTAB-deficient mice showed that osteoclasts derived from their bone marrow have increased secretion of TRAP and CTSK but not cathepsin D [24]. Another study used mucolipidosis type II-deficient mice, generated by a single-base insertion into the GNPTAB gene corresponding to a mutation detected in mucolipidosis type II patients [25], to show the increased formation of intact osteoclasts, combined with decreased activity of bone-forming osteoblasts [26]. The present study has tested the hypothesis that molecules commonly expressed by these two cell types such as GNPTAB serve as molecular switches differentially regulating osteoclast and osteoblast functions.

2. Materials and Methods

2.1. Human Carotid Arteries

Human carotid arteries (non-calcified arteries, n = 3; calcified atherosclerotic plaques, n = 6) were obtained from endarterectomy and autopsy specimens harvested following protocol approved by the Institutional Review Board of Brigham and Women's Hospital (protocol # 1999P001348). Human tissues were analyzed by immunohistochemistry and immunofluorescence. Cryosections of 6-µm thickness were stained for GNPTAB, CD68, TRAP, and CTSK. Adjacent sections were double labeled for GNPATB and CD68 for colocalization analysis. Sections with high expression of GNPTAB in calcified plaques or no expression of GNPTAB in non-calcified regions were submitted for laser-capture microdissection (LMD 6500, Leica, Wetzlar, Germany). Calcified GNPTAB-enriched areas as well as non-calcified areas were captured in four adjacent 20-µm sections and pooled for RNA extraction using TRIzol reagent (Invitrogen, Carlsbad, CA, USA).

2.2. Immunohistochemistry and Immunofluorescence for Human Tissues

Immunohistochemistry and immunofluorescence for human tissues were performed on fresh-frozen sections as previously described [27,28]. Tissue samples were frozen in OCT compound (Sakura Finetech, Torrance, CA, USA) and 6-µm sections were fixed in 4% paraformaldehyde, blocked in 4% horse serum and incubated with primary antibody for 90 min. Primary antibodies included GNPTAB (Novus Biologicals, Littleton, CO, USA), CD68 (Dako, Copenhagen, Denmark), TRAP (Abcam, Cambridge, MA, USA), and CTSK (Abcam, Cambridge, MA, USA). The avidin-biotin peroxidase method was used. The reactions were visualized with 3-amino-9-ethylcarbazole substrate (AEC substrate; Dako, Denmark). Sections treated with PBS without primary antibody were used as negative controls. The slides were scanned using 20× magnification for digital imaging on a GE Omnyx™ VL4 scanner (Omnyx LLC, Pittsburgh, PA, USA) and exported from the Omnyx™ Pathologist Work Station to view whole slide images. Areas of interest were also captured using 400× magnification with a charged-coupled device camera with a fixed aperture (Nikon DS-Fi1c, Nikon, Tokyo, Japan) on a Nikon ECLIPSE 50i microscope (Nikon, Tokyo, Japan).

For immunofluorescence, GNPATB and CD68 were labeled with streptavidin-conjugated Alexa Fluor 594 antibody and streptavidin-conjugated Alexa Fluor 488 antibody, respectively. Sections were mounted with mounting medium containing 4',6-diamidino-2-phenylindole (DAPI, Vector Laboratories, Burlingame, CA, USA). Images were then captured using confocal microscopy (A1, Nikon).

2.3. CD14-Immunoreactive Monocyte Isolation and Osteoclast Differentiation

CD14-immunoreactive monocytes were isolated from human peripheral blood mononuclear cells using Dynabeads® FlowComp™ Human CD14 Kit (Invitrogen, Carlsbad, CA, USA). Thirty milliliters of buffy coat (Research Blood Components, Boston, MA, USA) underwent lymphocyte separation using lymphocyte separation medium (LSM; MP Biomedicals, Santa Ana, CA, USA) and washed with Hank's balanced salt solution (HBSS; Corning Cellgro, Manassas, VA, USA), specifically purified by CD14 antibody. This protocols yields up to 30–60 million CD14-immunopositive monocytes.

These isolated CD14-immunoractive monocytes were maintained in alpha-MEM (Sigma, St Louis, MO, USA) supplemented with 10% fetal bovine serum (FBS; Life Technologies, Rockville, MD, USA), 1% L-glutamine, penicillin, and streptomycin (Sigma) and cultured on 6-well plate (2×10^6 cells/well) for mRNA and protein isolation, Corning Osteo Assay Surface 24-well plate for bone resorption analysis (0.5×10^6 cells/well; Corning Life Sciences, Lowell, MA), and 96-well plate for TRAP staining and immunofluorescence.

CD14-immunoractive monocytes underwent three following treatments: (1) macrophage colony-stimulating factor (MCSF, 25 ng/mL; PeproTech, Rocky Hill, NJ, USA) for macrophage control; (2) MCSF (25 ng/mL) + soluble human receptor activator of nuclear factor-κB ligand (RANKL, 30 ng/mL; PeproTech, Rocky Hill, NJ, USA) with non-targeting (NT) scrambled control siRNA (NT siRNA; SMARTpool siGENOME siRNA; GE Healthcare, Lafayette, CO, USA); and (3) MCSF followed by treatments with RANKL and GNPTAB siRNA (siGNPTAB; SMARTpool siGENOME siRNA; GE Healthcare, CO, USA). Group 1 served as negative control in which cells were maintained as macrophages; group 2 served as positive control in which cells were differentiated into osteoclasts, and group 3 represented differentiated osteoclasts treated with siRNA GNPTAB. The medium was changed twice a week and cells were maintained for 14 days.

2.4. siRNA Transfection Experiments

Small interfering RNA (siRNA) transfer to human CD14-immunoreactive monocytes used SilenceMag (Boca Scientific, Boca Raton, FL, USA). Fifty nanometers of siRNA was diluted in reduced-serum Opti-MEM® Medium (Life Technologies, Gaithersburg, MD, USA), mixed with the SilenceMag reagent, and incubated at RT. This mixture was added drop by drop onto the cells. Cell cultures were placed on the magnetic plates for 15 min. After 6 h, medium was changed. The siRNA transfection procedures were performed on day 4, day 7, and day 10. By the end of the experiment on day 14, efficiency of the knockdown was determined at both mRNA and protein levels. Cells were lysed using TRIzol reagent (Invitrogen, Carlsbad, CA, USA) and analyzed by RT-PCR. The protein expression was assessed by immunofluorescence.

2.5. Real-Time PCR Analysis

Total RNA from both human tissue and human CD14-immunoreactive monocytes were isolated by TRIzol reagent (Invitrogen, Carlsbad, CA, USA) and reversed transcribed using qScript™ cDNA Synthesis Kit (Quanta Biosciences, Gaithersberg, MD, USA). Real-time quantitative PCR was performed using Taqman® Gene Expression Assay probes (Applied Biosystems, Foster City, CA, USA; Supplemental Table S1) TaqMan® fast universal master kit (Applied Biosystems, Foster City, CA, USA) by Applied Biosystems® 7900HT Fast Real-Time PCR System and normalized by GAPDH. Relative fold changes were calculated by the $2^{-\Delta\Delta CT}$ method.

2.6. Immunofluorescence for Human Cells

Human CD14-immunoreactive monocytes were washed with PBS, fixed by 4% formaldehyde, blocked with 2% bovine serum albumin (BSA) and 0.05% Tween-20 in PBS. For silencing efficiency of GNPTAB, cells were incubated with rabbit anti-GNPTAB (Novus Biologicals, Littleton, CO, USA) for 90 minutes at room temperature, followed with AlexaFlour® 488-conjugated anti-rabbit IgG antibody (Life Technologies, Gaithersburg, MD, USA) for 60 min at room temperature and then processed for imaging. For cellular morphology study, cells were incubated with Alexa Fluor® 594 phalloidin (Life Technologies, Gaithersburg, MD, USA) for 30 min at room temperature. Cells were washed three times with PBS and mounted with mounting medium containing DAPI (Vector Laboratories). Images were captured with confocal microscope A1 (Nikon, Tokyo, Japan).

2.7. TRAP Staining and Quantification

TRAP staining and quantification used the TRAP staining kit (B-Bridge International, Sunnyvale, CA, USA). Cells on 96-well plates were washed by PBS, fixed by 10% formalin for 5 min at room temperature, stained by chromogenic substrate for up to 60 min until the best color condition was obtained. Images were taken After TRAP staining by light microscope and used to count the number of osteoclast-like cells. Detailed method is provided in online only Supplemental Materials (Figure S1). Briefly, TRAP-positive cells that had at least three nuclei were counted as differentiated osteoclasts [29,30] (Figure S1A). Five random-chosen areas were used to count osteoclast numbers followed by statistical analysis (Figure S1B). For quantification of TRAP activity, cell lysates or supernatant media were incubated with by chromogenic substrate for 3 h at 37 °C and then read in a microplate reader at 540 nm.

2.8. Resorption Assay for Osteoclast Functional Analysis

By the end of experiments (day 14), cells were removed with 10% bleach for 10 min at room temperature. The wells were washed twice with distilled water, dried for 3–5 h at room temperature and then resorption pit images were taken using a light microscope (Nikon ECLIPSE 50i microscope; Nikon, Tokyo, Japan). Images were converted to black and white binary images for quantification of pit resorption area using the image J [31].

2.9. CTSK Activity Assay

CTSK activity was measured using Cathepsin K activity assay kit (Abcam), a fluorescence-based assay that utilizes the preferred cathepsin-L substrate sequence LR labeled with AFC (amino-4-trifluoromethyl coumarin). The released AFC can easily be quantified using a fluorescence plate reader. Ten microliters of cell lysates or 50 μL of supernatant media were added with 50 μL of cathepsin K reaction buffer and 2 μL of the 10 mM Ac-LR-AFC substrate, incubated at 37 °C for 1–2 h then read in a microplate reader (400 nm excitation/505 nm emission).

2.10. Statistics

Results are expressed as means ± standard error of the mean (SEM). Statistical analyses used single-factor ANOVA. Data were considered significant with p value <0.05. Asterisks in figures denote statistical significance ($p < 0.05$) for each group compared with controls.

3. Results

3.1. Human Calcified Arteries Contain Enriched GNPTAB around Calcified Areas but Low Levels of Osteoclast Lysosomal Hydrolases

Regions around calcified areas of human carotid arteries contained many macrophages, detected by CD68, and prominent expression of GNPTAB (Table 1, Figure 1A and online only Supplemental Figure S2). The evidence has suggested the discrepancy between limited numbers of osteoclasts and abundance of macrophages, precursors of osteoclasts, in calcifying atherosclerotic plaques. The reason behind the lack of fully differentiated multinuclear cells that are able to resorb calcium deposition in cardiovascular tissues is unknown. Our histopathological observations showed that two major osteoclast lysosomal hydrolases, TRAP and CTSK, had negligible expression within GNPTAB-immunoreactive cells, surrounding calcifying regions, indicating that GNPTAB may affect TRAP and CTSK expression and thus suppress osteoclast function (Table 1, Figure 1A and online only Supplemental Figure S2). Double labeling for GNPTAB and CD68 showed that large populations of macrophages express GNPTAB (Figure 1B).

Table 1. An analysis for immunohistochemistry (IHC) studies including GNPTAB, CD68, TRAP, and CTSK expression in non-calcified ($n = 3$) and calcified ($n = 6$) human arteries. Our quantitative criteria for relative abundance of expression include "-" for 0% of positive cells; "+" for ≤25%; "++" for ≤50%; "+++" for ≤75%; and "++++" for ≤100%. C: calcified; NC: non-calcified; CAA: carotid artery from autopsy specimens; LCE: left carotid artery from endarterectomy specimens; RCE: right carotid artery from endarterectomy specimens.

Human Arteries ID	GNPTAB	CD68	TRAP	CTSK
Non-Calcified Human Carotid Arteries ($n = 3$)				
NC1-CAA5	-	+	-	+
NC2-CAA8	-	+	-	+
NC3-CAA11	-	+	-	+
Calcified Human Carotid Arteries ($n = 6$)				
C1-CAA2b	+++	++++	-	+
C2-LCE1	++	++++	+	+
C3-LCE4	++++	++++	+	-
C4-LCE11	++++	++++	+	-
C5-RCE7	+	++	-	-
C6-RCE10	++	++++	+	-

Laser-capture microdissection (LCM) allows rapid one-step collection from a section of complex and heterogeneous tissue [32], which is then can be used to extract DNA, RNA and proteins [33]. To further examine gene expression, we used this method to dissect GNPTAB-immunoreactive cells adjacent to calcified areas and GNPTAB-negative regions within non-calcified areas (Figure 2A). Calcified areas had significant increase of GNPTAB mRNA level *versus* non-calcified areas (Figure 2B; 2.28 ± 0.10 fold change, $p = 0.0029$, $n = 4$; two technical replicates) accompanied by a decrease of CTSK mRNA levels (Figure 2B; 0.42 ± 0.09 fold change, $p = 0.0109$, $n = 4$; two technical replicates).

Of note, TRAP mRNA levels were non-detectable in both calcified and non-calcified areas. These results indicate that GNPTAB expression around calcified regions inhibit secretion of lysosomal hydrolases such as TRAP and CTSK, which can cause the dysfunction of osteoclast-like cells in atherosclerotic plaques.

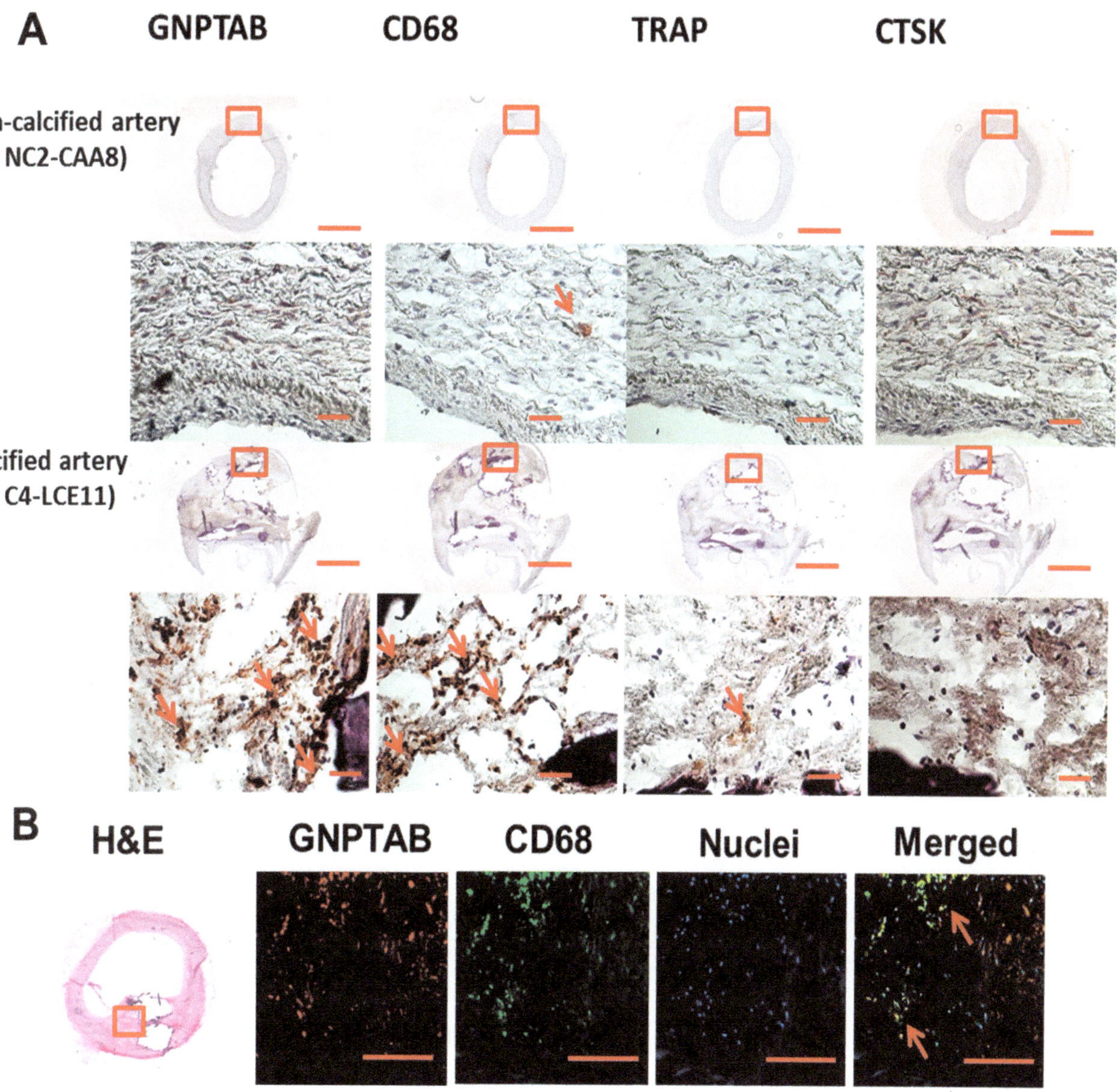

Figure 1. (**A**) Representative non-calcified and calcified arteries showed high expression of GNPTAB around and within CD68-immunopositive macrophages (red reaction product) but low expression of TRAP and CTSK in calcified arteries. No GNPTAB expression was observed in non-calcified arteries. Top row: bar = 2 mm; bottom row: bar = 500 μm. n = 3: non-calcified arteries; n = 6: calcified arteries; (**B**) Double fluorescence labeling for GNPTAB and CD68 identified a large population of macrophages co-expressing GNPTAB (arrows). Bars = 200 μm.

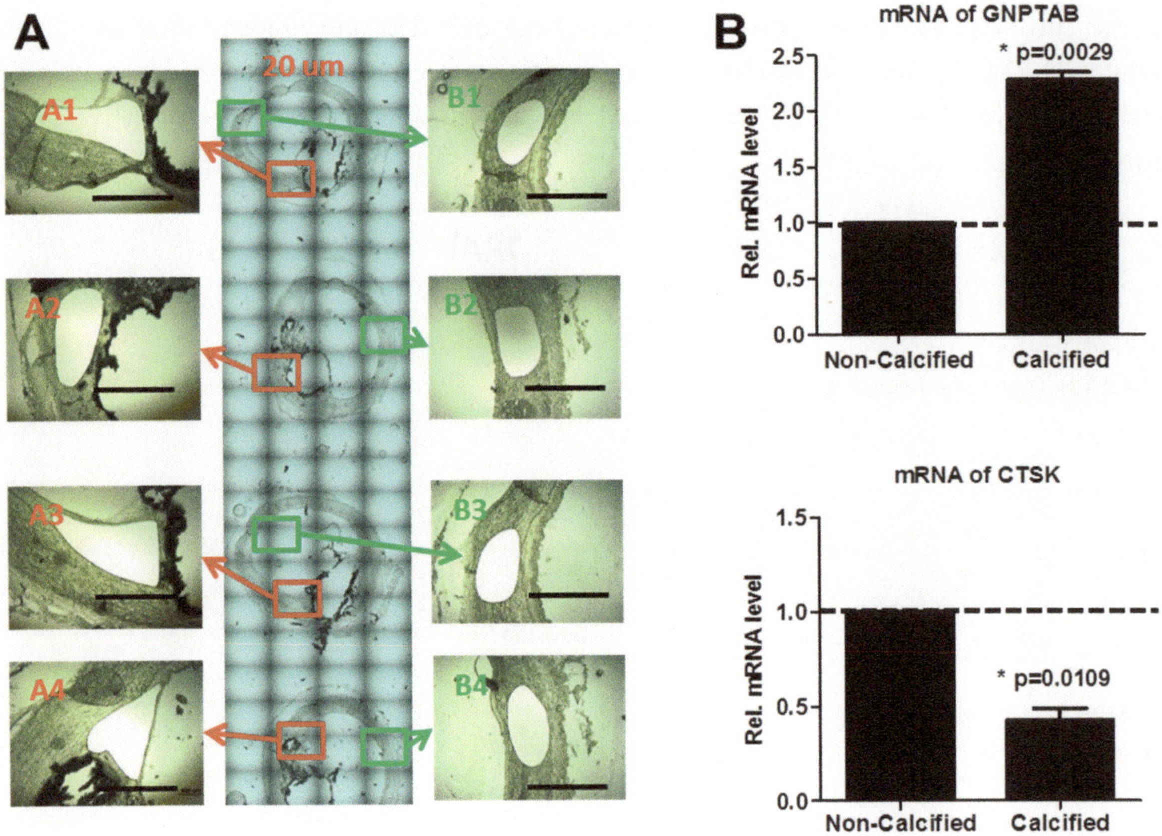

Figure 2. (**A**) Laser-capture microdissection-assisted mRNA analysis in human calcified carotid arteries. Four adjacent 20-μm sections both from GNPTAB-positive calcified areas (A1–A4) and GNPTAB-negative non-calcified areas (B1–B4) were pooled for RNA extraction. Bars = 500 μm; (**B**) mRNA levels of GNPTAB and CTSK in GNPTAB-positive calcified areas *versus* GNPTAB-negative non-calcified areas. (n = 4; two technical replicates each).

3.2. GNPTAB Silencing Increases Osteoclastogenesis and Resorption Pits Formed by Functional Osteoclast-Like Cells

To validate our proposed mechanisms on the role of GNPTAB in osteoclast differentiation, we used human peripheral blood mononuclear cells (PBMC), an established model for osteoclast differentiation [34]. The experimental design is shown in the schematic (Figure 3A). We used the following groups: (1) MCSF treatment group, a negative control for non-differentiated CD14-immunoreactive monocytes/macrophages; (2) MCSF, RANKL, and non-targeting (NT) scrambled control siRNA treatments group to induce osteoclast differentiation; (3) MCSF, RANKL and siRNA GNPTAB treatments group to test the effects GNPTAB on osteoclastogenesis and osteoclast bone resorption function. Efficiency of the knockdown experiments was determined at both mRNA and protein levels by immunofluorescence (Figure 3B,C). The concentration of 50 nM siRNA for GNPTAB showed sufficient silencing efficiency and therefore was used in all of the following experiments.

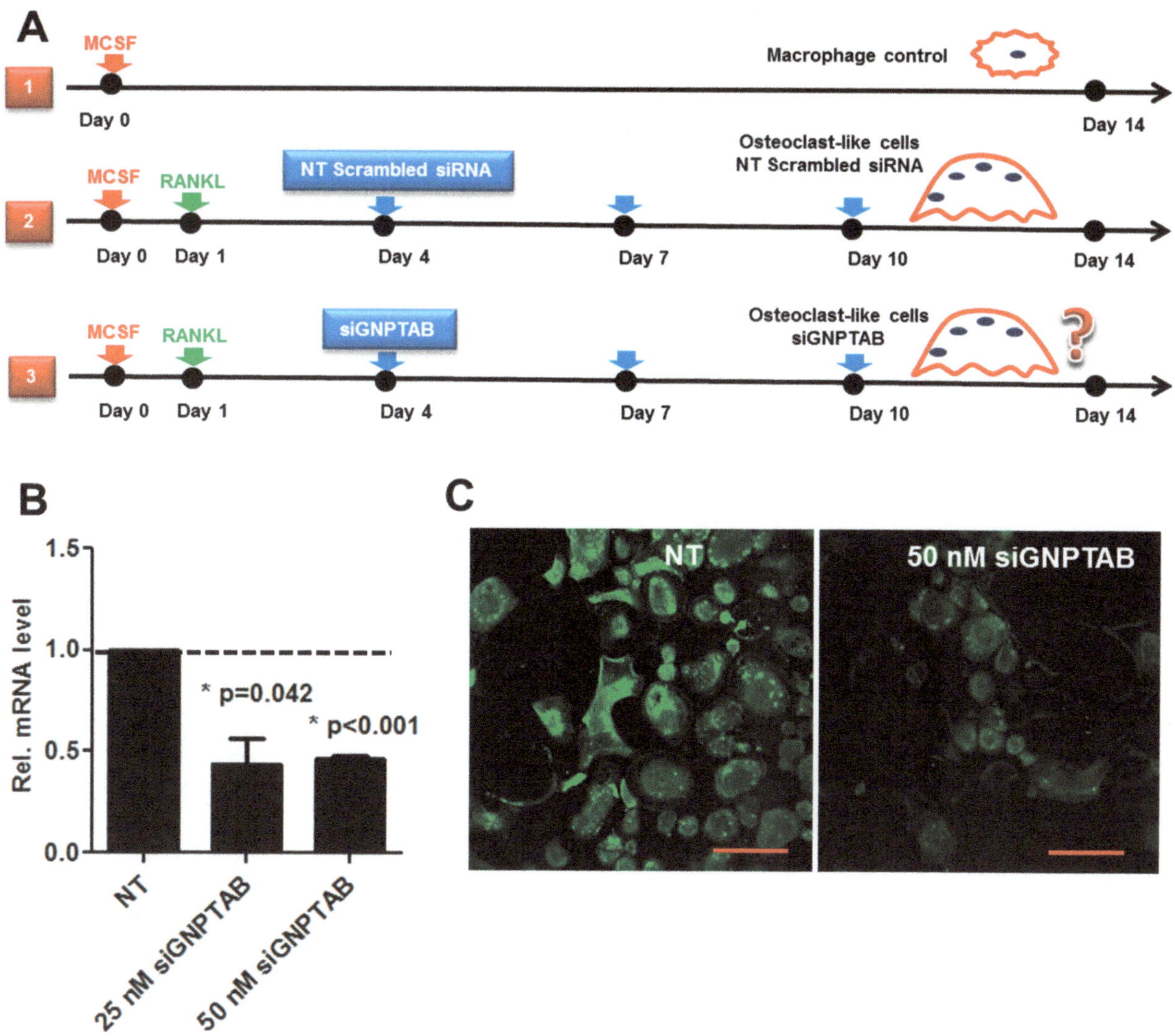

Figure 3. (**A**) Schematic illustrates the treatment protocol for isolated CD14-immunoreactive monocytes. Group 1, control group; group 2, differentiated osteoclasts treated with non-targeting (NT) scrambled control siRNA; and group 3, differentiated osteoclasts treated with siRNA GNPTAB; (**B**,**C**) Silencing efficiency was determined at both mRNA and protein levels by immunofluorescence. Bars = 200 µm (n = 4; two technical replicates each).

Our results showed that osteoclasts treated with siRNA GNPTAB were smaller in size and more numerous as compared to NT scrambled control siRNA treatments (Figure 4A). The number of multinucleated TRAP-positive osteoclasts increased in the siRNA GNPTAB group (Figure 4B; 62.61 ± 6.03 *versus* 37.64 ± 4.566, $p < 0.0001$; See online Supplemental Materials for raw images: Figure S3A). To demonstrate the functional activity of osteoclasts, untreated cells, NT scrambled control siRNA treated osteoclasts and siRNA GNPTAB-treated cells were grown on an inorganic crystalline calcium phosphate plates designed to mimic *in vivo* bone environment [35]. We found a significant increase in the areas of resorption pits formed by osteoclasts in the siRNA GNPTAB group as compared to NT scrambled control siRNA treated group (Figure 4C,D; 53.80 ± 3.11 *versus* 16.03 ±

6.59, $p < 0.0001$; See online Supplemental Materials for raw images: Figure S3B), suggesting that CNPTAB silencing increases osteoclast differentiation and functionality.

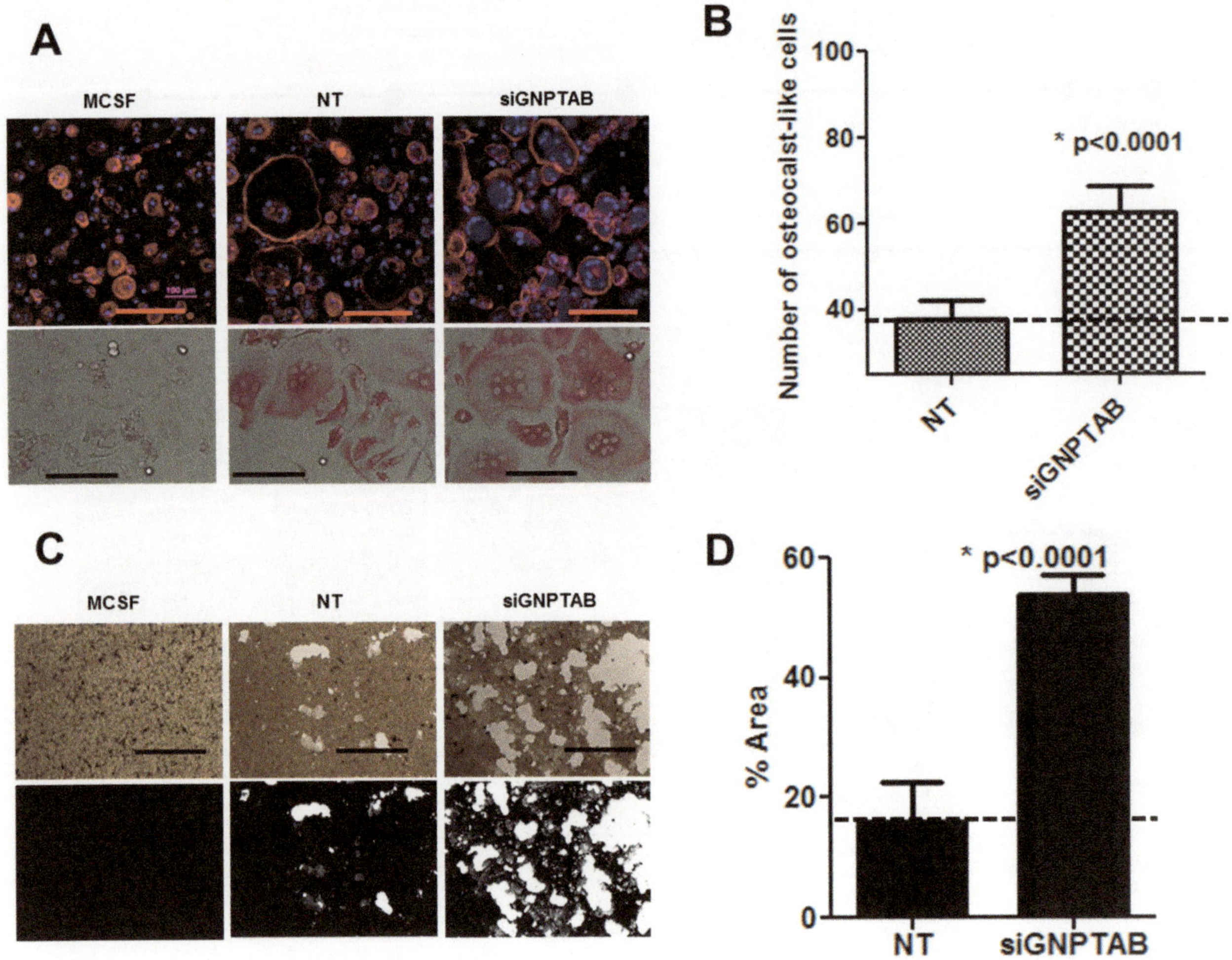

Figure 4. (**A**) Cellular morphology by F-actin immunofluorescence (top row) and TRAP staining (bottom row). F-actin rings were stained by Alexa Fluor® 594 phalloidin (Red) and Nuclei were stained by DAPI (Blue). TRAP activity assay showed increased numbers of multinucleated osteoclast-like cells. Top row: bars = 200 μm. Bottom row: bars = 200 μm. ($n = 4$, two or five technical replicates each); (**B**) Number of osteoclast-like cells counted based on TRAP staining ($n = 4$, two or five technical replicates each); (**C**) Pit resorption assays showed resorption pits (white color) formed by functional osteoclasts ($n = 4$, one or two technical replicates each). Black and white binary images converted by Image J. Bars = 50 μm; (**D**) Percentages of pit areas quantified by Image J ($n = 4$, one or two technical replicates each).

3.3. GNPTAB Silencing Increased Secretion of Lysosomal Hydrolases

To further elucidate the mechanisms of GNPTAB effects on osteoclastogenesis, we evaluated two major osteoclast lysosomal hydrolases, TRAP and CTSK, both at the mRNA and protein levels. The expression of both TRAP and CTSK increased at mRNA levels (2.00 ± 0.06, $p = 0.0015$; 2.51 ± 0.39, $p = 0.0313$-fold change; Figure 5A,D) and protein levels in cell lysates (2.44 ± 0.13, $p = 0.0041$;

1.31 ± 0.06, p = 0.0159-fold change; Figure 5C,F). We did not find changes in TRAP and CTSK mRNA levels in supernatant media (Figure 5B,E), suggesting that the secreted lysosomal hydrolases could be trapped in a sealed space formed by osteoclasts [14].

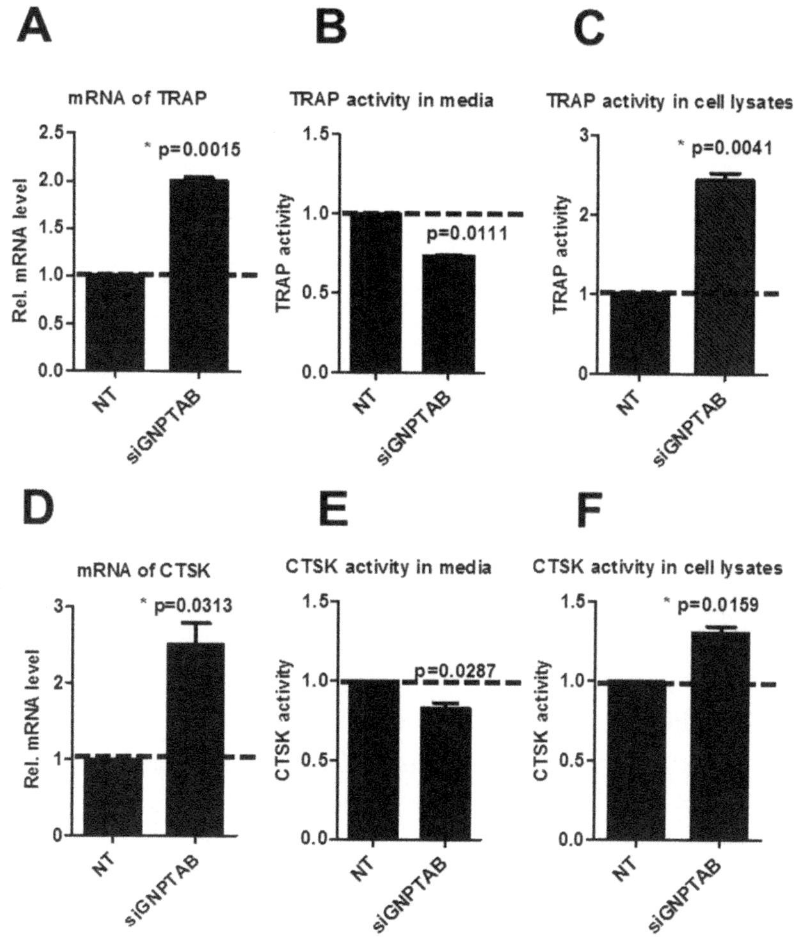

Figure 5. (**A–C**) mRNA levels of TRAP and TRAP activity in supernatant media and cell lysates ($n = 2$; two technical replicates each); (**D–F**) mRNA levels of CTSK and CTSK activity in supernatant media and cell lysates ($n = 2$; two technical replicates each).

4. Discussion

The findings of this study have provided evidence for the role of GNPTAB in vascular calcification. We found that human calcified atherosclerotic plaques contain higher protein and mRNA levels of GNPTAB around calcified areas than non-calcified plaques, associated with low expression of osteoclast lysosomal hydrolases. Based on previous studies and our own findings, we propose a link between GNPTAB, osteoclast lysosomal hydrolases, osteoclast functional activity, and vascular calcification in atherosclerotic plaques. Our experiments demonstrated that high expression of GNPTAB associates with a low CTSK and TRAP expression in calcified arteries, leading to our central hypothesis that GNPTAB inhibits secretion of lysosomal hydrolases and causes osteoclast dysfunction, which negatively affects resorption of calcium deposition in the arterial wall. Our *in vitro* loss-of-function mechanistic evidence that GNPTAB silencing by siRNA increases expression of lysosomal hydrolases and improves osteoclast function supports our hypothesis.

Numerous studies have investigated the osteoclast biology in skeletal system, but studies exploring the mechanisms for osteoclast dysfunctions in the vascular system are few. Multinuclear TRAP- and CSTK-positive osteoclast-like cells exist in calcified vascular tissues [4]. However, why osteoclast-like cells are sporadic in cardiovascular tissues and whether they have reduced ability to reverse calcification in calcified arteries remain unknown. The limited life span after implantation have reduced the effects of osteoclast-mediated therapies [5,36]. Studies also showed mechanisms of osteoclast dysfunction in osteopetrosis patients and found abnormal osteoclastogenesis and lack of osteoclast-specific adhesion structures [7]. Incomplete understanding of osteoclastogenesis in cardiovascular tissues has driven us to explore the specific molecules that can regulate osteoclast differentiation in the vasculature.

This study proposed the mechanism for GNPTAB-induced osteoclast dysfunction in vascular calcification (Figure 6). Our initial observations in human calcified carotid arteries demonstrated high expression of GNPTAB around calcified regions but low in non-calcified arteries. In osteoclast biology, many critical molecules control osteoclast differentiation and function. Two acid hydrolases highly expressed and secreted by differentiated osteoclasts are CTSK and TRAP. CTSK degrades type I collagen and osteonectin, two protein components of bone matrix [37]. TRAP is a metallophosphoesterase involved in bone matrix degradation. TRAP reacts with hydrogen peroxide to produce highly destructive reactive oxygen species (ROS) that can destroy collagen [38]. TRAP also participates in removing the M6P recognition receptor from lysosomal proteins [39]. GNPTAB modifies the M6P residues of CTSK and TRAP, allowing their recognition by M6P receptors in the Golgi apparatus and ensuring their transport to lysosomal system [23]. Disruption of the M6P pathway in GNPTAB-deficient osteoclasts from bone marrow-derived macrophages leads to dysregulated secretion of CTSK and TRAP [24].

To better model the physiological environment in the vascular system, we employed PBMC-derived macrophages stimulated with MCSF and RANKL, commonly used for osteoclast differentiation [34]. *In vitro* differentiation of human primary monocytes into mature macrophages requires MCSF [14]. Macrophage differentiation into osteoclasts commonly uses RANKL, a type 2 membrane protein of the tumor necrosis factor superfamily [40]. Previous studies showed that GNPTAB regulates osteoclastogenesis of bone marrow-derived cells [24]. Our findings supported similar mechanisms for the role of GNPTAB in regulating CTSK and TRAP in blood-derived osteoclasts. Silencing of GNPTAB by siRNA increased mRNA expression levels of lysosomal hydrolases in cell lysates but not in supernatant, indicating the possibility that these lysosomal hydrolases are trapped within a sealed space formed by ruffled border of osteoclasts or in intracellular space. Our findings agree with previously published results suggesting that bone matrix degradation occurs not only extracellularly in the resorption lacunae but also intracellularly in the transcytotic vesicles [38]. In GNPATB-deficient mice, GNPTAB increased osteoclastogenesis and decreased osteoblastogenesis [26]. However, we did not find significant changes in human SMC-derived osteoblast-like cells. Silencing of GNPTAB in human SMC exerted no effects on calcium deposition and tissue non-specific alkaline phosphatase (TNAP) activity (Online Supplemental Figure S4). GNPTAB silencing in human SMC did not affect their osteoblast differentiation, suggesting that the previously proposed role of GNPTAB in mouse osteoblasts may not represent the same mechanisms in humans.

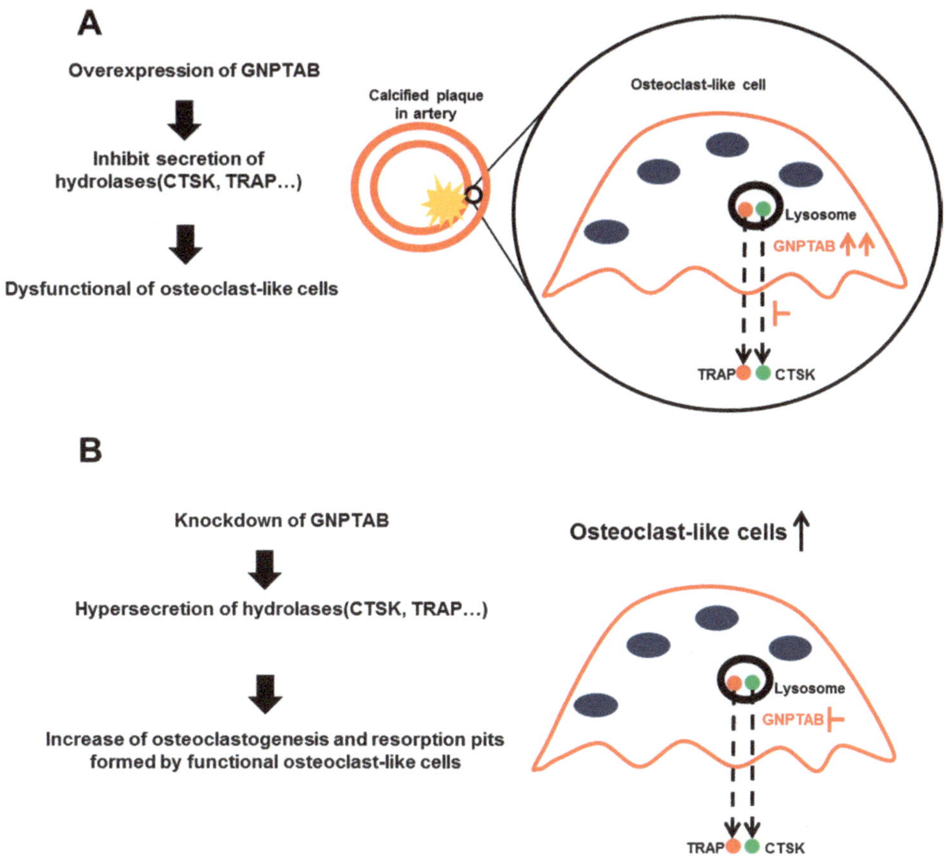

Figure 6. Proposed mechanisms of GNPTAB on regulating of osteoclast function. (**A**) High levels of GNPTAB around calcified areas in atherosclerotic plaques inhibit secretion of lysosomal hydrolases such as CTSK and TRAP, which causes dysfunction of osteoclast-like cells followed by lack of resolution of vascular calcification; (**B**) Silencing of GNPTAB enhances secretion of lysosomal hydrolases, resulting in improved osteoclast function.

Within the scope of the authors' knowledge, we for the first time reported enriched GNPATB around calcified arteries. The question as to how GNPTAB is upregulated in calcified area requires more investigation. We propose that in calcified atherosclerotic plaques, circulating monocytes/macrophages accumulate around the calcified areas and secrete lysosomal hydrolyses capable of degrading minerals, mainly hydroxyapatite. Since the majority of soluble acid hydrolases are modified by the M6P pathway, this triggers up-regulation of GNPTAB, which is one of the major functional components of the M6P pathway [22].

Taken together, our studies suggest that GNPTAB does not regulate both osteoclast and osteoblast functions in humans, while exhibiting this function in mice. However, this evidence supports the therapeutic potential of GNPTAB inhibition to promote calcification resorption in human calcified atherosclerotic plaques by improving osteoclast function without affecting SMC osteogenic potential. Since GNPTAB regulates the majority of more than 60 lysosomal enzymes besides CTSK and TRAP [22], more studies are needed to investigate the role of GNPTAB in both vascular and bone tissues.

5. Conclusions

We linked the GNPTAB to vascular calcification. Our GNPTAB siRNA silencing experiments supported the proposed mechanisms that GNPTAB regulates osteoclast function via increased CATK and TRAP production, facilitating osteoclast differentiation and improving their resorption function. In contrast, high expression levels of GNPTAB may delay macrophage differentiation into functional osteoclast-like cells characterized by low secretion levels of lysosomal hydrolases, which suppresses calcium deposition resorption in atherosclerotic plaques. Further investigation of GNPTAB and M6P pathway in vascular system may lead to the development of novel therapies for cardiovascular calcification.

Acknowledgments

The authors thank Brett Pieper for assistance with laser-dissection microscope. This study was supported by a research grant from Kowa Company, Ltd. (Nagoya, Japan, to M.A.). The Masanori Aikawa and Elena Aikawa laboratories are funded by the National Institutes of Health grants (R01HL107550 to M.A. and R01HL114805; R01HL109506 to E.A.).

Author Contributions

Study conception and design: Y.L., E.A.; acquisition of data: Y.L., M.I., J.C.; analysis and interpretation of data: Y.L., E.A., M.I., J.C.; drafting of manuscript: Y.L., M.I.; funding: M.A.; and critical revision and final approval of manuscript: Y.L., M.A., E.A.

Conflicts of Interest

The authors declare no conflict of interest.

References

1. Giachelli, C.M.; Bae, N.; Almeida, M.; Denhardt, D.T.; Alpers, C.E.; Schwartz, S.M. Osteopontin is elevated during neointima formation in rat arteries and is a novel component of human atherosclerotic plaques. *J. Clin. Investig.* **1993**, *92*, 1686–1696.
2. Levy, R.J.; Schoen, F.J.; Levy, J.T.; Nelson, A.C.; Howard, S.L.; Oshry, L.J. Biologic determinants of dystrophic calcification and osteocalcin deposition in glutaraldehyde-preserved porcine aortic valve leaflets implanted subcutaneously in rats. *Am. J. Pathol.* **1983**, *113*, 143–155.
3. Boström, K.; Watson, K.; Horn, S.; Wortham, C.; Herman, I.; Demer, L. Bone morphogenetic protein expression in human atherosclerotic lesions. *J. Clin. Investig.* **1993**, *91*, 1800–1809.
4. Boström, K.; Demer, L.L. Regulatory mechanisms in vascular calcification. *Crit. Rev. Eukaryot. Gene Expr.* **1999**, *10*, 151–158.

5. Simpson, C.L.; Lindley, S.; Eisenberg, C.; Basalyga, D.M.; Starcher, B.C.; Simionescu, D.T.; Vyavahare, N.R. Toward cell therapy for vascular calcification: Osteoclast-mediated demineralization of calcified elastin. *Cardiovasc. Pathol.* **2007**, *16*, 29–37.
6. Chellaiah, M.A.; Kizer, N.; Biswas, R.; Alvarez, U.; Strauss-Schoenberger, J.; Rifas, L.; Rittling, S.R.; Denhardt, D.T.; Hruska, K.A. Osteopontin deficiency produces osteoclast dysfunction due to reduced cd44 surface expression. *Mol. Biol. Cell* **2003**, *14*, 173–189.
7. Teti, A.; Migliaccio, S.; Taranta, A.; Bernardini, S.; De Rossi, G.; Luciani, M.; Iacobini, M.; de Felice, L.; Boldrini, R.; Bosman, C. Mechanisms of osteoclast dysfunction in human osteopetrosis: Abnormal osteoclastogenesis and lack of osteoclast-specific adhesion structures. *J. Bone Miner. Res.* **1999**, *14*, 2107–2117.
8. Luo, G.; Ducy, P.; McKee, M.D.; Pinero, G.J.; Loyer, E.; Behringer, R.R.; Karsenty, G. Spontaneous calcification of arteries and cartilage in mice lacking matrix gla protein. *Nature* **1997**, *386*, 78–81.
9. Rutsch, F.; Ruf, N.; Vaingankar, S.; Toliat, M.R.; Suk, A.; Höhne, W.; Schauer, G.; Lehmann, M.; Roscioli, T.; Schnabel, D. Mutations in enpp1 are associated with "idiopathic" infantile arterial calcification. *Nat. Genet.* **2003**, *34*, 379–381.
10. Tanimura, A.; McGregor, D.H.; Anderson, H.C. Matrix vesicles in atherosclerotic calcification. *Exp. Biol. Med.* **1983**, *172*, 173–177.
11. Giachelli, C.M. Vascular calcification mechanisms. *J. Am. Soc. Nephrol.* **2004**, *15*, 2959–2964.
12. Bini, A.; Mann, K.G.; Kudryk, B.J.; Schoen, F.J. Noncollagenous bone matrix proteins, calcification, and thrombosis in carotid artery atherosclerosis. *Arterioscler. Thromb. Vasc. Biol.* **1999**, *19*, 1852–1861.
13. Vaananen, H.; Zhao, H.; Mulari, M.; Halleen, J.M. The cell biology of osteoclast function. *J. Cell Sci.* **2000**, *113*, 377–381.
14. Teitelbaum, S.L. Bone resorption by osteoclasts. *Science* **2000**, *289*, 1504–1508.
15. Roberts, H.C.; Knott, L.; Avery, N.C.; Cox, T.M.; Evans, M.J.; Hayman, A.R. Altered collagen in tartrate-resistant acid phosphatase (trap)-deficient mice: A role for trap in bone collagen metabolism. *Calcif. Tissue Int.* **2007**, *80*, 400–410.
16. Gowen, M.; Lazner, F.; Dodds, R.; Kapadia, R.; Feild, J.; Tavaria, M.; Bertoncello, I.; Drake, F.; Zavarselk, S.; Tellis, I. Cathepsin K knockout mice develop osteopetrosis due to a deficit in matrix degradation but not demineralization. *J. Bone Miner. Res.* **1999**, *14*, 1654–1663.
17. Anderson, R.E.; Schraer, H.; Gay, C.V. Ultrastructural immunocytochemical localization of carbonic anhydrase in normal and calcitonin-treated chick osteoclasts. *Anat. Rec.* **1982**, *204*, 9–20.
18. Silverton, S.F.; Dodgson, S.J.; Fallon, M.D.; Forster, R. Carbonic anhydrase activity of chick osteoclasts is increased by parathyroid hormone. *Am. J. Physiol. Endocrinol. Metab.* **1987**, *253*, E670–E674.
19. Min, H.; Morony, S.; Sarosi, I.; Dunstan, C.R.; Capparelli, C.; Scully, S.; Van, G.; Kaufman, S.; Kostenuik, P.J.; Lacey, D.L. Osteoprotegerin reverses osteoporosis by inhibiting endosteal osteoclasts and prevents vascular calcification by blocking a process resembling osteoclastogenesis. *J. Exp. Med.* **2000**, *192*, 463–474.
20. Doherty, T.M.; Uzui, H.; Fitzpatrick, L.A.; Tripathi, P.V.; Dunstan, C.R.; Asotra, K.; Rajavashisth, T.B. Rationale for the role of osteoclast-like cells in arterial calcification. *FASEB J.* **2002**, *16*, 577–582.

21. Massy, Z.; Mentaverri, R.; Mozar, A.; Brazier, M.; Kamel, S. The pathophysiology of vascular calcification: Are osteoclast-like cells the missing link? *Diabetes Metab.* **2008**, *34*, 16–20.
22. Coutinho, M.F.; Prata, M.J.; Alves, S. Mannose-6-phosphate pathway: A review on its role in lysosomal function and dysfunction. *Mol. Genet. Metab.* **2012**, *105*, 542–550.
23. Braulke, T.; Bonifacino, J.S. Sorting of lysosomal proteins. *Biochim. Biophys. Acta* **2009**, *1793*, 605–614.
24. Van Meel, E.; Boonen, M.; Zhao, H.; Oorschot, V.; Ross, F.P.; Kornfeld, S.; Klumperman, J. Disruption of the man-6-p targeting pathway in mice impairs osteoclast secretory lysosome biogenesis. *Traffic* **2011**, *12*, 912–924.
25. Kollmann, K.; Damme, M.; Markmann, S.; Morelle, W.; Schweizer, M.; Hermans-Borgmeyer, I.; Röchert, A.; Pohl, S.; Lübke, T.; Michalski, J.-C. Lysosomal dysfunction causes neurodegeneration in mucolipidosis ii "knock-in" mice. *Brain* **2012**, *135*, 2661–2675.
26. Kollmann, K.; Pestka, J.M.; Kühn, S.C.; Schöne, E.; Schweizer, M.; Karkmann, K.; Otomo, T.; Catala-Lehnen, P.; Failla, A.V.; Marshall, R.P. Decreased bone formation and increased osteoclastogenesis cause bone loss in mucolipidosis II. *EMBO Mol. Med.* **2013**, *5*, 1871–1886.
27. New, S.E.; Goettsch, C.; Aikawa, M.; Marchini, J.F.; Shibasaki, M.; Yabusaki, K.; Libby, P.; Shanahan, C.M.; Croce, K.; Aikawa, E. Macrophage-derived matrix vesicles an alternative novel mechanism for microcalcification in atherosclerotic plaques. *Circ. Res.* **2013**, *113*, 72–77.
28. Aikawa, E.; Aikawa, M.; Libby, P.; Figueiredo, J.-L.; Rusanescu, G.; Iwamoto, Y.; Fukuda, D.; Kohler, R.H.; Shi, G.-P.; Jaffer, F.A. Arterial and aortic valve calcification abolished by elastolytic cathepsin s deficiency in chronic renal disease. *Circulation* **2009**, *119*, 1785–1794.
29. Alatalo, S.L.; Halleen, J.M.; Hentunen, T.A.; Mönkkönen, J.; Väänänen, H.K. Rapid screening method for osteoclast differentiation *in vitro* that measures tartrate-resistant acid phosphatase 5b activity secreted into the culture medium. *Clin. Chem.* **2000**, *46*, 1751–1754.
30. Takahashi, N.; Yamana, H.; Yoshiki, S.; Roodman, G.D.; Mundy, G.R.; Jones, S.J.; Boyde, A.; Suda, T. Osteoclast-like cell formation and its regulation by osteotropic hormones in mouse bone marrow cultures. *Endocrinology* **1988**, *122*, 1373–1382.
31. ImageJ. National Institute of Mental Health: Bethesda, MD, USA, 2010.
32. Emmert-Buck, M.R.; Bonner, R.F.; Smith, P.D.; Chuaqui, R.F.; Zhuang, Z.; Goldstein, S.R.; Weiss, R.A.; Liotta, L.A. Laser capture microdissection. *Science* **1996**, *274*, 998–1001.
33. Espina, V.; Wulfkuhle, J.D.; Calvert, V.S.; VanMeter, A.; Zhou, W.; Coukos, G.; Geho, D.H.; Petricoin, E.F.; Liotta, L.A. Laser-capture microdissection. *Nat. Protoc.* **2006**, *1*, 586–603.
34. Nicholson, G.C.; Malakellis, M.; Collier, F.M.; Cameron, P.U.; Holloway, W.R.; Gough, T.J.; Gregorio-King, C.; Kirkland, M.A.; Myers, D.E. Induction of osteoclasts from cd14-positive human peripheral blood mononuclear cells by receptor activator of nuclear factor kappab ligand (rankl). *Clin. Sci.* **2000**, *99*, 133–140.
35. Wood, R.M.; Rothenberg, M.; Kennebunk, M. Corning® Osteo Assay Surface 24 Well Plates with Transwell® Permeable Supports–A Useful Tool For Co-Culture Studies; Corning Life Sciences: Lowell, MA, USA, 2011.
36. Marks, S., Jr.; Seifert, M. The lifespan of osteoclasts: Experimental studies using the giant granule cytoplasmic marker characteristic of beige mice. *Bone* **1985**, *6*, 451–455.

37. Bossard, M.J.; Tomaszek, T.A.; Thompson, S.K.; Amegadzie, B.Y.; Hanning, C.R.; Jones, C.; Kurdyla, J.T.; McNulty, D.E.; Drake, F.H.; Gowen, M. Proteolytic activity of human osteoclast cathepsin K expression, purification, activation, and substrate identification. *J. Biol. Chem.* **1996**, *271*, 12517–12524.
38. Halleen, J.M.; Räisänen, S.; Salo, J.J.; Reddy, S.V.; Roodman, G.D.; Hentunen, T.A.; Lehenkari, P.P.; Kaija, H.; Vihko, P.; Väänänen, H.K. Intracellular fragmentation of bone resorption products by reactive oxygen species generated by osteoclastic tartrate-resistant acid phosphatase. *J. Biol. Chem.* **1999**, *274*, 22907–22910.
39. Sun, P.; Sleat, D.E.; Lecocq, M.; Hayman, A.R.; Jadot, M.; Lobel, P. Acid phosphatase 5 is responsible for removing the mannose 6-phosphate recognition marker from lysosomal proteins. *Proc. Natl. Acad. Sci. USA* **2008**, *105*, 16590–16595.
40. Wong, B.R.; Josien, R.; Lee, S.Y.; Sauter, B.; Li, H.-L.; Steinman, R.M.; Choi, Y. Trance (tumor necrosis factor [TNF]-related activation-induced cytokine), a new tnf family member predominantly expressed in T cells, is a dendritic cell–specific survival factor. *J. Exp. Med.* **1997**, *186*, 2075–2080.

5

Investigation of the Matrix Metalloproteinase-2 Gene in Patients with Non-Syndromic Mitral Valve Prolapse

Maëlle Perrocheau [1,2], Soto Romuald Kiando [1,2], Déwi Vernerey [1,2], Christian Dina [3,4], Pilar Galan [5], Albert Hagege [1,2,6], Xavier Jeunemaitre [1,2,7] and Nabila Bouatia-Naji [1,2,*]

1 Paris Cardiovascular Research Center, INSERM UMR970, 56 rue Leblanc, Paris F-75015, France; E-Mails: maelle.perrocheau@gmail.com (M.P.); romuald.kiando@inserm.fr (S.R.K.); dvernerey@chu-besancon.fr (D.V.); albert.hagege@aphp.fr (A.H.); xavier.jeunemaitre@inserm.fr (X.J.)

2 Paris Descartes University, Sorbonne Paris Cité, 12 rue de l'école de medicine, Paris F-75006, France

3 INSERM UMR1087, CNRS UMR 6291, Institut du Thorax, 8 Quai Moncousu, Nantes F-44007, France; E-Mail: Christian.Dina@univ-nantes.fr

4 Centre Hospitalier Universitaire (CHU) Nantes, Université de Nantes, 8 Quai Moncousu, Nantes F-44007, France

5 Equipe de Recherche en Epidémiologie Nutritionnelle (EREN), Centre d'Epidémiologie et Statistiques Sorbonne Paris Cité, Inserm (U1153), Inra (U1125), Cnam, Université Paris 13, COMUE Sorbonne Paris Cité, Bobigny F-93017, France; E-Mail: p.galan@uren.smbh.univ-paris13.fr

6 Department of Cardiology, Hôpital Européen Georges Pompidou, Assistance publique-Hôpitaux de Paris (AP-HP), 20 rue Leblanc, Paris F-75015, France

7 Department of genetics, Hôpital Européen Georges Pompidou, Assistance publique-Hôpitaux de Paris (AP-HP), 20 rue Leblanc, Paris F-75015, France

* Author to whom correspondence should be addressed; E-Mail: nabila.bouatia-naji@inserm.fr

Academic Editors: Russell Norris and Cheryl L. Maslen

Abstract: Non-syndromic mitral valve prolapse (MVP) is a common degenerative valvulopathy, predisposing to arrhythmia and sudden death. The etiology of MVP is suspected to be under genetic control, as supported by familial cases and its manifestation in genetic syndrome (e.g., Marfan syndrome). One candidate etiological mechanism is a perturbation of the extracellular matrix (ECM) remodeling of the valve. To test this hypothesis, we assessed the role of genetic variants in the matrix metalloproteinase 2 gene (*MMP2*) known to regulate the ECM turnover by direct degradation of proteins and for which transgenic mice develop MVP. Direct sequencing of exons of *MMP2* in 47 unrelated patients and segregation analyses in families did not reveal any causative mutation. We studied eight common single nucleotide polymorphisms (TagSNPs), which summarize the genetic information at the *MMP2* locus. The association study in two case controls sets ($N_{Cases} = 1073$ and $N_{Controls} = 1635$) provided suggestive evidence for the association of rs1556888 located downstream *MMP2* with the risk of MVP, especially in patients with the fibroelastic defiency form. Our study does not support the contribution of *MMP2* rare variation in the etiology to MVP in humans, though further genetic and molecular investigation is required to confirm our current suggestive association of one common variant.

Keywords: *MMP2*; mitral valve prolapse; Single Nucelotide Polymorphism; genetic association

1. Introduction

Mitral valve insufficiency is a major cause of morbidity and mortality worldwide [1]. One of the main mechanisms contributing to mitral insufficiency is mitral valve prolapse (MVP), characterized by the systolic displacement or billowing of the mitral leaflets into the left atrium. MVP is the clinical expression of degeneration of the mitral valve. This causes the displacement of one or both enlarged, thickened mitral leaflets into the left atrium during systole [2]. MVP results from the consequence of a degenerative process with variable morphological presentations such as billowing mitral leaflets with excess of connective tissue and myxomatous degeneration, also named Barlow disease or thin elongated leaflets and chordae with fibroelastic and acid mucopolysaccharide deficiency [3]. Many patients with MVP show few clinical symptoms, if any. Nonetheless, MVP is the most common cause of isolated mitral regurgitation requiring surgical repair and a confirmed risk factor of heart failure, arrhythmia, endocarditis, and sudden cardiac death [1].

The etiology of MVP is complex and this includes acquired (e.g., rheumatic, trauma and ischemic origin) and genetic causes, including several connective tissue genetic disorders (e.g., Marfan and Elhers-Danlos syndromes) [4]. Several efforts have attempted to decipher the genetics of MVP using linkage within families in the past two decades. We have previously reported linkage studies of large families where four loci were linked to MVP on Chr16p11-12, Chr11p15.4, Chr13q31-32 and ChrXq28 [5–8]. Mutations in the FLNA, the filamin A gene, were demonstrated to cause the X-linked myxomatous MVP [9], which is to date, the only known causative gene for rare familial MVP. Filamin A regulates reorganization of the actin cytoskeleton and is essential for matrix organization during fetal valve development [10]. On the other hand, MVP is also present in several rare connective tissue syndromes, (e.g., Marfan, Ehlers-Danlos) [11], which supports a role of the extracellular matrix biology and cytoskeleton cell cross talk in valve development and integrity. At the population level,

MVP prevalence is estimated ~3% [12] and thus presents a putative complex genetic pattern of inheritance where common genetic variants could be at play, especially in candidate genes and pathway.

The physiological function of metalloproteinases (MMPs) is the modulation and the regulation of extracellular matrix (ECM) turnover by direct proteolytic degradation of the ECM proteins, including collagen, fibronectin, and proteoglycans [13]. Previous studies suggested a role for the *MMP2* in the pathogenesis of MVP. In humans, a higher level of *MMP2* expression is reported in myxomatous valves compared to normal valves [14]. On the other hand, there is evidence for increased activity of *MMP2* in myxomatous valves compared to normal valves [15] and an ability *MMP2* to cleave collagen, elastin, and fibrillin [13,16]. In addition, although normal when young, 12–14 months mice with cardiac-specific constitutively active *MMP2* reproduce many of the features of the human MVP syndrome including mitral valve thickening and prolapse with severe myxomatous changes [17]. These data suggest the *MMP2* coding gene (*MMP2*) as a strong candidate gene for non-syndromic MVP.

The aim of this study is to investigate the link between genetic variants in *MMP2* and mitral valve prolapse, including mostly severe cases with mitral repair by surgery and Barlow, myxomatous disease. We first screened by direct sequencing all coding exons of *MMP2* in MVP patients and investigated the role of rare coding variants in genetic segregation in families. We have also performed a locus-based case-control association study to assess the role of common single nucleotide polymorphisms (SNPs) in and around *MMP2* in MVP genetic susceptibility in a case control study design. We have also performed stratified analysis in surgery cases and Barlow and fibroelastic deficiency-only forms of MVP.

2. Methods

2.1. Study Populations

2.1.1. Familial MVP Index Cases

Sequencing of the *MMP2* coding regions was performed on DNA from 47 index cases selected from families affected by mitral valve prolapse recruited at the Department of Cardiology and the Department of Genetics of the "Hôpital Européen Georges Pompidou: HEGP". Familial cases were defined as such when at least one additional member was affected in the family. The diagnosis of index cases (Familial cases, see Table 1) and relatives was determined by echocardiographic examination as previously described [5]. Patients were 54.4 years old on average; mostly men and 35% had already had surgery for valve repair or replacement (Table 1).

2.1.2. MVP-France Cases

The MVP-France study (Genetic polymorphisms in idiopathic mitral valve prolapse: A French prospective study) is a prospective multicenter nation-wide study promoted by the French Society of Cardiology. Adult (≥18 years) patients with idiopathic MVP were included after written informed consent if they presented either: (1) leaflet prolapse defined as the displacement within the left atrium of any part of the mitral valve leaflet(s) ≥ 2 mm beyond a line connecting the annular hinge points on the parasternal long-axis view of the left ventricle by two-dimensional (2D) echocardiography [18];

and either increased leaflet thickness ≥ 4 mm measured in diastole at the mid-portion of the leaflet or mitral regurgitation ≥ 2+ based on extension of the regurgitant jet within the left atrium on a scale of 1 to 4+ using color Doppler; or (2) previous surgery for pure severe mitral regurgitation due to MVP supported by an operative report and written confirmation of the diagnosis by the surgeon.

Table 1. Characteristics of mitral valve prolapse populations and controls.

Cohort	*n*	Age at Examination (Years)	Sex Ratio (F%)	BMI (kg/m^2)	Surgery (%)
Familial Cases	47	54.4 ± 15.6	45%	22.7 ± 2.7	35%
MVP-France (Set1)	625	62.7 ± 13.1	30%	24.3 ± 3.6	67%
Myxomatous (Barlow)	414	60.7 ± 13.5	30%	23.7 ± 3.2	64%
Non myxomatous (FED)	116	67.7 ± 10.7	33%	25.5 ± 4.1	67%
Surgery	421	63.7 ± 12.1	25%	24.5 ± 3.7	100%
MVP-France (Set2)	401	63.8 ± 12.2	26%	24.3 ± 3.7	80%
Myxomatous (Barlow)	255	62.5 ± 12.5	25%	23.9 ± 3.6	77%
Non myxomatous (FED)	57	67.6 ± 9.4	37%	25.6 ± 4.3	72%
Surgery	322	64.2 ± 11.8	24%	24.4 ± 3.6	100%
		Controls			
SU.VI.MAX (Set 1)	815	65.8 ± 6.3	60%	NA	NA
SU.VI.MAX (Set 2)	820	67.3 ± 6.1	61%	NA	NA

FED: Fibroelastic deficiency form; NA: Not available.

An echocardiographic core laboratory (AH) validated echo cardiac recordings and operative reports. MVP-France recruitment excluded patients with MVP associated to heart disease (coronary artery disease, hypertrophic cardiomyopathy, or rheumatic disease) or syndromes (e.g., Marfan and Ehlers-Danlos). Clinical data were collected on electronic case report forms. Genetic core laboratory (XJ) centralized the collection of blood samples. Genomic DNA was successfully extracted from peripheral blood lymphocytes of patients using a commercial isolation kit and following the provider's procedure (Qiagen®, Venlo, the Netherlands).

The study was approved by a local ethical committee (CPP Ile-de-France VI, approval n° 60-08, Paris, France, 25 June 2008), the "Commission Informatique et Libertés" (CNIL) (approval n° 908359, Paris, France, 14 October 2008) and the French Ministry of Health (ID-RCB: 2008-A00568-47, Paris, France) and was registered on the Clinical Trial Gov website (protocol ID: 2008-01).

2.1.3. Control Individuals

We defined two independent samples of controls with comparable sample sizes and age and sex distribution for the discovery and replication of case control analyses using a random sampling function (SPSS 16) on the SU.VI.MAX cohort (Table 1). SU.VI.MAX is a national sample of middle-age (women, aged 35–60, or men, aged 45–60 years) healthy volunteers living in France and enrolled between 1996 and 2001 in a randomized, placebo-controlled trial testing the benefit of anti-oxidant nutrients on the incidence of cancers and cardiovascular diseases [19]. We included 1635 individuals, aged 35–65 years at baseline who had genotyping available for the eight TagSNPs of *MMP2*. Cardiac echography was not performed in this population and the MVP status is unknown for all participants.

2.2. Sequencing of the MMP2 Gene

Genomic DNA was extracted from whole blood using a standard saline protocol. *MMP2* maps on chromosome 16q12.2 and extends on 47.72 kilobases (kb). The gene has 13 exons and encodes three transcripts of 27.72 kb, 25.11 kb, and 24.99 kb. Fifteen pairs of primers were necessary to amplify the whole coding sequences and the intron-exon boundaries (Table S1). Twelve of the 13 exons constituting the coding regions of the *MMP2* gene were successfully sequenced in 47 index cases of families affected by mitral valve prolapse. Genomic DNA from 47 familial cases and four DNAs of unaffected probands were amplified by PCR. Reactions were performed in 25 µL volumes containing 50 ng genomic DNA, 1X reaction buffer (Sigma-Aldrich, Saint-Louis, MO, USA), 1.5 mM $MgCl_2$ (Sigma-Aldrich), 0.2 mM each dNTP (Invitrogen, Thermo Fisher Scientific, Waltham, MA, USA), 0.25 µM each of both primers and 1.25 U Taq DNA polymerase (Sigma-Aldrich). The mix was then subjected to 30 cycles of PCR amplification under annealing temperature adapted for each primer with a C1000 thermal cycler (BioRad, Hercules, CA, USA). Primer excess was removed from the amplified fragments with the use of antarctic phosphatase and exonuclease I (Ozyme, St Quentin en Yvelines, France). Purified PCR products were then sequenced with a big dye terminator cycle-sequencing system (Applied Biosystems, Thermo Fisher Scientific) and amplified DNA fragments were separated using an ABI Prism 3730 DNA Analyzer Sequencer (Applied Biosystems, Thermo Fisher Scientific).

2.3. SNPs Selection and Genotyping

We extracted genotyping data at the *MMP2* locus for the HapMap population of Europeans (CEU, accessed May 2010, Build NCBI 35, Hg 17) and performed a linkage disequilibrium (LD) analysis and identified eight common TagSNPs as having a minor allele frequency (MAF) ≥ 0.05 and presenting low LD between each other (Figure 1). TagSNPs were genotyped in 625 MVP-France Set 1 and 47 familial cases. The LGC genomics company performed the genotyping using a homogeneous fluorescent FRET based system (lgcgenomics.com). Genotyping call rate was at least 99% for all SNPs.

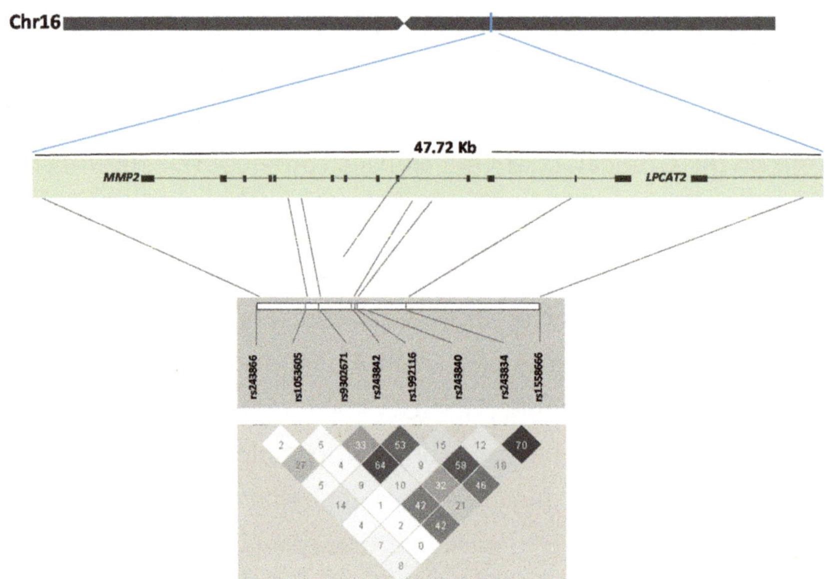

Figure 1. Structure of *MMP2* gene on chromosome 16, position of 8 polymorphisms across the *MMP2* locus and linkage disequilibrium (r^2) between SNPs.

At the replication stage, we used genotypes for rs1558666 that we have generated using genotyping arrays (Illumina 660W-Quad in MVP-France and Illumina Human Hap300 and imputation in SU.VI.MAX) for the purposes of an ongoing genome-wide association study.

2.4. Statistical Methods

The correlation between SNPs in HapMap individuals was assessed using Haploview [20]. The association with MVP at each stage was performed by logistic regression under the additive model using PLINK software [21]. Adjusted analyses were logistic regressions where sex and age were included as covariates. Dominant and recessive models were tested and did not provide better association than the additive model, and thus were not presented in the tables.

3. Results

3.1. Genetic Variation of the Coding Regions of MMP2 in Familial MVP

We did not succeed in amplifying the first exon, probably because of its high GC content (72%), and describe here the results for nine different exons where we identified genetic variants (Table S1). Using the DNAs from 47 patients, we identified 15 different SNPs including one indel and seven non-coding SNPs (six SNPs in the UTR3′ and one SNP in the exon-intron junction). Among the eight coding SNPs, seven are synonymous and one variant (rs368282133) is nonsynonymous and rare with no MAF in HapMap. This variant leads to a missense substitution of an Arginine residue into a Histidine residue (Arg222His) and was observed in two heterozygote patients (MAF in our sample is 0.021). This change occurs in a collagen-binding domain and is described as conserved among mammals and chicken. However, the conservation does not stand for other vertebrates where a Lys is reported for *Xenopus Tropicalis* and zebrafish for instance. On the other hand, the Arg222His is predicted as benign, according to two sequence homology—based tools (SIFT: Sort Intolerant from Tolerant [22] and PolyPhen2: Polymorphism Phenotype [23], score Grantham = 29), which allows a bioinformatics-based prediction of the potential impact of this non synonymous variation on the protein function. Given the limited potential functionality of this variant and the absence of additional affected members in the two families where Arg222His was described, the implication of this variation in the MVP was not further continued.

3.2. Association Analyses of Common Variants in MMP2 with MVP

Here we analyzed two sets of MVP-France cases with genetically confirmed European background, defined from an ongoing genome-wide association study (GWAS), to test the association of eight common SNPs with MVP risk in French clinical populations. The first sample (Set 1) corresponds to an intermediate recruitment freeze of MVP-France. This sample is 625 patients aged 62.7 ± 13.1 years, among which 67% had surgery, either valve repair or replacement.

3.2.1. Association Analyses of *MMP2* Common Variants with MVP

We analyzed eight TagSNPs with MAF ranging from 0.06 to 0.48 in the control population as summarizing the genetic information of common variants at the *MMP2 locus* (Figure 1, Table S2). The logistic regression analyses indicated a significant association with MVP for rs1558666 (OR = 0.86 95% CI (0.74–0.99), *p*-value = 0.033). MVP-France displayed an important sex ratio discrepancy compared to controls with 30% and 60% females in cases and controls, respectively (Table 1). To account for this putative confounding factor, we performed adjusted logistic regressions including age and sex as covariates for all SNPs (Table 2). The adjusted analyses strengthen the association of rs1558666 (OR_{adj} = 0.79, *p*-value = 0.003) with MVP and indicate an additional significant association for rs930271 (OR = 0.82 95% CI (0.70–0.96), *p*-value = 0.016). However, only rs158666 remains significantly associated with MVP risk after the application of the Bonferroni corrected *p*-value (p_{Adj} = 0.006), which takes into account for multiple testing.

Table 2. Association of *MMP2* common tagSNPs with mitral valve prolapse.

SNP	Minor Allele	MAF Cases *n* = 672	MAF Controls *n* = 815	OR [IC 95%]	*p*	OR_{Adj} [IC 95%]	p_{Adj}
rs1053605	T	0.07	0.06	1.23 [0.90–1.68]	0.196	1.22 [0.87–1.70]	0.251
rs1558666	A	0.45	0.49	0.86 [0.74–0.99]	0.033	0.79 [0.68–0.93]	0.003 *
rs1992116	A	0.41	0.43	0.93 [0.80–1.07]	0.291	0.87 [0.75–1.02]	0.080
rs243834	G	0.49	0.48	1.08 [0.93–1.24]	0.317	1.15 [0.99–1.34]	0.070
rs243840	G	0.20	0.19	1.12 [0.93–1.35]	0.220	1.13 [0.93–1.37]	0.237
rs243842	C	0.38	0.39	0.98 [0.85–1.14]	0.832	1.05 [0.90–1.23]	0.540
rs243866	A	0.23	0.24	0.96 [0.81–1.14]	0.637	0.95 [0.79–1.14]	0.584
rs9302671	T	0.33	0.36	0.88 [0.75–1.02]	0.091	0.82 [0.70–0.96]	0.016

OR: Odds ratios. *p*: *p*-value generated by the logistic regression test performed to compare the prevalence of minor alleles in cases and controls under the additive model. OR_{Adj} and p_{Adj} indicate ORs and *p*-values from the logistic regression analyses including age and sex are covariates. *: Significant associations after Bonferroni correction, with corrected *p*-value = 0.05/8 = 0.006.

The valve repair or valve replacement occurs when mitral regurgitation is established and patients are considered to be in a more severe stage of the disease. As a surrogate marker of mitral regurgitation, we tested the association of *MMP2* variants by comparing allele frequencies of MVP patients who had surgery (*n* = 421) to the total sample of SU.VI.MAX Set 2 (*n* = 815). All SNPs studied showed comparable effects on MVP risk, with rs1558666 showing a significant association with MVP when adjusted for age and sex but not below the corrected threshold (OR = 0.83, *p*-value = 0.036, Table S2).

3.2.2. Association Analyses of *MMP2* Common Variants Stratified on Myxomatous and Fibroelastic Deficiency MVP

Among the 672 MVP patients that we analyzed (Set 1), 414 patients were diagnosed a myxomatous valve phenotype or Barlow disease while 116 were defined as non-myxomatous valve prolapse. In two out of three patients, the myxomatous phenotype was defined during surgery intervention and was reported in the surgery report. On average, Barlow disease patients were seven years younger at examination and had similar sex ratio and surgery percentage to the non-myxomatous patients (Table 1).

The stratified association analyses show comparable results to the global analyses in term of effects and significance for *MMP2* SNPs except for rs1558666 with the non-myxomatous phenotype (OR_{adj} = 0.67 (0.51–0.89), *p*-value = 0.006, Table 3).

Table 3. Association of *MMP2* common tagSNPs with myxomatous (Barlow disease) and non-myxomatous mitral valve prolapse.

SNP	Minor Allele	MAF Cases	MAF Controls	OR [95% CI]	*p*	OR_{Adj} [95% CI]	p_{Adj}
			Myxomatous (Barlow) MVP				
rs1053605	T	0.06	0.06	1.10 [0.77–1.58]	0.599	1.01 [0.68–1.50]	0.968
rs1558666	A	0.46	0.49	0.88 [0.75–1.04]	0.130	0.83 [0.69–0.99]	0.036
rs1992116	A	0.40	0.43	0.91 [0.77–1.07]	0.237	0.84 [0.71–1.01]	0.065
rs243834	G	0.49	0.48	1.08 [0.92–1.27]	0.355	1.18 [0.99–1.41]	0.064
rs243840	G	0.21	0.19	1.16 [0.94–1.42]	0.163	1.17 [0.93–1.47]	0.171
rs243842	C	0.38	0.39	0.99 [0.84-1.16]	0.861	1.06 [0.89–1.27]	0.509
rs243866	A	0.23	0.24	0.93 [0.77–1.13]	0.484	0.96 [0.78–1.19]	0.716
rs9302671	T	0.34	0.36	0.89 [0.75–1.05]	0.170	0.83 [0.68–1.00]	0.049
			Non-Myxomatous (FED) MVP				
rs1053605	T	0.08	0.06	1.43 [0.84–2.46]	0.191	1.47 [0.85–2.54]	0.173
rs1558666	A	0.40	0.49	0.71 [0.54-0.93]	0.012	0.67 [0.51–0.89]	0.006 *
rs1992116	A	0.40	0.43	0.89 [0.68–1.18]	0.417	0.87 [0.65–1.15]	0.329
rs243834	G	0.55	0.48	1.33 [1.01–1.75]	0.042	1.37 [1.03–1.82]	0.029
rs243840	G	0.21	0.19	1.19 [0.85–1.67]	0.322	1.17 [0.83–1.66]	0.364
rs243842	C	0.38	0.39	0.99 [0.75–1.30]	0.929	1.02 [0.77–1.35]	0.888
rs243866	A	0.23	0.24	0.92 [0.67–1.27]	0.622	0.91 [0.66–1.26]	0.570
rs9302671	T	0.30	0.36	0.77 [0.57–1.03]	0.080	0.75 [0.55–1.02]	0.063

OR: Odds ratios. *p*: *p*-value associated to the logistic regression test performed to compare the prevalence of minor alleles in cases and controls. OR_{Adj} and p_{Adj} indicate ORs and *p*-values from the logistic regression analyses including age and sex are covariates.
*: Significant associations after Bonferroni correction, with corrected *p*-value = 0.006.

3.2.3. Validation of rs1558666 as a Genetic Susceptibility Variant for Non-Myxomatous MVP

At the end of the recruitment of the MVP-France protocol, additional patients were available (*n* = 401) with overall similar clinical characteristics to the first sample (Table 1) that we initially analyzed in the *MMP2* genetic investigation. We decided to use this sample of MVP cases to validate the suggestive association observed for rs1558666 and compared the allele frequencies to the SU.VI.MAX Set 2 as controls.

Table 4 summarizes the association of rs1558666 with MVP. In the initial association analyses, we observed a lower MAF of rs1558666 in the cases compared to the controls in all the samples analyzed, with the lowest frequency observed in the non-myxomatous group (MAF = 0.40) and the highest in the controls (MAF = 0.49, Table 4). In the validation analyses, while the MAF in the controls was almost identical (MAF = 0.49 in SU.VI.MAX Set 1 and MAF = 0.48 in SU.VI.MAX Set 2), we obtained higher frequency for the rs1558666 in MVP cases (MAF = 0.51). Thus, the association that we observed initially was not significantly replicated in the additional sample with an opposite effect (OR = 1.14, *p* = 0.169). Accordingly, the global analysis was also non conclusive (OR = 0.91, *p* = 0.126).

Interestingly, the stratified analysis in non-myxomatous MVP cases only showed consistent direction of the effect of the rs1558666 in the validation sample, with a MAF lower in the cases (MAF = 0.44) compared to the controls (MAF = 0.48), despite a lack of significance (OR = 0.84, $p = 0.38$) in this rather smaller and underpowered sample of patients ($n = 57$). Consequently, the association with the non myxomatous phenotype of MVP reached significance in the global sample (OR = 0.73, $p = 0.005$, $N_{Cases} = 173$).

4. Discussion

In our genetic investigation of metalloproteinase 2 gene (*MMP2*) we assessed the role of rare coding variants and discarded their implication in the etiology of familial, mainly early onset forms of MVP and described a suggestive association between rs1558666, a common variant near *MMP2*, and MVP risk in French populations.

In order to optimize the genetic coverage of the *MMP2* locus, we included all common genetic variants representative of the linkage disequilibrium (LD) block of *MMP2*, which also includes *LPCAT2* encoding lysophosphatidylcholine acyltransferase 2, putatively involved in membrane biosynthesis and production of platelet-activating factor in inflammatory cells (Figure 1). LPCAT2 function has no obvious biological link with valve integrity or development. According to our association result, the major allele (G) at rs1558666 is more prevalent in MVP patients compared to control participants. The rs1558666 maps downstream *MMP2*, in a sequence predicted *in silico* to be recognized by C/EBP and in interaction with nuclear proteins because protected in a DNase sequencing experiment in the endothelial cells model HUVEC, as reported by the ENCODE project (regulome.db.org and [24]). According to the recent data from the pilot study of the gene by tissue expression (GTEx) project [25], the MVP risk allele of rs1558666 tends to correlate with higher expression of *MMP2* in heart left ventricle human samples ($p = 0.07$). Because mitral valve tissue is not collected in the GTEx project, further investigation in this specific tissue is needed to confirm the putative effect of rs1558666 on MVP risk by increasing *MMP2* expression.

In support of this hypothesis is the increased *MMP2* activity reported in diseased mitral valves [15,26]. Histological analyses of myxomatous mitral valves show changes in the amount of collagen, elastin and fibrillin, and a disorganized distribution pattern and structural abnormalities of these components. These abnormalities include spiraling collagen fibrils and alterations in the pattern of arrangement of collagen bundles, structural changes in the organization of elastic fibers, an increase in the number and a decrease in size of the elastic fibers [27–29]. Myxomatous mitral valves are also characterized by an accumulation of proteoglycans, particularly in the spongiosa layer, and changes in their composition [30,31]. Moreover, the spongiosa contains an increased number of interstitial cells, which have properties of activated myofibroblasts. These cells express raised concentrations of various proteolytic enzymes including matrix metalloproteinases (MMPs) [14]. The physiological function of MMPs is the modulation and the regulation of extracellular matrix (ECM) turnover by direct proteolytic degradation of the ECM proteins, including collagen, fibronectin, and proteoglycans [13].

Table 4. Association of rs1558666 with mitral valve prolapse in the initial association studies, the validation and the global analyses.

rs1558666	Initial Associations					Validations					Global Analyses				
	N_{Cases}	MAF Cases	MAF Controls	OR_{Adj} [95% CI]	p_{Adj}	N_{Cases}	MAF Cases	MAF Controls	OR_{Adj} [95% CI]	p_{Adj}	N_{Cases}	MAF Cases	MAF Controls	OR_{Adj} [95% CI]	p_{Adj}
All forms	672	0.45	0.49	0.79 [0.68–0.93]	0.003	401	0.51	0.48	1.14 [0.95–1.37]	0.169	1077	0.47	0.48	0.91 [0.81–1.03]	0.126
Myxomatous (Barlow)	414	0.46	0.49	0.83 [0.69–0.99]	0.036	255	0.52	0.48	1.17 [0.94–1.46]	0.165	669	0.48	0.48	0.94 [0.82–1.08]	0.414
Non Myxmatous (FED)	116	0.40	0.49	0.67 [0.51–0.89]	0.006	57	0.44	0.48	0.84 [0.57–1.24]	0.385	173	0.41	0.48	0.73 [0.58–0.91]	0.005
Surgery Cases	421	0.46	0.49	0.83 [0.70–0.99]	0.036	322	0.51	0.48	1.16 [0.95–1.41]	0.147	743	0.48	0.48	0.96 [0.84–1.09]	0.502

OR_{Adj} and p_{Adj} indicate odds ratios and p-values from the logistic regression tests performed to compare the prevalence of minor alleles frequencies (MAF) in cases and controls, including age and sex are covariates. FED: Fibroelastic deficiency.

The overexpression of *MMP2* specifically in the heart of mice resulted in normal mice at ages four to six months [17]. This finding in the mouse is consistent with the lack of causative rare mutations in the more severe and early onset MVP phenotype that characterizes the familial patients. Thus, the overexpression of *MMP2* reported in diseased valves [15] is probably a secondary defect, not due to genetic defaults. Actually, the echocardiographic MVP manifests in transgenic mice at a later age (at 12 to 14 months) [17], which is consistent with the association of a common variant with sporadic forms of MVP more likely to be due to degenerative process overtime. Thus, *MMP2*'s role in the etiology of MVP is putatively a long process of susceptibility, genetic background, and aging and/or mechanical stress interactions. This hypothesis needs confirmation using a prospective genetic epidemiological setting to assess the extent to which the rs1558666 risk allele carriers are more prone to mitral valve degeneration, compared to non-carriers. On the other hand, the existence of rare coding variants that would result in the increase of *MMP2* levels of activity is unlikely. Only regulatory regions are susceptible to harbor such variants and their investigation would be warranted.

5. Conclusions

Our genetic investigation of *MMP2* suggests a limited implication of rare coding genetic variants in the inheritance of non-syndromic MVP in French families and suggests the association of common variants near this gene with sporadic MVP in two cases controls studies. More comprehensive genomic investigation such as exome sequencing and genome-wide association studies are more likely to decipher the genetic basis of MVP.

Acknowledgments

We thank Jean-Jacques Schott and Thierry Le Tourneau for providing DNA and phenotypes of patients from Nantes, Joël Cagnard for assistance with the DNA preparation and Mark Lathrop for coordinating the genotyping in the MVP-France cohort GWAS. This study was funded by the "Leducq Foundation MITRAL network". N. Bouatia-Naji is the recipient of a French young investigator fund (ANR-13-ISV1-0006-0). The MVP-France study was supported by the French Society of Cardiology and the French Federation of Cardiology for the financial support. MVP-France was promoted by the French Society of Cardiology help to the "Commission Promotion et Recherche Clinique" (Anissa Bouzamondo and Sophie Thevenin). We also acknowledge the participating centers and investigators of MVP-France (classified by the number of inclusions): ≥100 patients: Centre Hospitalo-Universitaire Pitié Salpêtrière, Paris (Christophe Acar); Groupement Hospitalier Est, Bron (Geneviève Derumeaux, Jean-François Obadia); Centre Hospitalo-Universitaire Pontchaillou, Rennes (Erwan Donal, Christophe Leclercq, Alain Leguerrier); Hôpital Européen Georges Pompidou, Paris (Jean-Noël Fabiani, Paul Achouh); Clinique Saint Augustin, Bordeaux (Eric Abergel, Christophe Chauvel, Patrick Dehant); ≥50 patients: Hôpital du Bocage, Dijon (Jean-Christophe Eicher, Jean-Eric Wolf); Hôpital Gabriel-Montpied, Clermont-Ferrand (Lionel Camilleri, Jean-René Lusson); ≥15 patients: Hôpital Sud,

Amiens (Dan Rusinaru, Christophe Tribouilloy); Hôpital Charles Nicolle, Rouen (Fabrice Bauer); Hôpital Cardiologique du Haut Lévêque, Pessac (Stéphane Lafitte, Patricia Reant, Raymond Roudaut); Hôpital de la Cavale Blanche, Brest (Jean-Jacques Blanc, Yves Etienne, Yannick Jobic); Hôpital Dupuytren, Limoges (Caroline Etchecopar); Centre Hospitalo-Universitaire Arnaud de Villeneuve, Montpellier (Catherine Sportouch-Dukhan); <15 patients: Hôpital Lariboisière, Paris (Damien Logeart); Hôpital Saint Antoine, Paris (Ariel Cohen, Stéphane Ederhy); Centre Hospitalo-Universitaire Ambroise Paré, Boulogne-Billancourt (Nacera Abbou, Nicolas Mansencal); Hôpital de la Timone, Marseille (Jean-François Avierinos, Gilbert Habib); Centre Hospitalo-Universitaire Henri Mondor, Créteil (Thibaud Damy, Jean-Luc Monin); Institut Cardiologique Paris Sud, Massy (Bertrand Cormier, Marie-Christine Malergue); Centre Hospitalo-Universitaire Bichat, Paris (Eric Brochet, Bernard Iung).

Author Contributions

M.P. performed the experiments and drafted parts of the manuscript. S.R.K., D.V. and C.D. performed statistical analyses and drafted parts of the manuscript. P.G. coordinated recruitments of controls. A.A.H. coordinated the MVP-France protocol and validated the diagnosis of patients. X.J. coordinated the genetic investigation and participated to prepare the manuscript. N.B.N. supervised the genetic and statistical analyses and wrote the manuscript.

Conflicts of Interest

The authors declare no conflict of interest.

References

1. Avierinos, J.F.; Gersh, B.J.; Melton, L.J., III; Bailey, K.R.; Shub, C.; Nishimura, R.A.; Tajik, A.J.; Enriquez-Sarano, M. Natural history of asymptomatic mitral valve prolapse in the community. *Circulation* **2002**, *106*, 1355–1361.
2. Hayek, E.; Gring, C.N.; Griffin, B.P.; Mitral valve prolapse. *Lancet* **2005**, *365*, 507–518.
3. Maslow, A.D.; Regan, M.M.; Haering, J.M.; Johnson, R.G.; Levine, R.A. Echocardiographic predictors of left ventricular outflow tract obstruction and systolic anterior motion of the mitral valve after mitral valve reconstruction for myxomatous valve disease. *J. Am. Coll. Cardiol.* **1999**, *34*, 2096–2104.
4. Guy, T.S.; Hill, A.C. Mitral valve prolapse. *Annu. Rev. Med.* **2012**, *63*, 277–292.
5. Disse, S.; Abergel, E.; Berrebi, A.; Houot, A.M.; Heuzey, J.Y.L.; Diebold, B.; Guize, L.; Carpentier, A.; Corvol, P.; Jeunemaitre, X. Mapping of a first locus for autosomal dominant myxomatous mitral-valve prolapse to chromosome 16p11.2-p12.1. *Am. J. Hum. Genet.* **1999**, *65*, 1242–1251.
6. Freed, L.A.; Acierno, J.S., Jr.; Dai, D.; Leyne, M.; Marshall, J.E.; Nesta, F.; Levine, R.A.; Slaugenhaupt, S.A. A locus for autosomal dominant mitral valve prolapse on chromosome 11p15.4. *Am. J. Hum. Genet.* **2003**, *72*, 1551–1559.

7. Kyndt, F.; Schott, J.J.; Trochu, J.N.; Baranger, F.; Herbert, O.; Scott, V.; Fressinaud, E.; David, A.; Moisan, J.P.; Bouhour, J.B.; *et al.* Mapping of X-linked myxomatous valvular dystrophy to chromosome Xq28. *Am. J. Hum. Genet.* **1998**, *62*, 627–632.
8. Nesta, F.; Leyne, M.; Yosefy, C.; Simpson, C.; Dai, D.; Marshall, J.E.; Hung, J.; Slaugenhaupt, S.A.; Levine, R.A. New locus for autosomal dominant mitral valve prolapse on chromosome 13: Clinical insights from genetic studies. *Circulation* **2005**, *112*, 2022–2030.
9. Kyndt, F.; Gueffet, J.P.; Probst, V.; Jaafar, P.; Legendre, A.; Le Bouffant, F.; Toquet, C.; Roy, E.; McGregor, L.; Lynch, S.A.; *et al.* Mutations in the gene encoding filamin A as a cause for familial cardiac valvular dystrophy. *Circulation* **2007**, *115*, 40–49.
10. Sauls, K.; de Vlaming, A.; Harris, B.S.; Williams, K.; Wessels, A.; Levine, R.A.; Slaugenhaupt, S.A.; Goodwin, R.L.; Pavone, L.M.; Merot, J.; *et al.* Developmental basis for filamin-A-associated myxomatous mitral valve disease. *Cardiovasc. Res.* **2012**, *96*, 109–119.
11. Pyeritz, R.E.; Wappel, M.A. Mitral valve dysfunction in the Marfan syndrome. Clinical and echocardiographic study of prevalence and natural history. *Am. J. Med.* **1983**, *74*, 797–807.
12. Freed, L.A.; Levy, D.; Levine, R.A.; Larson, M.G.; Evans, J.C.; Fuller, D.L.; Lehman, B.; Benjamin, E.J. Prevalence and clinical outcome of mitral-valve prolapse. *N. Engl. J. Med.* **1999**, *341*, 1–7.
13. Klein, T.; Bischoff, R. Physiology and pathophysiology of matrix metalloproteases. *Amino Acids* **2011**, *41*, 271–290.
14. Rabkin, E.; Aikawa, M.; Stone, J.R.; Fukumoto, Y.; Libby, P.; Schoen, F.J. Activated interstitial myofibroblasts express catabolic enzymes and mediate matrix remodeling in myxomatous heart valves. *Circulation* **2001**, *104*, 2525–2532.
15. Togashi, M.; Tamura, K.; Nitta, T.; Ishizaki, M.; Sugisaki, Y.; Fukuda, Y. Role of matrix metalloproteinases and their tissue inhibitor of metalloproteinases in myxomatous change of cardiac floppy valves. *Pathol. Int.* **2007**, *57*, 251–259.
16. Ashworth, J.L.; Murphy, G.; Rock, M.J.; Sherratt, M.J.; Shapiro, S.D.; Shuttleworth, C.A.; Kielty, C.M. Fibrillin degradation by matrix metalloproteinases: Implications for connective tissue remodelling. *Biochem. J.* **1999**, *340*, 171–181.
17. Mahimkar, R.; Nguyen, A.; Mann, M.; Yeh, C.C.; Zhu, B.Q.; Karliner, J.S.; Lovett, D.H. Cardiac transgenic matrix metalloproteinase-2 expression induces myxomatous valve degeneration: A potential model of mitral valve prolapse disease. *Cardiovasc. Pathol.* **2009**, *18*, 253–261.
18. Levine, R.A.; Handschumacher, M.D; Sanfilippo, A.J.; Hagege, A.A.; Harrigan, P.; Marshall, J.E.; Weyman, A.E. Three-dimensional echocardiographic reconstruction of the mitral valve, with implications for the diagnosis of mitral valve prolapse. *Circulation* **1989**, *80*, 589–598.
19. Hercberg, S.; Preziosi, P.; Briançon, S.; Galan, P.; Triol, I.; Malvy, D.; Roussel, A.M.; Favier, A. A primary prevention trial using nutritional doses of antioxidant vitamins and minerals in cardiovascular diseases and cancers in a general population: The SU.VI.MAX study—Design, methods, and participant characteristics. *Control. Clin. Trials* **1998**, *19*, 336–351.
20. Barrett, J.C.; Fry, B.; Maller, J.; Daly, M.J. Haploview: Analysis and visualization of LD and haplotype maps. *Bioinformatics* **2005**, *21*, 263–265.

21. Purcell, S.; Neale, B.; Todd-Brown, K.; Thomas, L.; Ferreira, M.A.; Bender, D.; Maller, J.; Sklar, P.; de Bakker, P.I.; Daly, M.J.; *et al.* PLINK: A tool set for whole-genome association and population-based linkage analyses. *Am. J. Hum. Genet.* **2007**, *81*, 559–575.
22. Ng, P.C.; Henikoff, S. Predicting deleterious amino acid substitutions. *Genome Res.* **2001**, *11*, 863–874.
23. Adzhubei, I.A.; Schmidt, S.; Peshkin, L.; Ramensky, V.E.; Gerasimova, A.; Bork, P.; Kondrashov, A.S.; Sunyaev, S.R. A method and server for predicting damaging missense mutations. *Nat. Methods* **2010**, *7*, 248–249.
24. Gerstein, M.B.; Kundaje, A.; Hariharan, M.; Landt, S.G.; Yan, K.K.; Cheng, C.; Mu, X.J.; Khurana, E.; Rozowsky, J.; Alexander, R.; *et al.* Architecture of the human regulatory network derived from ENCODE data. *Nature* **2012**, *489*, 91–100.
25. Consortium, G.T. Human genomics. The Genotype-Tissue Expression (GTEx) pilot analysis: Multitissue gene regulation in humans. *Science* **2015**, *348*, 648–660.
26. Soini, Y.; Satta, J.; Määttä, M.; Autio-Harmainen, H. Expression of *MMP2*, *MMP9*, *MT1-MMP*, *TIMP1* and *TIMP2* mRNA in valvular lesions of the heart. *J. Pathol.* **2001**, *194*, 225–231.
27. Akhtar, S.; Meek, K.M.; James, V. Ultrastructure abnormalities in proteoglycans, collagen fibrils, and elastic fibers in normal and myxomatous mitral valve chordae tendineae. *Cardiovasc. Pathol.* **1999**, *8*, 191–201.
28. Cole, W.G.; Chan, D.; Hickey, A.J.; Wilcken, D.E. Collagen composition of normal and myxomatous human mitral heart valves. *Biochem. J.* **1984**, *219*, 451–460.
29. Tamura, K.; Fukuda, Y.; Ishizaki, M.; Masuda, Y.; Yamanaka, N.; Ferrans, V.J. Abnormalities in elastic fibers and other connective-tissue components of floppy mitral valve. *Am. Heart J.* **1995**, *129*, 1149–1158.
30. Grande-Allen, K.J.; Griffin, B.P.; Ratliff, N.B.; Cosgrove, D.M.; Vesely, I. Glycosaminoglycan profiles of myxomatous mitral leaflets and chordae parallel the severity of mechanical alterations. *J. Am. Coll. Cardiol.* **2003**, *42*, 271–277.
31. Gupta, V.; Barzilla, J.E.; Mendez, J.S; Stephens, E.H.; Lee, E.L.; Collard, C.D.; Laucirica, R.; Weigel, P.H.; Grande-Allen, K.J. Abundance and location of proteoglycans and hyaluronan within normal and myxomatous mitral valves. *Cardiovasc. Pathol.* **2009**, *18*, 191–197.

6

Vascular Calcification and Stone Disease: A New Look towards the Mechanism

Allen J. Yiu [1], Daniel Callaghan [1,2], Razia Sultana [1] and Bidhan C. Bandyopadhyay [1,2,3,*]

[1] Calcium Signaling Laboratory, Research Service, Veterans Affairs Medical Center, 50 Irving Street, NW, Washington, DC 20422, USA; E-Mails: allen.yiu@va.gov (A.J.Y.); danieljcallaghan3@gmail.com (D.C.); razia8222@yahoo.com (R.S.)

[2] Department of Pharmacology and Physiology, Georgetown University, 3900 Reservoir Road, NW, Washington, DC 20007, USA

[3] Department of Pharmacology and Physiology, School of Medicine, George Washington University, Ross Hall 2300 Eye Street, NW, Washington, DC 20037, USA

* Author to whom correspondence should be addressed; E-Mail: bidhan.bandyopadhyay@va.gov

Academic Editor: Andy Wessels

Abstract: Calcium phosphate (CaP) crystals are formed in pathological calcification as well as during stone formation. Although there are several theories as to how these crystals can develop through the combined interactions of biochemical and biophysical factors, the exact mechanism of such mineralization is largely unknown. Based on the published scientific literature, we found that common factors can link the initial stages of stone formation and calcification in anatomically distal tissues and organs. For example, changes to the spatiotemporal conditions of the fluid flow in tubular structures may provide initial condition(s) for CaP crystal generation needed for stone formation. Additionally, recent evidence has provided a meaningful association between the active participation of proteins and transcription factors found in the bone forming (ossification) mechanism that are also involved in the early stages of kidney stone formation and arterial calcification. Our review will focus on three topics of discussion (physiological influences—calcium and phosphate concentration—and similarities to ossification, or bone formation) that may elucidate some commonality in the mechanisms of stone formation and calcification, and pave the way towards opening new avenues for further research.

Keywords: calcium phosphate; kidney; calcification; physiologic; calculi; ossification; ectopic

1. Introduction

Calcium ions (Ca^{2+}) are an abundant mineral inside the human body, stored as calcium phosphate (CaP) in the skeleton, where it serves to maintain healthy bones and teeth. Little amounts of calcium are also dissolved as ionized Ca^{2+} in the intra- and extracellular fluid of every cell, which is essential for the normal functioning of the heart, muscles, blood vessels, and nerves [1]. In order to achieve these functions, our body constantly regulates those Ca^{2+} levels [1]. Ca^{2+} can also act as signaling molecule by acting both as first [2] and second [3] messenger to drive many of the intracellular signal transduction pathways. However, Ca^{2+} can build up as CaP, either in the form of brushite, hydroxyapatite, or other apatites, in places where it does not belong, *i.e.*, in the soft tissue, called ectopic calcification, which can cause several life-threatening diseases including nephrolithiasis and atherosclerosis [4,5]. Interestingly, some of these CaP deposits originate in tubular microenvironments within a hollow tissue structure (such as in kidney tubule and in salivary duct), and thus there may be some common factors that can influence the process of CaP crystal deposits, leading to stone formation [5–7]. Moreover, CaP crystals, which can form within blood vessels and the kidney tubular system, involve bone-related factors such as bone morphogenetic proteins (BMPs) and osteopontin (OPN) in the crystal matrices through an upregulation of transcription factors runt-related transcription factor 2 (Runx2) and msh homeobox 2 (Msx-2) [8].

The core idea of the mechanism of calcium biomineralization remains centered on pH, and physiological phosphate and calcium concentrations. However, to date, the stimuli for CaP deposition and the precise mechanism by which these crystals grow into stones are still poorly understood. Some have suggested that preformed microcrystals attach to the surface of, for example, kidney tubular cells, which then leads to further deposition of crystals and the subsequent formation of full-sized stones [9,10]. Other researchers have emphasized the so-called free solution crystallization mechanism, whereby a continuous crystallization process, although periodically inhibited by organic molecules, eventually leads to the materialization of a nucleus from which stones form [9,10]. Moreover, different factors affect CaP deposition and stone formation, such as the supersaturation of unbound calcium and phosphate ions or the absence of inhibitors that prevent crystal formation, which pose a challenge to predict the biomineralization process [11].

Accordingly, our review examines the most recent research on CaP crystal deposition, a contributing factor in vascular calcification [12] and in the process of salivary and calcium kidney stone formation [13,14], and their potential commonalities, specifically: (1) physiological influences; (2) calcium and phosphate concentration; and (3) similarities to ossification or bone formation. For example, some studies have found that CaP nanocrystal deposition may induce the osteogenic transformation of vascular smooth muscle cells by upregulating *BMP2* and *OPN* expression, genes associated with vascular calcification [12,15,16], CaP crystal exposure to renal epithelial cells [8] and bone ossification [17]. Additionally, vascular calcification, which is now an accepted predictor of adverse cardiovascular events, such as myocardial infarction and stroke, and has been shown to lead to atherosclerosis, and cardiac valve calcification [18], is prevalent among the chronic kidney disease (CKD) patients [19]; interestingly, population studies have shown that symptomatic kidney stone formers are at an increased risk for CKD [20]. One study also demonstrated a possible association between the severity of CKD in young patients and the formation of dental calculus, an additional manifestation of disturbed calcium and phosphate (Ca/P) homeostasis in distant parts of the body [21]. Thus, we believe that a systematic analysis of parallel factors of CaP crystal formation may generate a new understanding of stone development and calcification, and lead to the development of focused research towards new treatment options.

2. Physiology Influences the Microenvironment

Physiological factors in the salivary/renal systems and vasculature may affect the microenvironment that could contribute to salivary and calcium kidney stone formation, and calcification. Salivary gland calculi (or sialolithiasis) can lead to the blockage of the gland, and result in persistent swelling and ductal dilation [22], secondary infections, abscess, salivary duct stenosis, and even Kuttner's tumour, a pseudo-tumour of the submandibular gland accompanied by calcification [23]. Interestingly, a vast majority of salivary calculi occur in the submandibular gland or its duct; the remaining salivary stones develop in the parotid and the sublingual gland [23,24]. The primary reason could be physiological: the submandibular gland has a long duct with two bends, traveling upward and forward, then initiates a radical turn toward the hilus of the gland [25,26]. This slow flow rate against gravity results in saliva stagnation, or "salivary stasis"; the relatively narrower tubule in the Wharton's duct of the submandibular gland than the Stensen's duct of the parotid gland also contributes [26]. This higher viscosity in submandibular saliva increases the likelihood of hydroxyapatite calculi and stone formation.

Similarly, differences in renal fluid flow may induce the formation of kidney stones, which have been associated with urinary tract obstruction with acute renal failure, infection, and end-stage renal disease [27]. A recent computer model may provide a clue as to a potential cause. The model incorporated a series of hydrodynamic factors which included the fact that: (1) CaP crystals travelling close to the walls of the descending loop of Henle move at slower velocities than the fluid at the central axis of the tubule; and (2) CaP nucleates as it travels down the renal tubules [28]. This model predicted that, under certain conditions, CaP crystals, which start in the descending loop of Henle, travelling close to the tubular epithelial wall may grow and accumulate [28]. Indeed, nephrocalcinosis, which may be defined as the retention of crystals in the renal tubules, occurs when the tubular epithelial cells become susceptible to crystal attachment [29]. Although under normal conditions, the possibility of crystals growing large enough to be trapped is very small due to the short transit time, hydrodynamic factors (for example, fluid drag close to tubule walls and the gravitational effect on particles travelling upward in the tubule) may lead to a delay of crystal passage long enough to grow and become trapped in the collecting duct, and lead to the formation of Randall's Plugs in the Ducts of Bellini [28], in which brushite and other CaP stones in primary hyperparathyroidism have been found attached [8].

Thus, the conventional approaches to studying CaP stone formation using two-dimensional cell cultures fail to consider the microenvironmental mechanisms of stone formation. Because such stone formation occurs in a dynamic microenvironment, which requires luminal properties with dynamic pressure-flow kinetics over the microenvironment, the absence of all these critical factors severely limits the capability of understanding the true mechanism underlying the biological process of stone formation. Moreover, stone formation is a multifactorial mechanism [30,31], therefore an *in situ* analysis with all of these factors, which are intertwined with each other, along with the overwhelming complexity of cellular behaviors, regulatory pathways, and differences in physiological interactions poses a grand challenge in understanding such biomineralization process. Since CaP crystal formation is also a multifactorial process, examining one factor alone with several unknowns would not be helpful in delineating the crystallization process. Therefore, a step-by-step analysis of the process in a defined system is vital to the understanding of CaP crystal formation and aggregation, which can lead to stone formation and calcification. A microfluidic (MF) approach, one that simulates an *in vivo*-like tubular system and achieves previously unattainable precision in analysis and control over the spatiotemporal biological conditions, have been described [32,33]. Among these establishing polarized epithelia with perfectly cylindrical scaffolds in MF offers an effective means for the recreation of 3D non-leaky polarized monolayer of renal/salivary tubular structures with *in vivo*-like permeability and barrier functions have recently been demonstrated, which can allow a systematic evaluation of the dynamic microenvironmental cues (e.g., cellular regulations, fluidic hydrodynamics) that are critical for CaP stone formation [33].

Additionally the physiological features of the vasculature play a role in stone formation and calcification. Interstitial CaP deposits (Randall's Plaque) were found to have been attached to a majority of calcium oxalate stones in human idiopathic calcium oxalate stone formers, who represent about 75% of all stone formers [34]. One theory regarding the development of Randall's plaque centers on the vasculature. Stoller and others have proposed that the flow of blood from an intact endothelium in the descending vasa recta to the fenestrated ascending vasa recta decreases both vascular resistance and flow velocity in the ascending vasculature, predisposing the renal papilla to injury [35]. Each descending vasa recta "approaches the papillary tip and makes a hairpin turn," bifurcating into four ascending vasa recta, changing the blood flow from laminar to turbulent, and increasing the likelihood of injury at the renal papilla's vascular environment [35]. This vascular injury may subsequently augment Randall's plaque precipitation [36]. It has also been proposed that the repair of renal papillary vasculature leads to calcification near the vessel walls and may ultimately form a calculus into the papilla [37]. Interestingly, it has been suggested that the repair of this injury to the renal papilla is similar to the atherosclerotic-like reaction in damaged vessel walls, which has shown to lead to the calcification of the vessel wall [35,37]. Additionally, some have proposed that atherosclerotic plaque, in which calcium deposits in the form of hydroxyapatite were found within [38,39] and the site where coronary arterial calcification occurs [39,40], form at the arteries that are most disposed to injury, *i.e.*, sites where arteries bifurcate, similar to vasa recta bifurcation in the kidneys.

3. Calcium and Phosphate Concentrations

3.1. Salivary

Salivary gland stones have been found to be composed of different CaP. Hydroxyapatite is traditionally thought to make up a large part of salivary gland stones. Recent studies also suggest that salivary calculi are made up of other apatites, including amorphous carbonated CaP and carbonated apatite and whitlockite. In addition to the CaP, these calculi are also composed of an organic matrix, including fibrous proteins that can be found in greater than 60% of calculi and in fact can make up 60% to 95% of a given stone, which accumulate around the CaP serving as a nucleus [41–43].

The build-up of CaP crystals is the nidus for the development of salivary gland stones. While the precise mechanism may not be understood, there are certain etiological factors that are known to contribute to the formation of salivary calculi, such as the deposition of calcium salts around a core comprised of shed epithelial cells [23]. This makes sense since higher concentrations of saliva calcium have been shown in patients who develop hydroxyapatite calculi [41]. Moreover, experimental and clinical studies strongly suggest a link between high calcium concentration ([Ca^{2+}]) in saliva and sialolithiasis. Sialolithiasis starts with the formation of calculi; patients with calculi and sialolithiasis are shown to have higher [Ca^{2+}] in their final saliva [44]. Additionally, total saliva [Ca^{2+}] levels have been shown to be higher (~20 mg/L) in patients with calculi [41]. Evidence also indicates that calcium is the major component of salivary stones [43,45,46]. This, therefore, suggests that [Ca^{2+}] in ductal saliva is critical in the development of salivary gland stones [47].

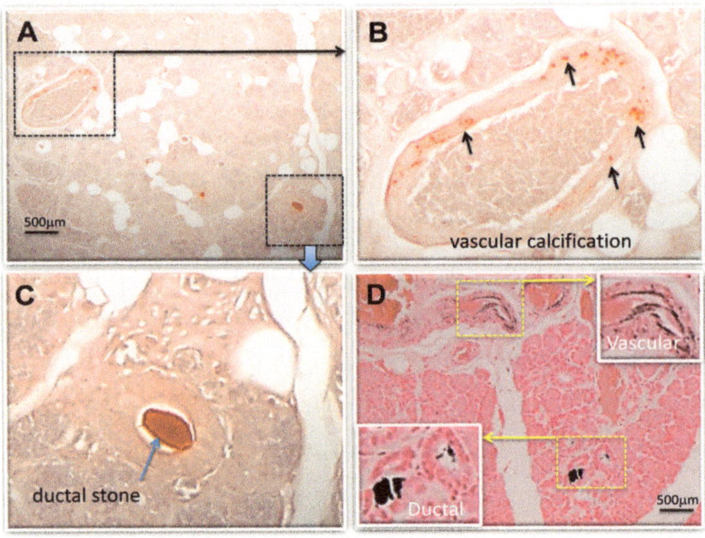

Figure 1. Vascular and ductal calcifications were found in salivary gland from stone patient. Human submandibular gland (SMG) sections from stone patient were used to detect calcified material. Calcified blood vessel and intra-ductal stones were stained with the: (**A**) alizarin red method [48] for examining the calcified deposits; enlarged in (**B**) showing vascular calcification; and (**C**) showing intra-ductal stone (pictures are representative of n = 6); no such staining was found in control SMG (n = 4). Von Kossa [49] stained SMG (**D**) confirms the presence of calcification, both vascular and stone, in same SMG tissue. Specimens are formalin fixed paraffin embedded (FFPE) de-identified tissue section (biopsy sample, not individually identifiable to any person) from tissue bank through an exempt Institutional Review Board (IRB) protocol.

Interestingly, we have identified vascular calcifications in human submandibular (SMG) salivary gland section from a stone patient (Figure 1). Indeed, both vascular calcification and intra-ductal stones are detected in the salivary gland tissue sections (Figure 1), indicating an organ specific deregulation of both Ca^{2+} and PO_4^{3-} in salivary stone conditions. CaP, in the form of hydroxyapatite, is the major inorganic component in salivary stones [44] and CaP deposition is critical to vascular calcification [12]; this indicates that the overall levels of Ca^{2+} and PO_4^{3-} in serum and the saliva could play in the calcification/stone forming mechanism. In support of this view, researchers already found that saliva Ca^{2+} of sialolithiasis patients is higher [44], which favors the crystallization mechanisms. However, what triggers the vascular calcification in such case is unknown. Additional mechanistic research is needed to provide further understanding of the molecular mechanism of calcium stone formation and calcification.

3.2. Kidneys

Research has shown that increases in calcium and phosphate concentration may contribute to the formation of CaP crystals that eventually lead to stone development. A recent computer model has indicated that a possible cause of spontaneous tubular CaP crystal formation, specifically at the descending loop of Henle, may either be due to an increase in plasma phosphate, or a decrease in phosphate fractional reabsorption in the proximal tubule [28]. Additionally, in a recent study that found a greater incidence of tubular plugging, in which CaP stone formers (brushite and apatite) exhibited severe plugging, CaP supersaturation was one factor that was associated to these plug formations [50]. Indeed, hypercalciuria is considered the most common abnormality in calcium nephrolithiasis patients [51] and has been frequently associated with Randall's plaque formation [52].

In animal models, sodium–hydrogen exchanger regulatory factor-1 (NHERF-1) null mice, which are hypercalciuric and hyperphosphaturic, produced interstitial CaP deposits in the form of apatite in the renal papilla [8,51]. Although the site of these depositions in NHERF-1 null mice were similar to those found in human idiopathic calcium oxalate stone formers [53], no direct evidence of NHERF-1 mutation has shown to cause kidney stones in humans. However, a clinical study observed that humans with a loss-of-function NHERF-1 mutation exhibited hypophosphatemia, indicating decreased capacity for kidney tubule reabsorption of phosphate, which increases the risk of renal calcium lithiasis [54]. Hypophosphatemia can then lead to an increase in intestinal phosphate and calcium absorption through increased 1,25-dihydroxyvitamin D [$1,25(OH)_2$ D] production [55], leading to hypercalcemia and hypercalciuria, a risk factor for calcium renal stone formation [56].

Another animal model has shown that kidney type-IIa sodium-phosphate (Na-Pi) co-transporter (Npt2a) null mice exhibited a production of CaP crystal deposits in the kidney tubules and interstitium [8,57]. It is possible that CaP crystals may have originated in the tubular lumen but was eventually displaced to the interstitium, as has been shown in certain Npt2a null mice models, and suggested by clinical and other animal studies [58]. However, no evidence has been found of this to occur in human cases; indeed, the pathogenesis of interstitial CaP deposits of Npt2a null mice are seemingly different from Randall's Plaque in humans [58]. Interestingly, though, disrupted Npt2a null mice exhibited an adaptive increase in $1,25(OH)_2$ D serum concentration, and associated hypercalciuria and renal calcification [59]. The same may also occur in humans with Npt2a mutations. One study in humans showed that Npt2a mutations led to the impairment of phosphate reabsorption, causing hypophosphatemia [60]. This may eventually result in low phosphate concentration in the serum and the expected increase in $1,25(OH)_2$ D serum concentration [61,62], hypercalciuria [60,63,64], and the formation of different CaP complexes [55]. Indeed, the combination of hypercalciuria, whether from increased intestinal calcium absorption [55,63] or idiopathic hypercalciuria [64], and hyperphosphaturia may lead to the formation of calcium phosphate complexes, and subsequently, nephrolithiasis.

3.3. Vascular

Elevated levels of calcium and phosphate in the serum can increase the deposition of CaP in the vasculature. For example, calcification found in the vascular system has been linked to hyperphosphatemia and increased calcium-phosphate products [65–67]. Also, *in vitro* studies have found that in response to elevated extracellular calcium ($[Ca^{2+}]_o$), the expression of the calcium sensing receptor (CSR), a G-protein coupled receptor that evokes signaling pathways according to changes in $[Ca^{2+}]_o$ concentration, had been downregulated in vascular smooth muscle cells induced to calcify, suggesting that ablation of CSR function was associated with increased calcification in vascular smooth muscle cells [67,68]. It is believed that, without the function of CSR, vascular smooth muscle cells are unable to respond to the increase in calcium, and produce the necessary inhibitory proteins to prevent calcification [68]. Moreover, one study has shown that elevated calcium concentrations, even under normal phosphate levels, induced the mineralization of human smooth muscle cells, and then was accelerated by increased phosphate levels [69]. Increases in calcium and phosphate also induced calcification in human vascular smooth muscle cells [70]. In both cases, the presence of elevated calcium and phosphate exacerbated calcification [71].

Intriguingly, in both animal and clinical studies, it has been shown that elevated phosphate levels indeed played a role in osteogenic and chondrogenic differentiation, which eventually leads to the formation of a complex and highly structured extracellular matrix [68] found in calcified vasculature. It has been shown that inorganic phosphate uptake by vascular smooth muscle cells induces transcription factors related to bone ossification, *i.e.*, Core-binding factor α(1), Cbfα1, also known as Runt-related transcription factor 2 (Runx2) [72,73]. Moreover, studies have shown that high phosphate cultured with vascular smooth muscle cells *in vitro* can calcify, and contain phenotypic transitions to several types of cells association with bone formation, such as osteoblasts and chondrocytes [18,73–78]. Thus, increasing evidence such as these indicates that arterial calcification is also an active process that shares many similarities with bone formation [16].

Interestingly, hypercalcemia and hyperphosphatemia can further exacerbate vascular calcification initiated by lipids. Indeed, Demer noted that lipids have an in important role in both bone calcification and calcification in atherosclerosis [79]. For example, researchers noticed through confocal microscopy that there was cholesterol within the calcified granules of atherosclerotic plaque, which suggest that lipids may nucleate calcium crystals [79,80]. Similarly, within the matrix vesicles, the nidus for crystallization is phospholipids, which are purposed to initiate and regulate hydroxyapatite formation [81].

4. Vascular Calcification and Stone Formation Similarities to Bone Mineralization

4.1. Overview of Bone Formation

There are two types of ossification: intramembranous and endochondral. Intramembranous ossification involves the formation of bone directly from mesenchymal tissue, primarily forming bones of the skull, clavicle, and mandible [17], and has been noted to be essential in the healing of compound fractures [81]. In endochondral ossification, mesenchymal cells are converted to bone through a cartilage intermediate [17], and are involved in the formation of long bones such as the femur, tibia, humerus, and radius [81].

Intramembranous ossification is initiated by mesenchymal stem cells and involves BMPs and transcription factor Cbfα1/Runx2. BMPs, such as BMP2, BMP4, and BMP7, activate the *Cbfα1* gene in mesenchymal cells to transform them into osteoblasts [17]. A study has shown that Runx2/Cbfα1 not only regulates osteoblast differentiation by activating major bone matrix genes [82] but also is necessary to induce osteoblastic differentiation in undifferentiated mesenchymal cells into osteoblasts [83], where Cbfα1 expression requires the activation by BMP2 [84]. BMP2 has shown to induce ectopic bone formation *in vivo* [85], regulate osteogenic differentiation *in vitro* [85], and mediate bone fracture repair [86]. Conversely, Runx2 null mice did not demonstrate intramembranous or endochondral ossification [87,88], and BMP blocking antibodies inhibited Runx2 osteoblastic differentiation [89]. Thus, Runx2/Cbfα1 [90] and BMP2 [86] have been shown to be integral in osteoblastic bone formation. In fact, $Bmp2^{+/-}$, $Bmp6^{-/-}$ mice displayed a reduction in bone formation in primary spongiosa, which Kugimiya and others believed was probably due to reduced bone formation [85]. Furthermore, BMP ligand deletion has shown to weaken chondrogenic or osteogenic differentiation [91]. Interestingly, one study found that BMP2 stimulates vascular smooth muscle cell differentiation into an osteoblastic phenotype; moreover, the BMP2 effect was reversed by β-catenin knockout, which implies that a second major pathway in osteoblastogenesis, the Wnt/β-catenin signaling pathway, is involved in BMP2 induced vascular smooth muscle cell differentiation into an osteogenic phenotype and subsequent calcification [92].

In endochondral ossification, rather than differentiating directly into osteoblastic phenotype, mesenchymal cells form cartilage tissue as an intermediate [17]. Transcription factors, Pax1 and Scleraxis, activate cartilage-specific genes [93,94] to commit the mesenchymal cells into differentiating into chondrocytes [17]. In fact, *Sox9* gene has been expressed in these precartilaginous condensations, and is quintessential in the regulation of chondrocyte development [95–97]. Studies have shown that a defect in the *Sox9* gene results in bone deformities in the body [17]. Interestingly, the repression of *Sox9* suppresses reprogramming of descending aorta vascular smooth muscle cells into chondrogenic phenotype, and the potential calcification of the vascular wall [98]. Continuing in the endochondral ossification process, chondrocytes then rapidly proliferate and enlarge their volume by secreting an extracellular matrix; the enlarged chondrocytes add collagen X and fibronectin to ensure it is mineralized by calcium carbonate [17]. All of the cartilage is eventually replaced by bone.

4.2. Kidney

The previous discussion of the kidneys highlighted that the physiological features of the vasculature, and high calcium and phosphate concentrations, may lead to the deposits of CaP in the interstitium. Interstitial CaP deposits, which are found in calcium oxalate stones in idiopathic calcium oxalate stone formers [4], may subsequently lead to the development of Randall's plaque, initially formed when a CaP spherule is deposited in the loops of Henle, collecting ducts, or vasa recta [99]. However, not all of Randall's plaque can lead to stone formation [99]. Interestingly, it has even been proposed that

Randall's plaque may be an example of nephrocalcinosis [100]. Nevertheless, the formation of stones requires the complex integration of numerous factors, for example, the formation, retention, and accumulation of crystals; mineral (*i.e.*, calcium and phosphate) supersaturation; urinary pH; and a disruption, reduction, or abnormalities in crystallization inhibitors [99]. Interestingly, in a recent retrospective study, one specific type of papillary stone (calcium oxalate monohydrate, COM) was found to have developed from crystals or organic matter that was attached to the renal papilla [101]. Indeed, it is believed that renal subepithelial papillary hydroxyapatite calcification is involved in COM stone formation [102], with recent evidence showing that hydroxyapatite crystals in the papillary, which can form into Randall's Plaque, can certainly become the nidus of a COM papillary stone [103].

Thus, the formation of Randall's plaque is particularly interesting, made more so because the involvement of membranous vesicles and collagen is similar to the mechanisms of other forms of ectopic calcification [104]. This may help to explain the association between kidney stones and subclinical atherosclerosis in young adults and the observation that these diseases share many of the same factors [105]. A new retrospective, matched case-control study by Shavit and others has found that patients who recurrently formed calcium kidney stones had higher incidences of aortic calcification, which suggests that stone formation and vascular calcification are linked [106]. Moreover, these [105] and other authors [107–111] found that patients who formed calcium kidney stones exhibited lower bone mineral density, suggesting that bone demineralization, which often accompanies hypercalcemia [112], may be linked to calcium stone formation. In fact, a previous study found increased occurrences of osteopenia and osteoporosis in patients with recurrent calcium nephrolithiasis and hypercalciuria [113]. Interestingly, as Gambaro *et al.* has pointed out, lower bone density has also been linked to abnormal arterial stiffness, partially due to calcification, which is a strong indicator of cardiovascular mortality [114]. These studies seemingly provide a link between bone, kidney calcium stone formation, and arterial calcification.

Moreover, a number of studies have found bone-related proteins, and transcription factors related to bone ossification, in kidney calcium stone formation. For example, evidence has shown that kidney epithelial cells can de-differentiate into an osteoblastic phenotype, increasing production of bone-specific proteins such as OSN, OPN and bone sialoprotein (BSP), supporting the nucleation of CaP crystals [8,115]. Moreover, increased levels of BMP2 and transcription factors has been linked to osteoblastic differentiation and bone formation, such as Runx2, to kidney CaP deposits in idiopathic hypercalcuria, where 1,25(OH)$_2$ D$_3$/vitamin D receptor (VDR) plays an important role in its regulation [116]. These connections provide a potentially novel relationship between bone formation, and crystal deposition and formation in the kidneys. Furthermore, new research has found that Ca^{2+} augments the response of transforming growth factor β1 (TGF-β1) to produce BMP2 and OPN in human kidney proximal tubule epithelial cell line, HK2, and in primary renal epithelial cells (PRECs) of nephrolithiasis patients with idiopathic hypercalciuria [117]. It has even been suggested that serum BMP2 levels, in combination with cystatin C, may be a potential biochemical marker for stone formation [118]. These findings suggest the important role of increased Ca^{2+} in the pathogenesis of stone formation and accentuate the potential relationship between kidney stone formation and bone mineralization/de-mineralization.

4.3. *Vascular*

Although vascular calcification was believed to be a passive process, it is now accepted that arterial calcification are active and highly regulated forms of calcification [119], similar to bone formation [16] (Figure 2). Indeed, magnetic resonance spectroscopy studies indicate that the hydroxyapatite structure in calcified vessels were similar to the hydroxyapatite in bone [120]. It has been proposed that vascular calcification is initiated when the cells de-differentiate into osteoblast-like phenotypes [121]. Indeed, cells (*i.e.*, pericytes in microvessels; pericyte-like, calcifying vascular cells in the aortic intima; smooth muscle cells in media; and myofibroblasts in the adventitia) have been isolated from vascular tissue and have been found to undergo osteoblastic de-differentiation [121]. These cells may originate from similar mesenchymal stem cells as osteoblasts, which themselves are induced with the transcription factor Runx2 or Msx-2 [122]. Although this is believed to be a common mechanism in both types of calcification, the factors that initiate this de-differentiation may differ [122].

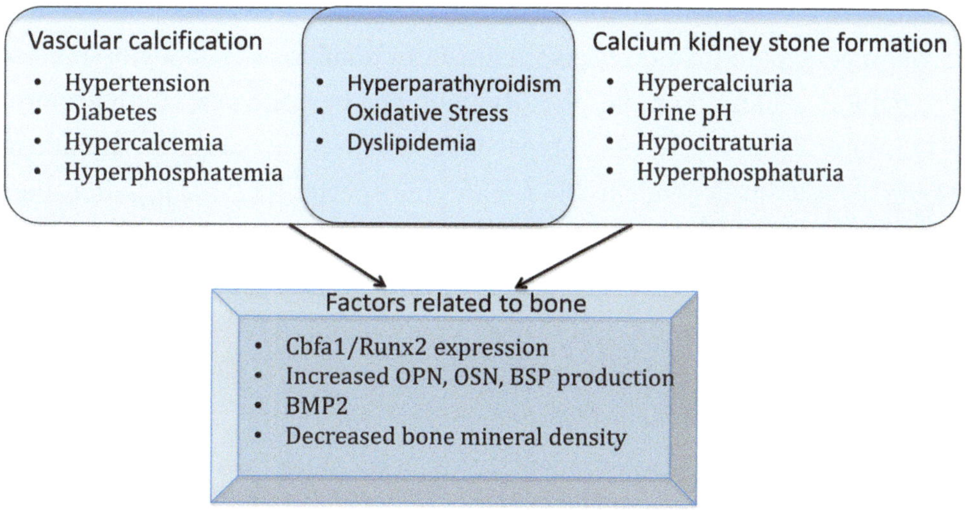

Figure 2. Identified instigators of vascular calcification and stone formation, highlighting common factors, and several commonalities related to bone mineralization/de-mineralization. Risk factors for vascular calcification include both the "traditional" (such as hypertension and diabetes) and the "non-traditional" (*i.e.*, abnormal mineral metabolism such as hypercalcemia and hyperphosphatemia) [123]. A majority of calcium kidney stones are predominantly calcium oxalate, with CaP admixed in small amounts [4]. Thus, factors associated with the predominant form of calcium stone formation include: hypercalciuria; urine pH, high (pH > 6.3) for CaP stone formation, and for CaP deposits that may be the initial nidus for calcium oxalate stones, and low for calcium oxalate stone formation; and hypocitraturia, which increases the chance for calcium to bind with oxalate or phosphate [4]. Hyperphosphaturia may increase the risk of calcium kidney stone formation by urinary calcium excretion and urinary saturation [56]. Common risk factors for both vascular calcification and calcium kidney stone formation include hyperparathyroidism [4,123], oxidative stress [99,123], and dyslipidemia [37,123]. Interestingly, studies have found bone related proteins and other bone related factors in vascular calcification, calcium deposits and calcium kidney stone formation as discussed in the review.

Specific factors that lead to intimal calcification in atherosclerosis include inflammatory factors produced within the actual atherosclerotic plaque, including modified lipoproteins and cytokines [121,124]. Notably, patients with homozygous familial hypercholesterolemia, due to mutations in the LDL receptor (LDL-R), develop aortic calcification independent of the levels of total cholesterol [121]. This has led to the hypothesis that LDL-R modulates the osteogenic signaling pathways, such that a mutation at the LDL-R gene locus leads to the dysregulation of the calcification signaling pathways in the osteoblast-like cells and the activation of Msx-2 and Runx2 [121]. Additionally, hydroxyapatite crystals within atherosclerotic plaques themselves may promote further calcification by inducing monocytes that ingest them to produce inflammatory cytokines [119]. Ultimately, in arterial intimal calcification, the Runx2/Cbfa-1 and Sox9 pathways predominate, although Msx-2 expression has been found in arterial specimens that include diabetic patients [125].

Whereas the Runx2/Cbfa-1 pathway predominates in intimal calcification, the early stages of medial calcification have been that the Msx-2 and Wnt pathways predominate [121]. Hyperglycemia also promotes calcification via enhanced alkaline phosphatase expression via the Runx2/Cbfa-1 pathway [121]. Arterial medial calcification is also induced in renal insufficiency by high serum levels of phosphate and calcium, which promote the Runx2/Cbfa-1 pathways. Furthermore, inorganic phosphate directly promotes osteoblastic phenotype transformation in vascular smooth muscle cells (VSMCs) by inducing a sodium-dependent phosphate transporter [12,121]. After the phenotype change, the osteoblastic cells also induce calcification via expression of other bone-regulating proteins include OPN, osteocalcin, OSN and type II collagen [126]. Additionally, these osteoblastic cells secrete matrix proteins, which serve as the foundation upon which calcification occurs both through the secretion of matrix vesicles containing preformed apatite [127,128] or through further apoptosis [124,127,129,130]. Apoptotic cell death increases membranous debris rich in phospholipids that can be the conduit to nucleate apatite, particularly in individuals with atherosclerosis and other diseases with widespread necrosis and apoptosis.

Once the matrix vesicles are secreted, increased levels of phosphorus and calcium can increase their mineralizing potential, which may explain why calcification is more prominent in individuals with chronic kidney disease and thus causes disturbances in mineral (*i.e.*, calcium and phosphate) metabolism [122]. Normally, mineralization through said matrix vesicles is prevented through mineralization inhibitors (such as matrix Gla protein and fetuin-A), but in cases where there are diminished or ineffective mineralization inhibitors, the matrix vesicles can then serve as niduses for further calcification [127,128].

Interestingly, aortic valve (valvular) calcification has been suggested to possess similar characteristics of arterial (vascular) calcification [126]. Indeed, similar to VSMC, valvular interstitial myofibroblast-like cells showed expression of OPN, osteocalcin, and Runx2, which suggests an active mineralization process prior to the development of end-stage calcification (*i.e.*, macrocalcification) [126] involving valvular endothelial cells, valve interstitial cells, inflammatory cells, and the extracellular matrix [131]. Some studies have associated valvular calcification with a faster progression of aortic stenosis which clinically manifests into exertional angina, syncope, and heart failure [131], and worse morbidity and mortality [132]. Additionally, vascular calcification is common in end-stage renal disease (ESRD) patients [133], due to their elevated risk of mineral metabolism disturbances [134]. Interestingly, it has been proposed that valvular calcification may be marker of arterial calcification in ESRD patients [134].

4.4. Breast

Ectopic calcification in the breast is a telltale sign of breast cancer, and is one of the distinguishing features examined for on diagnostic mammography. It has been reported that microcalcifications can be found in up to 88% of non-palpable tumors [135], and up to 93% of ductal carcinoma *in situ* (DCIS) cases are presented alongside microcalcification [136]. Thus, these microcalcifications can be used to detect breast cancer in its early stages. However, studies have shown that microcalcification is being associated with worse prognoses; indeed breast cancer presenting with microcalcification are more associated with lymph node invasion and HER-2 positivity [136]. Similar to kidney calcification, breast microcalcification comes in two forms, known as Type I and II crystals. Type I crystals are composed of calcium oxalate and are more frequently associated with benign ductal cysts [137]. Type II crystals are composed of hydroxyapatite and are associated with both benign and breast cancer lesions [138]. Furthermore, as the carbonate content of the hydroxyapatite crystals decreases, the grade of the lesion increased [139]. Indeed, it is hypothesized that the hydroxyapatite itself increased the grade of the cancer because hydroxyapatite has been found to increase the mitogenesis of the cancer cells [140].

Until recently, very little information was known about the mechanism of hydroxyapatite formation in breast cancer, largely because of a lack of a reproducible, high-penetrance animal model available to study this process [141]. It was not even known whether the calcification was a result of an active or passive process. However Cox and others developed a reproducible *in vitro* model using the metastatic mammary adenocarcinoma 4T1 cell line that ultimately allowed them to propose a mechanism for hydroxyapatite calcification [136]. They hypothesized that alkaline phosphatase (ALP) not only hydrolyses β-glycerophosphate to glycerol and phosphate (Pi) [136], which is similar to the initial osteoblastic differentiation process in ossification [142], but ALP also dephosphorylates OPN and hydrolyzes pyrophosphate (PPi) to Pi on the surface of mammary cells [143]. The produced Pi is then believed to be transported into the 4T1 cells by type II Na-Pi co-transporters, which have been found to be expressed in higher levels in cancer tissue as opposed to normal tissue [136]. When inside the cell, the Pi combines with calcium to ultimately produce hydroxyapatite crystals [136]. However, further research will be necessary to ascertain how these crystals eventually are transported out of the cell to the extracellular matrix. Mineralization was prevented when these Na-Pi co-transporters were inhibited [143], which suggests that this calcification is an active process in the breast cancer cells. Interestingly, β-glycerophosphate was found to cause elevated OPN expression and calcification in bovine vascular smooth muscle cells, which were prevented by the inhibition of type III Na-Pi co-transporters [144]. This suggests that Na-Pi co-transporters play a role in the calcification and CaP (in the form of hydroxyapatite) deposition process in vascular and mammary cells, respectively (Figure 3).

Moreover, Cox and others later determined that, during this process of mineralization, there is no change in the amount of Runx2 mRNA [143], which also a role in bone ossification and is seen in vascular calcification. With that said, other transcription factors do exist and their involvement cannot be ruled out at this time. A separate study also suggests that BMP2 may be involved after determining that BMP2 can induce microcalcification in adenocarcinoma cells while at the same time sparing normal tissues, possible through the formation of osteoblast-like cells being derived from pericytes [141]. Additionally, studies have determined that both *in situ* and invasive breast carcinomas had increased levels of OSN, OPN, and BSP, which were also associated with higher levels of microcalcification [145,146]. Increased expression of OPN mRNA further suggests that this process is similar to physiological osteoblasts [143]. Indeed, one recent study suggested breast epithelial cells may acquire mesenchymal characteristics, where osteoblast-like cells secrete microcalcifications in the form of hydroxyapatite into the extracellular space [147].

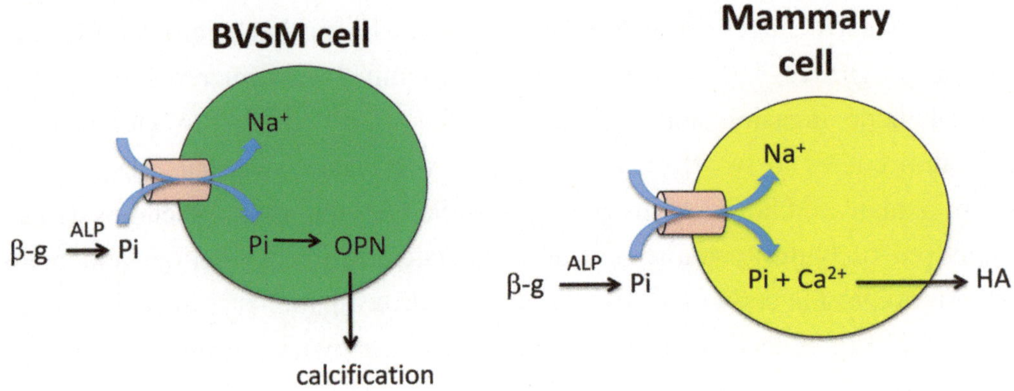

Figure 3. In bovine vascular smooth muscle (BVSM) cell and mammary cells, studies have suggested that Na-Pi co-transporters can induce calcification and hydroxyapatite (HA) crystal production, respectively. In BVSM and mammary cells, β-glycerophosphate (β-g) via alkaline phosphatase (ALP) hydrolyzes pyrophosphate (Ppi) into Pi, where Pi is transported into the cell via Na-Pi co-transporters [136,144]. In BVSM cells, the increase in Pi induces osteopontin (OPN) expression and calcification [144]. In mammary cells, increased in intracellular Pi combines with Ca^{2+} to product HA crystals; however, further research is needed to determine the mechanism in which HA crystals are transported into the extracellular matrix [136].

5. Conclusions

CaP crystal deposition has been identified to be the source of calcification and stone formation, both of which may lead to potential adverse conditions. Thus, a comparative review of the mechanism in which CaP crystal aggregates may provide important insights. For one, because such stone formation occurs due to changes within similar hollow tubular structures, it intimates an avenue of commonality among other sites of crystal formation [5–7,9,35]. Thus, further studies are needed, whether *in vivo*, or *ex vivo* utilizing microfluidics, to determine whether changes in the spatiotemporal compositions of the biological fluids may impact other sites of hollow tubular structures, such as the breast and pancreatic ducts.

Secondly, as suggested in this review, high $[Ca^{2+}]$ levels, for example, in the saliva and in kidney luminal fluid, may potentially develop into salivary calculi and CaP crystals [8,57,59], respectively. Studies have shown an association between increased $[Ca^{2+}]_o$ with increased expression of bone-specific proteins involving Ca^{2+} signaling. Elevated $[Ca^{2+}]_o$ levels have been shown to stimulate osteoblastic differentiation, but one study performed by Koori and others has shown that increased $[Ca^{2+}]_o$ levels also increase bone-related gene expression and calcification [148]. Interestingly, inhibiting the CSR induced greater bone-related gene expression and calcification; further antagonizing CSR had shown to enhance the role of calcium in osteogenic differentiation [148]. Additionally, one study has indicated that BMP2 may inhibit transient receptor potential canonical (TRPC) 1, TRPC4, and TRPC6 expression, thereby regulating Ca^{2+} signaling and decreasing intracellular Ca^{2+} levels in pulmonary arterial smooth muscle cells [149]. Interestingly, it has also been proposed that the dysregulation of Ca^{2+} homeostasis and the disruption of the coordinated action of calcium pumps, channels, sensors and buffers in breast epithelial cells may be involved in the formation of the mesenchymal cell type that has been associated with breast cancer metastasis [150]. Thus, more studies are needed to determine the molecular mechanism that leads to calcification and stone formation due to high [Ca^{2+}] levels.

Third, as Khan and others have suggested, studies have shown an increasing role of bone-specific proteins in calculi formation in the kidneys and cardiovascular system [8]. Studies have also shown that OPN can induce hydroxyapatite development [151]. A high phosphate diet has been found to induce OSN expression in the kidney tubules, suggesting that increased OSN expression is involved in the kidney formation of calcium deposits initiated by a high phosphate diet [152]. These same bone-specific proteins are linked to ectopic microcalcification in adenocarcinoma cells as well, suggesting similar mechanisms of crystallization formation in different parts of the body. Thus, there could be a potential link between microcalcification in adenocarcinoma cells, initiated by bone-specific proteins, and carcinoma. Accordingly, further research is required.

Additionally, research has indicated that BMPs, and transcription factors Runx2/Cbfα1, are involved in the deposition of CaP crystals in the kidney, which can eventually lead to stone formation, and in the initial formative stages of vascular calcification. This interesting link to ossification begs to ask whether other CaP deposits in the ducts of the salivary gland, breasts, and pancreas (all which lead to microcalcification and stone formation) are similar to the ossification mechanism. Further research may provide subtle clues that could enhance our understanding of the early stages of stone formation and calcification.

Acknowledgments

We thank Dr. Robert Redman, DCVAMC, for helpful discussions in calcium staining methods. We also thank Ivan Lau, Calcium Signaling Lab and Kathy Kalinyak, Pathology Laboratory Services, DCVAMC, for technical assistance. Our research is supported by intramural grants from Institute of Clinical Research Inc. and DCVAMC, Washington DC. This work is also supported in part by grants from NIH (DE 019524) and National Kidney Foundation of the National Capital Area to BCB.

Conflicts of Interest

The authors declare no conflict of interest.

References

1. Metheny, N.M. *Fluid and Electrolyte Balance: Nursing Considerations*, 5th ed.; Jones & Bartlett Learning: St. Louis, MO, USA, 2010.
2. Clapham, D.E. Calcium signaling. *Cell.* **2007**, *131*, 1047–1058.

3. Hopkins, C.R.; Walker, A.M. Calcium as a second messenger in the stimulation of luteinizing hormone secretion. *Mol. Cell. Endocrinol.* **1978**, *12*,189–208.
4. Worcester, E.M.; Coe, F.L. Nephrolithiasis. *Prim. Care* **2008**, *35*, 369–391.
5. Moe, S.M.; Chen, N.X. Mechanisms of vascular calcification in chronic kidney disease. *J. Am. Soc. Nephrol.* **2008**, *1*, 213–216.
6. Schepers, M.S.J.; van Ballegooijen, E.S.; Bangma, C.H.; Verkoelen, C.F. Crystals cause acute necrotic cell death in renal proximal tubule cells, but not in collecting tubule cells. *Kidney Int.* **2005**, *68*, 1543–1553.
7. Coe, F.L; Evan, A.P.; Worcester, E.M.; Lingeman, J.E. Three pathways for human kidney stone formation. *Urol. Res.* **2010**, *38*, 147–160.
8. Khan, S.R.; Canales, B.K. Unified theory on the pathogenesis of Randall's plaques and plugs. *Urolithiasis* **2015**, *43*, S109–S123.
9. Canales, B.K.; Anderson, L.; Higgins, L; Ensrud-Bowlin, K.; Roberts, K.P.; Wu, B.; Kim, I.W.; Monga, M. Proteome of Human Calcium Kidney Stones. *Urology* **2010**, *76*, e13–e20.
10. Parks, J.H.; Coe, F.L.; Evan, A.P.; Worcester, E.M. Urine pH in renal calcium stone formers who do and do not increase stone phosphate content with time. *Nephrol. Dial. Transpl.* **2009**, *24*, 130–136.
11. Callaghan, D.; Bandyopadhyay, B.C. Calcium Phosphate Kidney Stone: Problems and Perspectives. *Anat. Physiol.* **2012**, *2*, e118. doi:10.4172/2161-0940.1000e118.
12. Villa-Bellosta, R.; Millan, A.; Sorribas, V. Role of calcium-phosphate deposition in vascular smooth muscle cell calcification. *Am. J. Physiol. Cell. Physiol.* **2011**, *300*, C210–C220.
13. Tiselius, H.G. The role of calcium phosphate in the development of Randall's plaques. *Urolithiasis* **2013**, *41*, 369–377.
14. Kumar, V.; Farell, G.; Yu, S.; Harrington, S.; Fitzpatrick, L.; Rzewuska, E.; Miller, V.M.; Lieske, J.C. Cell biology of pathologic renal calcification: contribution of crystal transcytosis, cell-mediated calcification, and nanoparticles. *J. Investig. Med.* **2006**, *54*, 412–424.
15. Sage, A.P.; Lu, J, Tintut, Y., Demer, L.L. Hyperphosphatemia-induced nanocrystals upregulate the expression of bone morphogenetic protein-2 and osteopontin genes in mouse smooth muscle cells *in vitro*. *Kidney Int.* **2011**, *79*, 414–422.
16. Shroff, R.; Long, D.A. Shanahan, C.M. Mechanistic insights into vascular calcification in CKD. *J. Am. Soc. Nephrol.* **2013**, *24*, 179–189.
17. Gilbert, S.F. Osteogenesis: The development of bones. In *Developmental Biology*, 6th ed.; Sinauer Associates: Sunderland, UK, 2000. Available online: http://www.ncbi.nlm.nih.gov/books/NBK10056/ (accessed on 12 January 2015).
18. Zhu, D.; Mackenzie, N.C.; Farquharson, C.; Macrae, V.E. Mechanisms and clinical consequences of vascular calcification. *Front. Endocrinol.* **2012**, *3*, 95, doi:10.3389/fendo.2012.00095.
19. Moe, S.M. Vascular Calcification: The Three-Hit Model. *J. Am. Soc. Nephrol.* **2009**, *20*, 1162–1164.
20. Rule, A.D.; Krambeck, A.E.; Lieske, J.C. Chronic kidney disease in kidney stone formers. *Clin. J. Am. Soc. Nephrol.* **2011**, *6*, 2069–2075.

21. Davidovich, E.; Davidovits, M.; Peretz, B.; Shapira, J.; Aframian, D.J. The correlation between dental calculus and disturbed mineral metabolism in paediatric patients with chronic kidney disease. *Nephrol. Dial. Transpl.* **2009**, *24*, 2439–2445.
22. Pastor-Ramos, V.; Cuervo-Díaz, A.; Aracil-Kessler, L.; Sialolithiasis. Proposal for a new minimally invasive procedure: Piezoelectric surgery. *J. Clin. Exp. Dent.* **2014**, *6*, e295–e298. doi:10.4317/jced.51253.
23. Rzymska-Grala, I.; Stopa, Z.; Grala, B.; Gołębiowski, M.; Wanyura, H.; Zuchowska, A.; Sawicka, M.; Zmorzyński, M. Salivary gland calculi—contemporary methods of imaging. *Pol. J. Radiol.* **2010**, *75*, 25–37.
24. Kraai, J.S.; Karagozoglu, K.H.; Forouzanfar, T.; Veerman, E.C.I.; Brand, H.S. Salivary stones: Symptoms, aetiology, biochemical composition and treatment. *Br. Dent. J.* **2014**, *217*, E23. doi:10.1038/sj.bdj.2014.1054.
25. Mimura, M.; Tanaka, N.; Ichinose, S.; Kimijima, Y.; Amagasa, T.; Possible etiology of calculi formation in salivary glands: biophysical analysis of calculus. *Med. Mol. Morphol.* **2005**, *38*, 189–195.
26. Baurmash, H.D. Submandibular salivary stones: current management modalities. *J. Oral Maxillofac. Surg.* **2004**, *62*, 369–378.
27. Fink, H.A.; Wilt, T.J.; Eidman, K.E.; Garimella, P.S.; MacDonald, R.; Rutks, I.R.; Brasure, M.; Kane, R.L.; Monga, M. *Recurrent Nephrolithiasis in Adults: Comparative Effectiveness of Preventive Medical Strategies*; Executive Summary; Agency for Healthcare Research and Quality; Rockville, MD, USA, July 2012. Available online: http://www.ncbi.nlm.nih.gov/books/NBK99757/ (accessed on 24 May 2015).
28. Robertson, W.G.; Potenstial role of fluctuations in the composition of renal tubular fluid through the nephron in the initiation of Randall's plugs and calcium oxalate crystalluria in a computer model of renal function. *Urolithiasis* **2015**, *43*, S93–S107.
29. Verkoelen, C.F. Crystal retention in renal stone disease: A crucial role for the glycosaminoglycan hyaluronan? *J. Am. Soc. Nephrol.* **2006**, *17*, 1673–1687.
30. Arcidiacono, T.; Mingione, A.; Macrina, L.; Pivari.; Soldati, L.; Vezzoli, G. Idiopathic Calcium Nephrolithiasis: A Review of Pathogenic Mechanisms in the Light of Genetic Studies. *Am. J. Nephrol.* **2014**, *40*, 499–506.
31. Koul, H.K. Koul, S.; Fu, S.; Santosham, V.; Seikhon, A.; Menon, M. Oxalate: from crystal formation to crystal retention. *J. Am. Soc. Nephrol.* **1999**, *10*, S417–S421.
32. Benedetto, A.; Accetta, G.; Fujita, Y.; Charras, G. Spatiotemporal control of gene expression using microfluidics. *Lab. Chip.* **2014**, *14*, 1336–1347.
33. Wei, Z.; Amponsah, P.K.; Al-Shatti, M.; Nie, Z. Bandyopadhyay, B.C. Engineering of polarized tubular structures in a microfluidic device to study calcium phosphate stone formation. *Lab. Chip.* **2012**, *12*, 4037–4040.
34. Evan, A.P. Physiopathology and etiology of stone formation in the kidney and the urinary tract. *Pediatr. Nephrol.* **2010**, *25*, 831–841, doi:10.1007/s00467-009-1116-y.
35. Stoller, M.L.; Meng, M.V.; Abrahams, H.M.; Kane, J.P. The primary stone event: a new hypothesis involving a vascular etiology. *J. Urol.* **2004**, *171*, 1920–1924.

36. Taylor, E.R.; Stoller, M.L. Vascular theory of the formation of Randall plaques. *Urolithiasis* **2015**, *43*, S41–S45. doi:10.1007/s00240-014-0718-4.
37. Bagga, H.S.; Chi, T.; Miller, J.; Stoller, M.L. New Insights Into the Pathogenesis of Renal Calculi. *Urol. Clin. North. Am.* **2013**, *40*, 1–12.
38. Fitzpatrick, L.A.; Severson, A.; Edwards, W.D.; Ingram, R.T. Diffuse calcification in human coronary arteries. Association of osteopontin with atherosclerosis. *J. Clin. Invest.* **1994**, *94*, 1597–1604.
39. Sangiorgi, G.; Rumberger, J.A.; Severson, A; Edwards, W.D.; Gregoire, J.; Fitzpatrick, L.A.; Schwartz, R.S. Arterial Calcification and Not Lumen Stenosis Is Highly Correlated With Atherosclerotic Plaque Burden in Humans: A Histologic Study of 723 Coronary Artery Segments Using Nondecalcifying Methodology. *J. Am. Coll. Cardiol.* **1998**, *31*, 126–133.
40. Blankenhorn, D.H. Coronary Arterial Calcification A Review. *Am. J. Med. Sci.* **1961**, *242*, 1–9.
41. Grases, F.; Santiago, C.; Simonet, B.M.; Costa-Bauzá, A. Sialolithiasis: mechanism of calculi formation and etiologic factors. *Clin. Chim. Acta.* **2003**, *334*, 131–136.
42. Sabot, J.F.; Gustin, M.P.; Delahougue, K.; Faure, F.; Machon, C.; Hartmann, D.J. Analytical investigation of salivary calculi, by mid-infrared spectroscopy. *Analyst*. **2012**, *137*, 2095–2100.
43. Lee, L.T.; Wong, Y.K. Pathogenesis and diverse histologic findings of sialolithiasis in minor salivary glands. *J. Oral Maxillofac. Surg.* **2010**, *68*, 465–470.
44. Su, Y.X.; Zhang, K.; Ke, Z.F.; Zheng, G.S.; Chu, M.; Liao, G.Q. Increased calcium and decreased magnesium and citrate concentrations of submandibular/sublingual saliva in sialolithiasis. *Arch. Oral Biol*. **2010**, *55*, 15–20.
45. Westhofen, M.; Schäfer, H.; Seifert G. Calcium redistribution, calcification and stone formation in the parotid gland during experimental stimulation and hypercalcaemia. Cytochemical and X-ray microanalytical investigations. *Virchows. Arch. A Pathol. Anat. Histopathol*. **1984**, *402*, 425–438.
46. Waseem, Z.; Forte, V. An unusual case of bilateral submandibular sialolithiasis in a young female patient. *Int. J. Pediatr. Otorhinolaryngol.* **2005**, *69*, 691–694.
47. Bandyopadhyay, B.C.; Swaim, W.D.; Sarkar, A.; Liu, X.; Ambudkar, I.S. Extracellular Ca^{2+} sensing in salivary ductal cells. *J. Biol. Chem*. **2012**, *287*, 30305–30316.
48. Proia, A.D.; Brinn, N.T. Identification of calcium oxalate crystals using alizarin red S stain. *Arch. Pathol. Lab. Med.* **1985**, *109*, 186–189.
49. Luna, L.G. Gross, M.A. Artifacts simulating calcification associated with improper buffering of formalin fixative. *Am. J. Med. Technol*. **1965**, *31*, 412–416.
50. Linnes, M.P.; Krambeck, A.E.; Cornell, L.; Williams, J.C., Jr.; Korinek, M.; Bergstralh, E.J.; Li, X.; Rule, A.D.; McCollough, C.M.; Vrtiska, T.J.; *et al*. Phenotypic characterization of kidney stone formers by endoscopic and histological quantification of intrarenal calcification. *Kidney Int.* **2013**, *84*, 818–825.
51. Frick, K.K, Bushinsky, D.A. Molecular mechanisms of primary hypercalciuria. *J. Am. Soc. Nephrol.* **2003**, *14*, 1082–1095.
52. Daudon, M.; Bazin, D.; Letavernier, E. Randall's plaque as the origin of calcium oxalate kidney stones. *Urolithiasis* **2015**, *43* (Suppl 1), 5–11. doi:10.1007/s00240-014-0703-y.

53. Evan, A.P.; Weinman, E.J.; Wu, X.R.; Lingeman, J.E.; Worcester, E.M.; Coe, F.L. Comparison of the pathology of interstitial plaque in human ICSF stone patients to NHERF-1 and THP-null mice. *Urol. Res.* **2010**, *38*, 439–452.
54. Karim, Z.; Gérard, B.; Bakouh, N.; Alili, R.; Leroy, C.; Beck, L.; Silve, C.; Planelles, G.; Urena-Torres, P.; Grandchamp, B. *et al.* NHERF1 mutations and responsiveness of renal parathyroid hormone. *N. Engl. J. Med.* **2008**, *359*, 1128–1135.
55. Levi, M.; Breusegem, S. Renal phosphate-transporter regulatory proteins and nephrolithiasis. *N. Engl. J. Med.* **2008**, *359*, 1171–1173.
56. Prié, D.; Ravery, V.; Boccon-Gibod, L.; Friedlander G. Frequency of renal phosphate leak among patients with calcium nephrolithiasis. *Kidney Int.* **2001**, *60*, 272–276.
57. Khan, S.R.; Glenton, P.A. Calcium oxalate crystal deposition in kidneys of hypercalciuric mice with disrupted type IIa sodium-phosphate cotransporter. *Am. J. Physiol. Renal Physiol.* **2008**, *294*, F1109–1115.
58. Khan, S.R.; Canales, B.K. Ultrastructural Investigation of Crystal deposits in Npt2a knockout mice: Are they similar to Human Randall's plaques? *J. Urol.* **2011**, *186*, 1107–1113.
59. Chau, H.; El-Maadawy, S.; McKee, M.D. Tenenhouse, H.S. Renal calcification in mice homozygous for the disrupted type IIa Na/Pi cotransporter gene Npt2. *J. Bone Miner. Res.* **2003**, *18*, 644–657.
60. Prié, D.; Huart, V.; Bakouh, N.; Planelles, G.; Dellis, O.; Gérard, B.; Hulin, P.; Benqué-Blanchet, F.; Silve, C.; Grandchamp, B.; *et al.* Nephrolithiasis and osteoporosis associated with hypophosphatemia caused by mutations in the type 2a sodium-phosphate cotransporter. *N. Engl. J. Med.* **2002**, *347*, 983–991.
61. Gray, R.W.; Wilz, D.R.; Caldas, A.E.; Lemann, J., Jr. The importance of phosphate in regulating plasma 1,25-$(OH)_2$-vitamin D levels in humans: Studies in healthy subjects, in calcium-stone formers and in patients with primary hyperparathyroidism. *J. Clin. Endocrinol. Metab.* **1977**, *45*, 299–306.
62. Portale, A.A.; Halloran, B.P.; Morris, R.C.Jr. Physiologic regulation of the serum concentration of 1,25-dihydroxyvitamin D by phosphorus in normal men *J. Clin. Invest.* **1989**, *83*, 1494–1499.
63. Lederer, E.; Miyamoto, K. Clinical consequences of mutations in sodium phosphate cotransporters. *Clin. J. Am. Soc. Nephrol.* **2012**, *7*, 1179–1187.
64. Williams, C.P.; Child, D.F.; Hudson, P.R.; Soysa, L.D.; Davies, G.K.; Davies, M.G.; de Bolla, A.R. Inappropriate phosphate excretion in idiopathic hypercalciuria: The key to a common cause and future treatment? *J. Clin. Pathol.* **1996**, *49*, 881–888.
65. Block, G.A.; Hulbert-Shearon, T.E.; Levin, N.W.; Port, F.K. Association of serum phosphorus and calcium x phosphate product with mortality risk in chronic hemodialysis patients: A national study. *Am. J. Kidney Dis.* **1998**, *31*, 607–617.
66. Ganesh, S.K.; Stack, A.G.; Levin, N.W. Hulbert-Shearon, T.; Port, F.K. Association of elevated serum PO_4, Ca_xPO_4 product, and parathyroid hormone with cardiac mortality risk in chronic hemodialysis patients. *J. Am. Soc. Nephrol.* **2001**, *12*, 2131–2138.
67. Alam, M.U.; Kirton, J.P.; Wilkinson, F.L.; Towers, E.; Sinha, S.; Rouhi, M.; Vizard, T.N.; Sage, A.P.; Martin, D.; Ward, D.T.; *et al.* Calcification is associated with loss of functional calcium-sensing receptor in vascular smooth muscle cells. *Cardiovasc. Res.* **2009**, *81*, 260–268.

68. Shanahan, C.M.; Crouthamel, M.H.; Kapustin, A.; Giachelli, C.M. Arterial calcification in chronic kidney disease: Key roles for calcium and phosphate. *Circ. Res.* **2011**, *109*, 697–711.
69. Parks, J.H.; Worcester, E.M.; Coe, F.; Evan, A.P. Lingeman J.E. Clinical implications of abundant calcium phosphate in routinely analyzed kidney stones. *Kidney Int.* **2004**, *66*, 777–785.
70. Reynolds, J.L.; Joannides, A.J. Skepper, J.N.; McNair, R.; Schurgers, L.J.; Proudfoot, D.; Jahnen-Dechent, W.; Weissberg, P.L.; Shanahan, C.M. Human vascular smooth muscle cells undergo vesicle-mediated calcification in response to changes in extracellular calcium and phosphate concentrations: A potential mechanism for accelerated vascular calcification in ESRD. *J. Am. Soc. Nephrol.* **2004**, *15*, 2857–2867.
71. Cozzolino, M.; Brancaccio, D.; Gallieni, M.; Slatopolsky, E. Pathogenesis of vascular calcification in chronic kidney disease. *Kidney Int.* **2005**, *68*, 429–436.
72. Jono, S.; McKee, M.D.; Murry, C.E.; Shioi, A.; Nishizawa, Y.; Mori, K.; Morii, H.; Giachelli, CM. Phosphate regulation of vascular smooth muscle cell calcification. *Circ. Res.* **2000**, 87, E10–E17.
73. Li, X.; Yang, H.Y.; Giachelli, C.M. BMP-2 promotes phosphate uptake, phenotypic modulation, and calcification of human vascular smooth muscle cells. *Atherosclerosis* **2008**, *199*, 271–277.
74. Steitz, S.A.; Speer, M.Y.; Curinga, G.; Yang, H.Y.; Haynes, P.; Aebersold, R.; Schinke, T.; Karsenty, G.; Giachelli, C.M. Smooth muscle cell phenotypic transition associated with calcification: upregulation of Cbfα1 and downregulation of smooth muscle lineage markers. *Circ. Res.* **2001**, *89*, 1147–1154.
75. Johnson, K.; Polewski, M.; Van, E.D.; Terkeltaub, R. Chondrogenesis mediated by PPi depletion promotes spontaneous aortic calcification in NPP1$^{-/-}$ mice. *Arterioscler. Thromb. Vasc. Biol.* **2005**, *25*, 686–691.
76. Speer, M.Y.; Yang, H.Y; Brabb, T.; Leaf, E.; Look, A.; Lin, W.L.; Frutkin, A.; Dichek, D.; Giachelli, C.M. Smooth muscle cells give rise to osteochondrogenic precursors and chondrocytes in calcifying arteries. *Circ. Res.* **2009**, *104*, 733–741.
77. Zavaczki, E.; Jeney, V.; Agarwal, A.; Zarjou, A.; Oros, M.; Katkó, M.; Varga, Z.; Balla, G.; Balla, J. Hydrogen sulfide inhibits the calcification and osteoblastic differentiation of vascular smooth muscle cells. *Kidney Int.* **2011**, *80*, 731–739.
78. Zhu, D.; Mackenzie, N.C.; Millán, J.L.; Farquharson, C.; MacRae, V.E. The appearance and modulation of osteocyte marker expression during calcification of vascular smooth muscle cells. *PLoS ONE.* **2011**, *6*, e19595.
79. Demer, L.L. Lipid Hypothesis of Cardiovascular Calcification. *Circulation.* **1997**, *95*, 297–298.
80. Sarig, S.; Weiss, T.A.; Katz, I.; Kahana, F.; Azoury, R.; Okon, E.; Kruth, H.S. Detection of cholesterol associated with calcium mineral using confocal fluorescence microscopy. *Lab. Invest.* **1994**, *71*, 782–787.
81. Kini, U.; Nandeesh, B.N. Physiology of bone formation, remodeling and metabolism. In *Radionuclide and Hybrid Bone Imaging*; Fogelman, I., Gnanasegaran, G., van der Wall, H., Eds;. Springer-Verlag: Berlin, Germany, 2012; pp. 29–57.
82. Komori, T. Regulation of osteoblast differentiation by Runx2. *Adv. Exp. Med. Biol.* **2010**, *658*, 43–49.

83. Dong, S.; Ying, D.; Duan, X.; Zhu, C.; Liu, G.; Mi, J. Effect of core-binding factor α1 on the expression of osteoblast gene marker mesenchymal stem cells. *Zhongguo Xiu Fu Chong Jian Wai Ke Za Zhi* **2005**, *19*, 746–750. Available online: http://www.ncbi.nlm.nih.gov/pubmed/16206768 (accessed on 22 May 2015).

84. Nishimura, R.; Hata, K.; Harris, S.E.; Ikeda, F.; Yoneda, T. Core-binding factor α1 (Cbfα1) induces osteoblastic differentiation of C_2C_{12} cells without interactions with Smad1 and Smad5. *Bone* **2002**, *31*, 303–312.

85. Kugimiya, F.; Kawaguchi, H.; Kamekura, S.; Chikuda, H.; Ohba, S.; Yano, F.; Ogata, N.; Katagiri, T.; Harada, Y.; Azuma, Y.; *et al.* Involvement of endogenous bone morphogenetic protein $(BMP)_2$ and BMP6 in bone formation. *J. Biol. Chem.* **2005**, *280*, 35704–35712.

86. Tsuji, K.; Bandyopadhyay, A.; Harfe, B.D.; Cox, K.; Kakar, S.; Gerstenfeld, L; Einhorn, T.; Tabin, C.J.; Rosen, V. BMP2 activity, although dispensable for bone formation, is required for the initiation of fracture healing. *Nat. Genet.* **2006**, *38*, 1424–1429.

87. Komori, T.; Yagi, H.; Nomura, S.; Yamaguchi, A.; Sasaki, K.; Deguchi, K.; Shimizu, Y.; Bronson, R.T.; Gao, Y.H.; Inada, M.; *et al.* Targeted disruption of Cbfα1 results in a complete lack of bone formation owing to maturational arrest of osteoblasts. *Cell* **1997**, *89*, 755–764.

88. Otto, F.; Thornell, A.P.; Crompton, T.; Denzel, A.; Gilmour, K.C.; Rosewell, I.R.; Stamp, G.W.; Beddington, R.S.; Mundlos, S.; Olsen, B.R.; *et al.* Cbfα1, a candidate gene for cleidocranial dysplasia syndrome, is essential for osteoblast differentiation and bone development. *Cell* **1997**, *30*, 765–771.

89. Phimphilai, M.; Zhao, Z.; Boules, H.; Roca, H.; Franceschi, R.T. BMP signaling is required for RUNX2-dependent induction of the osteoblast phenotype. *J. Bone Miner. Res.* **2006**, *21*, 637–646.

90. Lin, G.L.; Hankenson, K.D. Integration of BMP, Wnt, and Notch signaling pathways in osteoblast differentiation. *J. Cell. Biochem.* **2011**, *112*, 3491–3501.

91. Bandyopadhyay, A.; Tsuji, K.; Cox, K.; Harfe, B.D.; Rosen, V.; Tabin, C.J. Genetic analysis of the roles of BMP2, BMP4, and BMP7 in limb patterning and skeletogenesis. *PLoS Genet.* **2006**, *2*, e216.

92. Rong, S.; Zhao, X.; Jin, X.; Zhang, Z.; Chen, L.; Zhu, Y.; Yuan, W. Vascular calcification in chronic kidney disease is induced by bone morphogenetic protein-2 via a mechanism involving the Wnt/β-catenin pathway. *Cell. Physiol. Biochem.* **2014**, *34*, 2049–2060.

93. Cserjesi, P.; Brown, D.; Ligon, K.L.; Lyons, G.E.; Copeland, N.G.; Gilbert, D.J.; Jenkins, N.A.; Olson, E.N. Scleraxis: A basic helix-loop-helix protein that prefigures skeletal formation during mouse embryogenesis. *Development* **1995**, *121*, 1099–1110.

94. Sosic, D.; Brand-Saberi, B.; Schmidt, C.; Christ, B.; Olson, E. Regulation of paraxis expression and somite formation by ectoderm- and neural tube-derived signals. *Dev. Biol.* **1997**, *185*, 229–243.

95. Oh, C.D. Lu, Y.; Liang, S.; Mori-Akiyama, Y.; Chen, D.; de Crombrugghe, B.; Yasuda, H. SOX9 regulates multiple genes in chondrocytes, including genes encoding ECM proteins, ECM modification enzymes, receptors, and transporters. *PLoS ONE* **2014**, *17*, e107577.

96. Lefebvre, V.; de Crombrugghe, B. Toward understanding SOX9 function in chondrocyte differentiation. *Matrix Biol.* **1998**, *16*, 529–540.

97. Akiyama, H.; Chaboissier, M.C.; Martin, J.F.; Schedl, A.; De, C.B. The transcription factor Sox9 has essential roles in successive steps of the chondrocyte differentiation pathway and is required for expression of Sox5 and Sox6. *Genes Dev.* **2002**, *16*, 2813–2828.

98. Briot, A.; Jaroszewicz, A.; Warren, C.M.; Lu, J.; Touma, M.; Rudat, C.; Hofmann, J.J.; Airik, R.; Weinmaster, G.; Lyons, K.; *et al*. Repression of sox9 by jag1 is continuously required to suppress the default chondrogenic fate of vascular smooth muscle cells. *Dev. Cell* **2014**, *31*, 707–721.

99. Khan, S.R. Reactive oxygen species, inflammation and calcium oxalate nephrolithiasis. *Transl. Androl. Urol.* **2014**, *3*, 256–276.

100. Gambaro, G.; Abaterusso, C.; Fabris, A.; Ruggera, L.; Zattoni, F.; Del Prete, D.; D'Angelo, A.; Anglani, F. The origin of nephrocalcinosis, Randall's plaque and renal stones: A cell biology viewpoint. *Arch. Ital. Urol. Androl*. **2009**, *81*, 166–170.

101. Grases, F.; Costa-Bauzá, A.; Prieto, R.M.; Conte, A.; Servera, A. Renal papillary calcification and the development of calcium oxalate monohydrate papillary renal calculi: A case series study. *BMC Urol.* **2013**, *13*, 14, doi:10.1186/1471-2490-13-14.

102. Grases, F.; Costa-Bauzá, A.; Gomila, I.; Conte, A. Origin and types of calcium oxalate monohydrate papillary renal calculi. *Urology* **2010**, *76*, 1339–1345.

103. Grases, F.; Costa–Bauzá, A.; Bonarriba, C.R.; Pieras, E.C.; Fernández, R.A.; Rodríguez, A. On the origin of calcium oxalate monohydrate papillary renal stones. *Urolithiasis* **2015**, *43*, S33–S39.

104. Khan, S.; Rodriguez, D.E.; Gower, L.B.; Monga, M. Association of Randall plaque with collagen fibers and membrane vesicles. *J. Urol.* **2012**, *187*, 1094–1100.

105. Tiselius, H.G. A hypothesis of calcium stone formation: an interpretation of stone research during the past decades. *Urol. Res.* **2011**, *39*, 231–243.

106. Shavit, L.; Girfoglio, D.; Vijay, V.; Goldsmith, D.; Ferraro, P.M.; Moochhala, S.H.; Unwin, R. Vascular calcification and bone mineral density in recurrent kidney stone formers. *Clin. J. Am. Soc. Nephrol*. **2015**, *10*, 278–285.

107. Lauderdale, D.S.; Thisted, R.A.; Wen, M.; Favus, M.J. Bone mineral density and fracture among prevalent kidney stone cases in the Third National Health and Nutrition Examination Survey. *J. Bone Miner. Res.* **2001**, *16*, 1893–1898.

108. Bataille, P.; Achard, J.M.; Fournier, A.; Boudailliez, B.; Westeel, P.F.; el Esper, N.; Bergot, C.; Jans, I.; Lalau, J.D.; Petit, J.; *et al.* Diet, vitamin D and vertebral mineral density in hypercalciuric calcium stone formers. *Kidney Int*. **1991**, *39*, 1193–1205.

109. Pietschmann, F.; Breslau, N.A.; Pak, C.Y. Reduced vertebral bone density in hypercalciuric nephrolithiasis. *J. Bone Miner. Res.* **1992**, *7*, 1383–1388.

110. Jaeger, P.; Lippuner, K.; Casez, J.P.; Hess, B.; Ackermann, D.; Hug, C. Low bone mass in idiopathic renal stone formers: magnitude and significance. *J. Bone Miner. Res.* **1994**, *9*, 1525–1532.

111. Asplin, J.R.; Bauer, K.A.; Kinder, J.; Müller, G.; Coe, B.J.; Parks, J.H.; Coe, F.L. Bone mineral density and urine calcium excretion among subjects with and without nephrolithiasis. *Kidney Int.* **2003**, *63*, 662–669.

112. Sella, S.; Cattelan C, Realdi G, Giannini S. Bone disease in primary hypercalciuria. *Clin. Cases Miner. Bone Metab.* **2008**, *5*,118–126.

113. Arrabal-Polo, M.A.; Del, C.C.M.; Canales, B.K.; Arrabal-Martín, M. Calcium nephrolithiasis and bone demineralization: pathophysiology, diagnosis, and medical management. *Curr. Opin. Urol.* **2014**, *24*, 633–638.

114. Gambaro, G.; Ferraro, P.M.; Capasso, G. Calcium nephrolithiasis, metabolic syndrome and the cardiovascular risk. *Nephrol. Dial. Transplant*. **2012**, *27*, 3008–3010.

115. Gambaro, G.; Fabris, A.; Abaterusso, C.; Cosaro, A.; Ceol, M.; Mezzabotta, F.; Torregrossa, R.; Tiralongo, E.; del Prete, D.; D'Angelo, A.; *et al.* Pathogenesis of nephrolithiasis: recent insight from cell biology and renal pathology. *Clin. Cases Miner. Bone Metab.* **2008**, *5*, 107–109.
116. Jia, Z.; Wang, S.; Tang, J.; He, D.; Cui, L.; Liu, Z.; Guo, B.; Huang, L.; Lu, Y.; Hu, H. Does crystal deposition in genetic hypercalciuric rat kidney tissue share similarities with bone formation? *Urology* **2014**, *83*, e7–e14.
117. He, D.; Wang, S.; Jia, Z.; Cui, L.; Lu, Y.; Hu, H.; Qin, B. Calcium ions promote primary renal epithelial cell differentiation into cells with bone-associated phenotypes via transforming growth factor-β1-induced epithelial-mesenchymal transition in idiopathic hypercalciuria patients. *Mol. Med. Rep.* **2015**, *11*, 2199–2206.
118. Salama, R.H.; Alghasham, A.; Mostafa, MS.; El-Moniem, A.E. Bone morphogenetic protein-2 will be a novel biochemical marker in urinary tract infections and stone formation. *Clin. Biochem.* **2012**, *45*, 766–769.
119. Shao, J.S.; Cheng, S.L.; Sadhu, J.; Towler, D.A.; Inflammation and the osteogenic regulation of vascular calcification: A review and perspective. *Hypertension* **2010**, *55*, 579–592.
120. Duer, M.J.; Friscić, T.; Proudfoot, D.; Reid, D.G.; Schoppet, M.; Shanahan, C.M.; Skepper, J.N.; Wise, E.R. Mineral surface in calcified plaque is like that of bone: further evidence for regulated mineralization. *Arterioscler. Thromb. Vasc. Biol.* **2008**, *28*, 2030–2034.
121. Demer, L.L.; Tintut, Y. Vascular calcification: pathobiology of a multifaceted disease. *Circulation* **2008**, *117*, 2938–2948.
122. Sun, Y.; Byon, C.H.; Yuan, K.; Chen, J.; Mao, X.; Heath, J.M.; Javed, A.; Zhang, K.; Anderson, P.G.; Chen, Y. Smooth muscle cell-specific runx2 deficiency inhibits vascular calcification. *Circ. Res.* **2012**, *111*, 543–552.
123. Chen, N.X.; Moe, S.M. Vascular calcification: Pathophysiology and risk factors. *Curr. Hypertens. Rep.* **2012**, *14*, 228–237.
124. Fantus, D.; Awan, Z.; Seidah, N.G.; Genest, J. Aortic calcification: Novel insights from familial hypercholesterolemia and potential role for the low-density lipoprotein receptor. *Atherosclerosis* **2013**, *226*, 9–15.
125. Al-Aly, Z.; Shao, J.S.; Lai, C.F.; Huang, E.; Cai, J.; Behrmann, A.; Cheng, S.L.; Towler, D.A. Aortic Msx2-Wnt calcification cascade is regulated by TNF-α-dependent signals in diabetic $Ldlr^{-/-}$ mice. *Arterioscler. Thromb. Vasc. Biol.* **2007**, *27*, 2589–2596.
126. New, S.E.; Aikawa, E. Molecular imaging insights into early inflammatory stages of arterial and aortic valve calcification. *Circ. Res.* **2011**, *108*, 1381–1391.
127. Kapustin, A.N.; Davies, J.D.; Reynolds, J.L.; McNair, R.; Jones, G.T.; Sidibe, A.; Schurgers, L.J.; Skepper, J.N.; Proudfoot, D.; Mayr, M.; *et al.* Calcium regulates key components of vascular smooth muscle cell-derived matrix vesicles to enhance mineralization. *Circ. Res.* **2011**, *109*, e1–e12.
128. Shroff, R.C.; McNair, R.; Skepper, J.N.; Figg, N.; Schurgers, L.J.; Deanfield, J.; Rees, L.; Shanahan, C.M. Chronic mineral dysregulation promotes vascular smooth muscle cell adaptation and extracellular matrix calcification. *J. Am. Soc. Nephrol.* **2010**, *21*, 103–112.
129. Lieske, J.C.; Norris, R.; Toback, F.G.; Adhesion of hydroxyapatite crystals to anionic sites on the surface of renal epithelial cells. *Am. J. Physiol.* **1997**, *273*, F224–F233.

130. Moe, S.M.; Chen, N.X. Vascular calcification in end stage renal disease. *Clin. Calcium.* **2002**, *12*, 1417–1422.
131. Czarny, M.J.; Resar, J.R. Diagnosis and management of valvular aortic stenosis. *Clin. Med. Insights Cardiol.* **2014**, *8*, S15–S24.
132. Aksoy, O.; Cam, A.; Agarwal, S.; Ige, M.; Yousefzai, R.; Singh, D.; Griffin, B.P.; Schoenhagen, P.; Kapadia, S.R.; Tuzcu, M.E. Significance of aortic valve calcification in patients with low-gradient low-flow aortic stenosis. *Clin. Cardiol.* **2014**, *37*, 26–31.
133. Goodman, W.G. Vascular calcification in end-stage renal disease. *J. Nephrol.* **2002**, *15*, S82–S85.
134. Wang, A.Y.; Ho, S.S.; Wang, M.; Liu, E.K.; Ho, S.; Li, P.K.; Lui, S.F.; Sanderson, J.E. Cardiac valvular calcification as a marker of atherosclerosis and arterial calcification in end-stage renal disease. *Arch. Intern. Med.* **2005**, *165*, 327–332.
135. Ferranti, C.; Coopmans, D.Y.G.; Biganzoli, E.; Bergonzi, S.; Mariani, L.; Scaperrotta, G.; Marchesini, M. Relationships between age, mammographic features and pathological tumour characteristics in non-palpable breast cancer. *Br. J. Radiol.* **2000**, *73*, 698–705.
136. Cox, R.F.; Hernandez-Santana, A.; Ramdass, S.; McMahon, G.; Harmey, J.H.; Morgan, M.P. Microcalcifications in breast cancer: Novel insights into the molecular mechanism and functional consequence of mammary mineralisation. *Br. J. Cancer* **2012**, *106*, 525–537.
137. Morgan, M.P.; Cooke, M.M.; McCarthy, G.M. Microcalcifications associated with breast cancer: An epiphenomenon or biologically significant feature of selected tumors? *J. Mammary Gland Biol. Neoplasia* **2005**, *10*, 181–187.
138. Haka, A.S.; Shafer-Peltier, K.E.; Fitzmaurice, M.; Crowe, J.; Dasari, R.R.; Feld, M.S. Identifying microcalcifications in benign and malignant breast lesions by probing differences in their chemical composition using Raman spectroscopy. *Cancer Res.* **2002**, *62*, 5375–5380.
139. Baker, R.; Rogers, K.D.; Shepherd, N.; Stone, N. New relationships between breast microcalcifications and cancer. *Br. J. Cancer* **2010**, *103*, 1034–1039.
140. Morgan, M.P.; Cooke, M.M.; Christopherson, P.A.; Westfall, P.R.; McCarthy, G.M. Calcium hydroxyapatite promotes mitogenesis and matrix metalloproteinase expression in human breast cancer cell lines. *Mol. Carcinog.* **2001**, *32*, 111–117.
141. Liu, F.; Bloch, N.; Bhushan, K.R.; De Grand, A.M.; Tanaka, E.; Solazzo, S.; Mertyna, P.M.; Goldberg, N.; Frangioni, J.V.; Lenkinski, R.E. Humoral bone morphogenetic protein 2 is sufficient for inducing breast cancer microcalcification. *Mol. Imaging* **2008**, *7*, 175–186.
142. Shobeiri, N.; Adams, M.A.; Holden, R.M. Phosphate: An old bone molecule but new cardiovascular risk factor. *Br. J. Clin. Pharmacol.* **2014**, *77*, 39–54.
143. Cox, R.F.; Jenkinson, A.; Pohl, K.; O'Brien, F.J.; Morgan, M.P. Osteomimicry of Mammary Adenocarcinoma Cells *in Vitro*; Increased Expression of Bone Matrix Proteins and Proliferation within a 3D Collagen Environment. *PLoS ONE* **2012**, *7*, e41679. doi:10.1371/journal.pone.0041679.
144. Chen, N.X.; O'Neill, K.D.; Duan, D.; Moe, S.M. Phosphorus and uremic serum up-regulate osteopontin expression in vascular smooth muscle cells. *Kidney Int.* **2002**, *62*, 1724–1731.
145. Bellahcène, A.; Merville, M.P.; Castronovo, V. Expression of bone sialoprotein, a bone matrix protein, in human breast cancer. *Cancer Res.* **1994**, *54*, 2823–2826.

146. Bellahcène, A.; Castronovo, V. Increased expression of osteonectin and osteopontin, two bone matrix proteins, in human breast cancer. *Am. J. Pathol.* **1995**, *146*, 95–100.
147. Scimeca, M.; Giannini, E.; Antonacci, C.; Pistolese, C.A.; Spagnoli, L.G.; Bonanno, E. Microcalcifications in breast cancer: an active phenomenon mediated by epithelial cells with mesenchymal characteristics. *BMC Cancer.* **2014**, *14*, 286, doi:10.1186/1471-2407-14-286.
148. Koori, K.; Maeda, H.; Fujii, S.; Tomokiyo, A.; Kawachi, G.; Hasegawa, D.; Hamano, S.; Sugii, H.; Wada, N.; Akamine, A. The roles of calcium-sensing receptor and calcium channel in osteogenic differentiation of undifferentiated periodontal ligament cells. *Cell. Tissue Res.* **2014**, *357*, 707–718.
149. Zhang, Y.; Lu, W.; Yang, K.; Lai, N.; Zhong, N.; Wang, J. Bone morphogenetic protein 2 decreases TRPC expression, store-operated Ca^{2+} entry, and basal $[Ca^{2+}]_i$ in rat distal pulmonary arterial smooth muscle cells. *Am. J. Physiol. Cell. Physiol.* **2013**, *304*, C833–C843.
150. Cross, B.M.; Breitwieser, G.E.; Reinhardt, T.A.; Rao, R. Cellular calcium dynamics in lactation and breast cancer: from physiology to pathology. *Am. J. Physiol. Cell. Physiol.* **2014**, *306*, C515–C526, doi:10.1152/ajpcell.00330.2013.
151. Pampena, D.A.; Robertson, K.A.; Litvinova, O.; Lajoie, G.; Goldberg, H.; Hunter, G.K. Inhibition of hydroxyapatite formation by osteopontin phosphopeptides. *Biochem. J.* **2004**, *378*, 1083–1087.
152. Matsuzaki, H.; Katsumata, S.; Uehara, M.; Suzuki, K.; Miwa, M. High-phosphorus diet induces osteopontin expression of renal tubules in rats. *J. Clin. Biochem. Nutr.* **2007**, *41*, 179–183.

7

Altered Hemodynamics in the Embryonic Heart Affects Outflow Valve Development

Vinal Menon [1], John F. Eberth [1,2], Richard L. Goodwin [3] and Jay D. Potts [1,2,*]

[1] Department of Cell Biology and Anatomy, School of Medicine, University of South Carolina, Columbia, SC 29209, USA; E-Mails: vinal.menon@uscmed.sc.edu (V.M.); john.eberth@uscmed.sc.edu (J.F.E.)

[2] Biomedical Engineering Program, College of Engineering and Computing, University of South Carolina, Columbia, SC 29208, USA

[3] Biomedical Sciences, School of Medicine, University of South Carolina, Greenville, SC 29605, USA; E-Mail: goodwirl@greenvillemed.sc.edu

* Author to whom correspondence should be addressed; E-Mail: jay.potts@uscmed.sc.edu

Academic Editors: Cheryl L. Maslen and Russell Norris

Abstract: Cardiac valve structure and function are primarily determined during early development. Consequently, abnormally-formed heart valves are the most common type of congenital heart defects. Several adult valve diseases can be backtracked to abnormal valve development, making it imperative to completely understand the process and regulation of heart valve development. Epithelial-to-mesenchymal transition (EMT) plays an important role in the development of heart valves. Though hemodynamics is vital to valve development, its role in regulating EMT is still unknown. In this study, intracardiac hemodynamics were altered by constricting the outflow tract (OFT)/ventricle junction (OVJ) of HH16–17 (Hamilton and Hamburger (HH) Stage 16–17) chicken embryos, *ex ovo* for 24 h. The constriction created an increase in peak and time-averaged centerline velocity along the OFT without changes to volumetric flow or heart rate. Computational fluid dynamics was used to estimate the level of increased spatially-averaged wall shear stresses on the OFT cushion from AMIRA reconstructions. OFT constriction led to a significant decrease in OFT cushion volume and the number of invaded mesenchyme in the OFT cushion. qPCR analysis revealed altered mRNA expression of a representative panel of genes, vital to valve development, in the OFT cushions from banded hearts. This study indicates the importance of hemodynamics in valve development.

Keywords: valvular disease; cardiac valve development; endocardial cushions; EMT; hemodynamics

1. Introduction

Valves in healthy adult four-chambered hearts allow for unidirectional flow of blood to both the pulmonary and systemic circuits. The structure and function of these cardiac valves are primarily determined during early embryonic development. Consequently, abnormally-formed heart valves, especially defective outflow valves, are the most common type of congenital heart defects (CHDs) [1]. Abnormal cardiac valve structure may be present at birth; however, this may be asymptomatic and could predispose the individual to valve disease later in life. Thus, several adult valve diseases may be backtracked to abnormal valve development. This makes it imperative to understand the molecular basis of heart valve development and the effect that hemodynamics has on these processes.

The heart is the first organ to develop and function during embryogenesis. It initially forms as a tubular blood vessel comprised of endocardial endothelial cells surrounded by myocardium [2]. An acellular layer of extracellular matrix (ECM), known as cardiac jelly, separates the two heart tube layers [3]. Myocardial cells secrete most of the ECM, which is composed primarily of glycosaminoglycans, chondroitin sulfate and hyaluronan [4]. After the onset of rightward looping, the cardiac jelly expands at two distinct foci—the atrio-ventricular (AV) canal and the outflow tract (OFT)—forming endocardial cushions (valve primordia) that eventually develop into the AV and OFT valves [3,5]. The mechanisms of cushion development are conserved in both the AV canal and the OFT. In addition to the endocardially-derived cells, neural crest cells also contribute to the OFT valves [2].

The regulated process of epithelial-to-mesenchymal transition (EMT) plays a crucial role in embryonic differentiation and development [6]. In response to local stimuli, a subset of AV and OFT endocardial cells delaminate into the cardiac jelly, due to loss of cell-cell contact, and adopt a migratory, mesenchymal phenotype leading to the onset of EMT [5]. In an *in vitro* model, it was shown that chick AV canal explants (consisting of endocardial cushion cells and myocardium) cultured on collagen gels exhibit EMT [7]. Furthermore, it has been shown that only the endothelium of the AV canal and OFT, but not that of the ventricle, undergoes EMT to produce the mesenchyme, thus demonstrating a requirement for specialized spatial signaling to induce EMT [8,9].

As blood flows through a vessel, shear stress is produced due to friction between the flowing blood and the vessel wall [10]. It is known that endothelial cells sense and respond to hemodynamics by means of mechanotransducer proteins and initiate the rearrangement of the cytoskeleton, leading to these cells being aligned parallel to the direction of flow [10]. Hemodynamics has been shown to play an important role in regulating embryonic cardiogenesis [11,12]. We have previously shown that in an *in vitro* 3D culture system, the expression and deposition of fibrous ECM proteins in AV and OFT cushions were affected by shear stress [13,14]. However, it is not clearly understood how hemodynamics regulates (initiates and eventually terminates) EMT during heart valve development. The purpose of this study was to alter the hemodynamics in the embryonic chicken heart by constricting the OFT and to study the effects of this intervention on early developmental processes. We hypothesize that changes in hemodynamics influence both EMT and OFT valve development, resulting in altered ECM production.

2. Materials and Methods

2.1. OFT Banding to alter Intracardiac Hemodynamics

Fertilized Bovan chicken eggs (Clemson University, Clemson, SC, USA) were incubated in a rocker incubator at 37 °C till they reached Hamilton and Hamburger (HH) Stage 17. After sterilizing the outside of the egg with 70% ethanol, the shell was gently cracked with a scalpel handle, and the embryo, positioned on top of the yolk, was then gently transferred to a petri dish containing Tyrode's buffer (Sigma, St. Louis, MO, USA) supplemented with sodium bicarbonate (1 g/L). The OFT was banded (constricted), *ex ovo*, using a 10-0 nylon suture at the OFT/ventricle junction (OVJ). Control embryos were also transferred to a Tyrode's-containing petri dish, but were not subjected to the banding intervention. Banded and control embryos were then placed in a humidified incubator at 37 °C for 24 h.

2.2. Analysis of Change in Flow Velocity

Changes in blood flow velocity at the OVJ of banded (n = 5) and control (n = 5) embryos were determined by ultrasound using the Vevo 770 imaging system (VisualSonics, Toronto, ON, Canada). The petri dish containing the embryo to be imaged was placed on a heating pad and carefully filled to the brim with Tyrode's buffer, making sure that the yolk sac was intact. A 708 scan head, operating in B mode, was used to obtain a 2D image of the beating heart, and the stage was moved till the OVJ was clearly visible. The pulsed-wave (PW) mode, at a pulse repetition frequency of 20 kHz, was used to obtain a waveform. For each embryo, peak velocities at the OVJ were measured for ten heartbeats. From the resulting data, the heart rate in beats-per-minute (BPM) was calculated by measuring the foot-to-foot time of the velocity wave, so that heart rate (HR) = 60/T. Time-dependent centerline and spatially-averaged velocities were measured from the PW Doppler waveforms using built-in software algorithms, and these waveforms were digitized using the ImageJ figure calibration plugin, so that the time-averaged and peak velocities could be found [15]. Embryos with a slowing heart rate during the test were not used for analysis. Embryos subjected to ultrasound imaging were not used for any other experiment.

2.3. Three-Dimensional OFT Reconstruction and Determination of the Extent of EMT

Banded (n = 3) and control (n = 3) embryos were carefully excised from the yolk sac and fixed overnight in 2% paraformaldehyde. Extra embryonic membranes were left intact, so as to prevent sectioning artifacts. Fixed embryos were dehydrated through an alcohol series, cleared with xylene, and penetrated with and embedded in paraffin. Five-micrometer serial sections were obtained on a microtome and stained with hematoxylin and eosin (H&E). Individual nuclei were counted from the

H&E images of banded and control OFTs to determine the number of cells that invaded the cushions by EMT. TIFF images of the complete OFT were captured using a Nikon Optiphot-2 light microscope at a total magnification of 40× and loaded into the AMIRA software package (FEI Visualization Science Group, Burlington, MA, USA). All sections were aligned, and the OFT and myocardium was segmented. A 3D model of the OFT was then generated from which the volume of the OFT cushion was determined. Models were reduced to 2500 faces to improve manageability and exported as stereolithography (.stl) files to Geomagic Studio (3D Systems, Rock Hill, SC, USA) for smoothing and anatomical measurements of cross-sectional area and perimeter at the OVJ. These reconstructions were then converted into the Initial Graphics Exchange Specification (IGES) file format for finite element analysis.

2.4. Computational Fluid Dynamics

IGES files were imported as a continuous geometry into COMSOL Multiphisics 4.3b (Comsol, Burlington, MA, USA). In COMSOL, faces perpendicular to the axis of blood flow were generated at the proximal (ventricle) and distal (OFT) sides to act as inlet and outlet conditions. A single representative 3D model was generated for the control, and a single representative 3D model was generated for the banded hearts. From these models, the cross-sectional areas at the OVJ were measured using Geomagic (Control: A = 14,491; Banded: A = 1714 μm^2). Unique volumetric flow inlet boundary conditions were applied for each of the control (n = 5) and banded hearts (n = 5). At a given cross-section, the time-averaged, peak and late retrograde flow velocities were calculated from the spatially-averaged velocity and used to calculate the inlet time-averaged, peak and late retrograde volumetric flow rates. A zero-pressure boundary condition was applied at the distal location for all samples. Despite the importance of a changing geometry during the cardiac cycle, our analyses are limited by the available imaging modalities to tissue arrested under physiological loading. Accordingly, a rigid wall assumption and no-slip boundary conditions were assigned for the remaining surfaces. Using a hematocrit of 19.4% for HH Stage 16–17 chick embryos, we assumed that blood, at high shear rates, behaved as a Newtonian fluid; therefore, the density $\rho = 1025$ kg/m^3 and apparent dynamic viscosity $\mu = 0.0015$ Pa·s remained constant in our simulations. Accordingly, the lowest time-averaged shear rate from our simulations was $\gamma = 424 \pm 113$ s^{-1}. Similarly, low peak Reynolds numbers (Re = 7.08 ± 1.06) indicated laminar flow behavior, while a rough estimate of the Womersley numbers ($\alpha = 0.18 \pm 0.02$), a metric used to relate pulsatile-inertial to viscous effects, yields a low value, as well. Collectively, these results suggest that quasi-static conditions are sufficient for analysis [16]. Wall shear stresses were calculated on the surface of the blood-tissue interfaces and spatially averaged for each of the flow conditions (time-averaged, peak and late cardiac cycle retrograde flow). The time-averaged pressure drop across the stenosis was calculated as the difference between the inlet and outlet (P = 0 mmHg) pressures.

2.5. Extraction of Total RNA from OFTs

OFTs (cushion + myocardium) were dissected after whole hearts were carefully excised from banded and control embryos. Each sample (n = 3–4) consisted of OFT tissue from about 20–22 pooled hearts. Total RNA was extracted using the GeneJET RNA purification kit (Thermo Scientific, Waltham, MA, USA) according to the manufacture's protocol. RNA was eluted from the columns with

50 μL of nuclease-free water (provided in the kit). The concentration and purity of the eluted RNA samples were determined using the NanoPhotometer Pearl (Implemen, GmbH, Munich, Germany). RNA samples were stored at −80 °C until further analysis.

2.6. Complementary DNA Synthesis

cDNA was synthesized from total RNA using the iScript cDNA Synthesis Kit (BioRad, Hercules, CA, USA) according to the protocol provided. Five hundred nanograms of RNA were used in each reaction. Each cDNA sample was diluted 5× with nuclease-free water before being used for qPCR.

2.7. Quantitative Real-Time Polymerase Chain Reaction

Table 1. Primers used for qPCR.

Gene	Forward (F) and Reverse (R) Primers
Arbp2	F: 5′-GCTTTGCTTCGGTCTTTGAG-3′ R: 5′-AACAACTTTCCGATCACCAC-3′
klf2	F: 5′-GCTTCTACCAGACAAACCCG-3′ R: 5′-CAGGACTGGCCCATAACTGT-3′
rhoA	F: 5′-CAGCACCCTGCACTTGAGTA-3′ R: 5′GCATCCTGTGAGTGCAGAAA-3′
collagen 1α1	F: 5′-TACCACTGCAAGAACAGCGT-3′ R: 5′-TCGGTGACCCCATAGGTGAA-3′
vinculin	F: 5′-CAGGTAGTATCGGCTGCTCG-3′ R: 5′-CCACCAGCCCTGTCATCTTT-3′
elastin	F: 5′-GTATCCCATCAAAGCTCCCA-3′ R: 5′-CAGCTCCGTATTTAGCTGCC-3′
periostin	F: 5′-GGATGGTATGAGAGGATGTC-3′ R: 5′GCAAAGAAAGTGAATGAACC-3′
tenascinC	F: 5′-AGGACACAGCCTCTGCAAGT-3′ R: 5′-TACTGCCCCTGAGAGCTGAT-3′
CDH11	F: 5′-AAGACACTGGACCGAGAGGA-3′ R: 5′-TTCTGAGGGCGGTTCCAAAG-3′
filamin A	F: 5′-CGGCGACTACACCATCAACA-3′ R: 5′-GTCACTTTGGTGGGGTCGAA-3′
TGFβRIII	F: 5′-CTCTTACCGTCGTGGGCATT-3′ R: 5′-CTGCTTCCCCTGTGTGAGAG-3′
TGFβ2	F: 5′-GAGAAAGCCAACCACAGAGC-3′ R: 5′-GGTACAGCTCTATCCGCTGC-3′
TGFβ3	F: 5′-CACAATGAGTTGGGCATTTG-3′ R: 5′-GGAACTCTGCTCGAAACAGG-3′
snai2	F: 5′-CACGCTCCTTCCTGGTCAAG-3′ R: 5′-GGCTGCGGTATGATAGGGAC-3′
has2	F: 5′-CACCGCTGCTTACATTGTGG-3′ R: 5′-TGTGATGCCAGGATAGCACC-3′
mmp2	F: 5′-TGATGATGACCGCAAGTGGG-3′ R: 5′-TGTAGATCGGGGCCATGAGA-3′

qPCR was carried out using Fast SYBR Green Master Mix (Applied Biosystems, Foster City, CA, USA) on a BioRad CFX connect system. The following run conditions were used: enzyme activation at 95 °C for 3 min, denaturation at 95 °C for 10 s and annealing/extension at 60 °C for 30 s (40 cycles). A melt curve analysis was performed on each run. Each sample was run in triplicate, and qPCR was carried out on each gene three times. Relative gene expression was quantified using the Pfaffl method [17] with Arbp2 as the housekeeping (normalizing) gene. Primer sequences used for qPCR are listed in Table 1.

2.8 Statistical Analysis

Student's *t*-test was used for analysis between groups, with α set to 0.05. All statistics and graphs were generated using Microsoft Excel 2011. Data in figures and in the text are reported as the means ± SD.

3. Results

3.1. Effect of OFT Banding on Blood Flow Velocity

Ultrasound imaging was performed to investigate whether the constriction of the OFT (Figure 1a,b) resulted in a change in flow velocity across the OVJ.

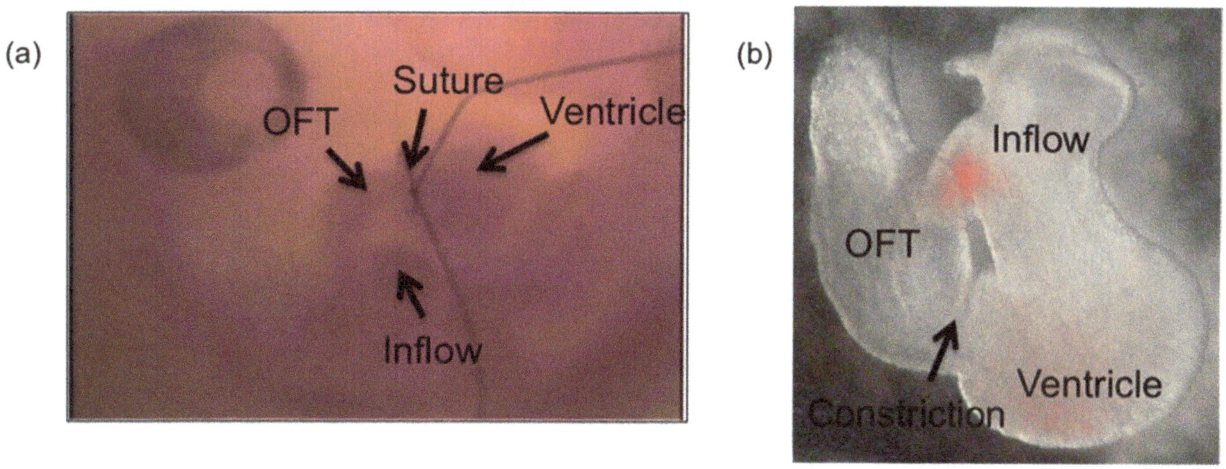

Figure 1. Our *in vivo* (ex ovo) chicken embryonic system. (**a**) Whole chicken embryo with the outflow tract (OFT) banded, imaged after 24 h; (**b**) isolated chick embryonic heart, 24 h after OFT banding.

The suture placed around the OVJ was clearly visible in a B-mode 2D image of the beating heart (Figure 2a). As expected, centerline flow velocity, measured with PW Doppler (Figure 2b,c), yielded higher time-averaged (control = 2.54 ± 0.68 cm/s, banded = 17.6 ± 6.32 cm/s; p = 0.002) and peak velocities (control = 8.57 ± 2.54 cm/s, banded = 51.5 ± 17.16 cm/s; p = 0.0018) at the banded OVJ relative to the control OVJ (Figure 2d). No statistical differences were found between heart rates of control (95.8 ± 21.4 BPM) and banded (108 ± 23.0 BPM) embryonic chick hearts (Figure 2e) (p = 0.19) or between the late cycle retrograde flow velocities (control = −1.44 ± 1.55 cm/s, banded = −2.74 ± 2.43 cm/s; p = 0.44) (Figure 2d).

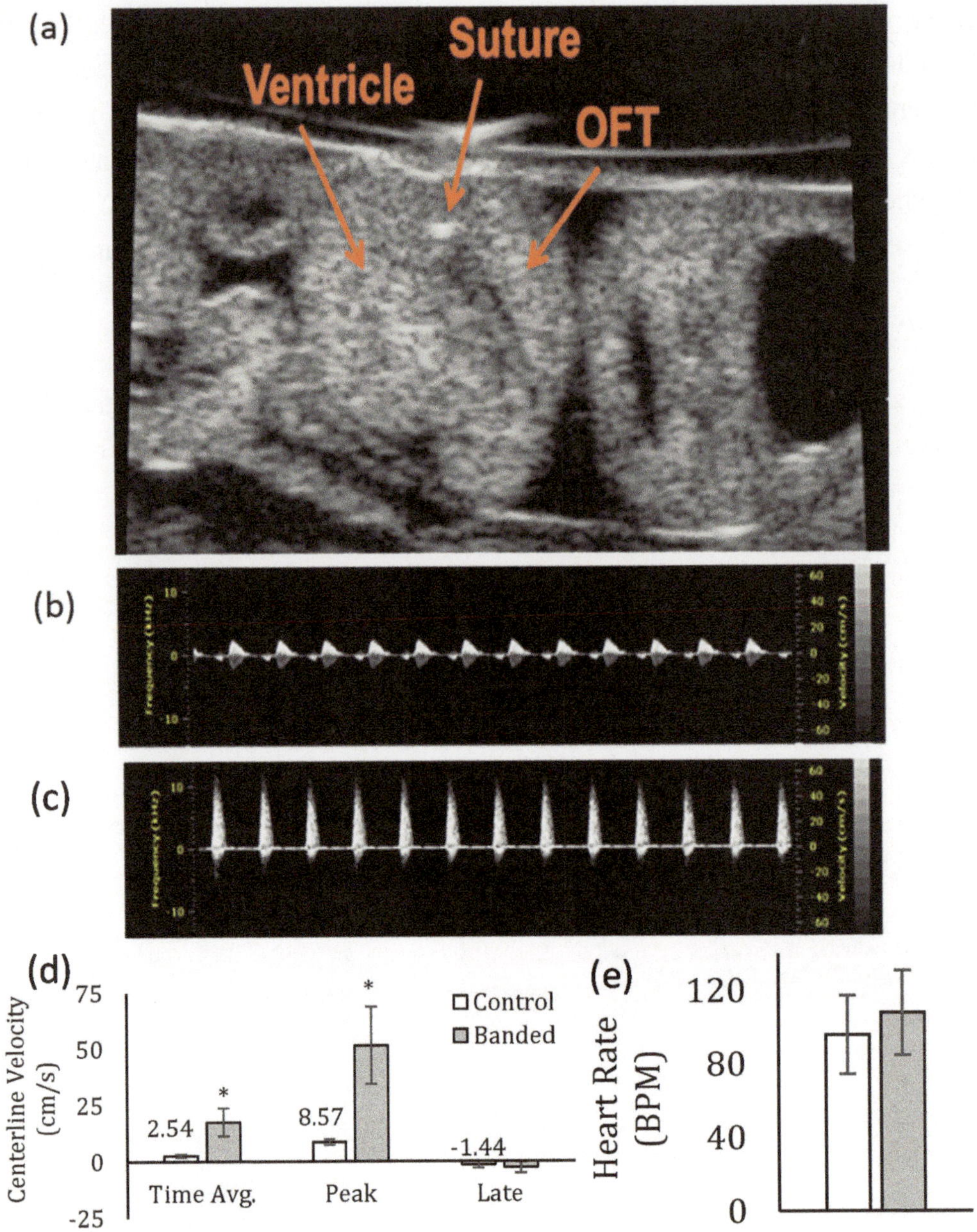

Figure 2. Ultrasound imaging. (**a**) B mode of a banded embryo showing the suture at the ventricle junction (OVJ). Pulsed-wave Doppler (PWD) at the OVJ for the (**b**) control and (**c**) banded hearts; (**d**) OFT banding caused significant changes in the time-averaged (avg) and peak centerline velocities, but not for velocities measured late in the cardiac cycle during retrograde flow measured at the OVJ; (**e**) the heart rate remained unchanged between controls and banded chick hearts. * $p < 0.05$.

3.2. Effect of OFT Banding on OFT Cushion Volume and Extent of EMT

To determine whether the alteration in hemodynamics in the embryonic heart caused any change in the volume of the OFT cushions, the OFTs of banded and control hearts were 3D reconstructed from H&E TIFF images of the OFTs (Figure 3a) using AMIRA (Figure 3b). A comparison of the AMIRA-generated volume data revealed a significant decrease in the OFT cushion volume of banded hearts compared to the control hearts (Figure 3c) ($p = 0.01$).

Individual cells that invaded the OFT cushions were counted from H&E images (Figure 3a), which revealed that OFT banding led to a significant decrease in the number of cells that entered the OFT cushion tissue, by means of EMT, in the banded relative to control OFT (Figure 3d) ($p = 0.002$).

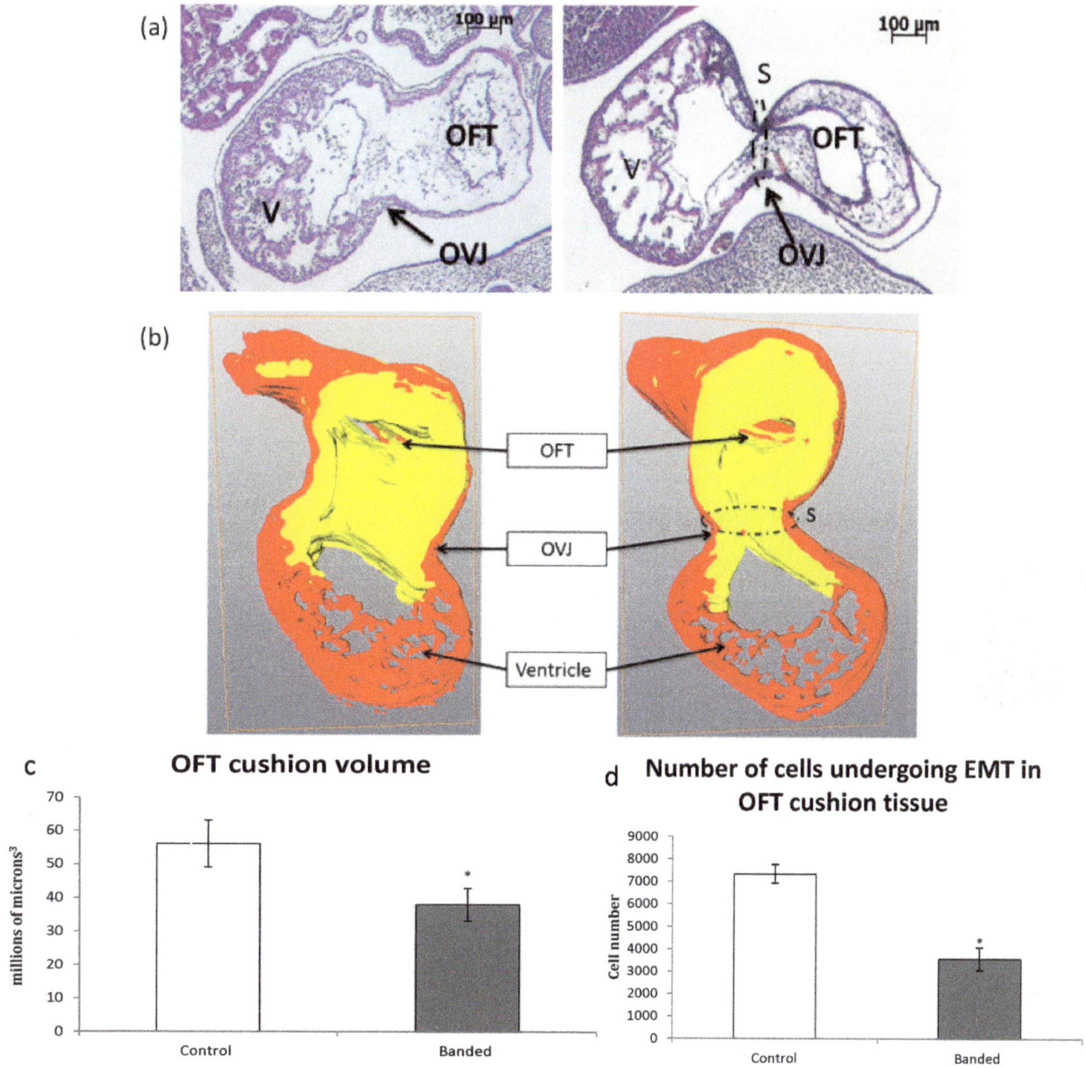

Figure 3. 3D reconstructed OFT. (**a**) Representative H&E-stained images of a control (left) and banded OFT (right); (**b**) cut-away view of a control (left) and banded (right) 3D reconstructed OFT showing cushion (yellow) and myocardium (red). The effect of OFT banding on (**c**) OFT cushion volume and (**d**) the number of cells undergoing EMT. V, ventricle; S, position of suture. * $p < 0.05$.

3.3. Effect of OFT Banding on Computed Hemodynamics

A 3D streamline velocity plot was generated from computational fluid dynamics (CFD) simulations to show the path and velocity magnitude within the developing embryonic chick heart. Consistent with the Doppler studies, the highest velocity occurred at the OVJ banding site (Figure 4). Consequently, this location experienced the highest time-averaged and peak wall shear stresses (Figure 5).

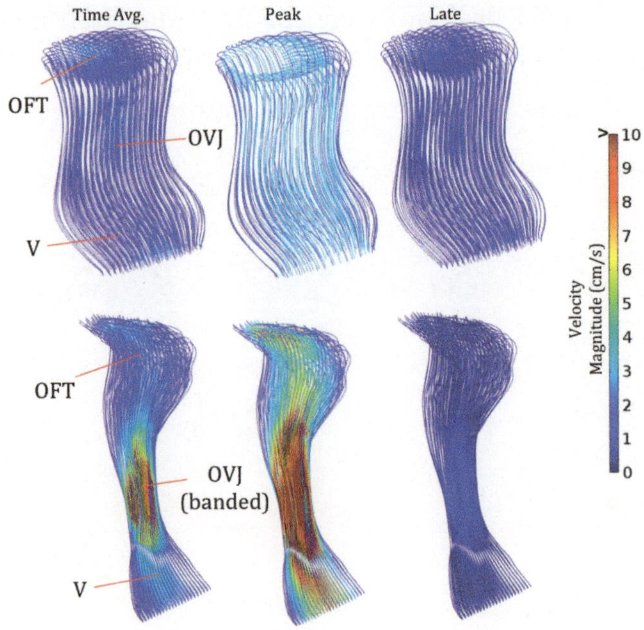

Figure 4. Velocity magnitude streamlines for (top) control chick hearts and (bottom) OFT banded chick hearts at the time-averaged flow velocity, peak flow conditions and late in the cardiac cycle during retrograde flow. V, ventricle; OVJ, OFT/ventricle junction; OFT, outflow tract.

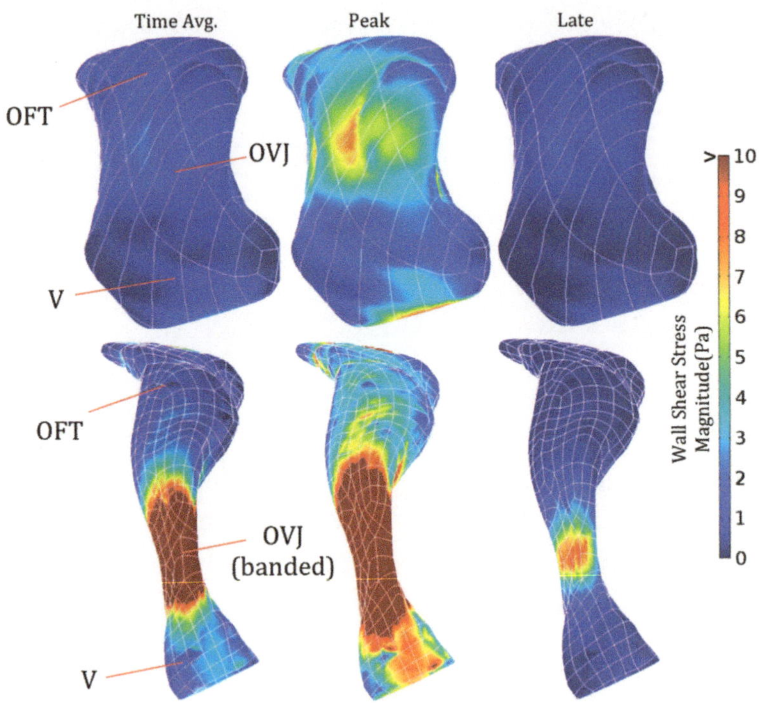

Figure 5. Wall shear stress magnitude for (top) control chick hearts and (bottom) OFT banded chick hearts at the time-averaged flow condition, during peak flow conditions and late in the cardiac cycle during retrograde flow. V, ventricle; OVJ, OFT/ventricle junction; OFT, outflow tract.

When spatially averaged, significant differences were found between the time-averaged control (0.97 ± 0.26 Pa) and banded (6.1 ± 2.19 Pa) wall shear stresses (p = 0.002) (Figure 6a). Peak spatially-averaged wall shear stresses were also found to be significantly different between control (3.30 ± 0.50 Pa) and banded (17.8 ± 5.96 Pa) hearts ($p = 0.002$) (Figure 6a). No statistical differences in shear stresses were found at the late retrograde flow condition (control = −0.71 ± 0.49 Pa, banded = −0.95 ± 0.88 Pa; $p = 0.32$). Banding generated a 5.32 ± 1.19-mmHg pressure gradient across the banding site, whereas normal hearts experienced a pressure drop of 0.20 ± 0.05 mmHg through this section (Figure 6b) ($p < 0.001$). Overall, no statistical differences were found between the volumetric flow rates in the control (0.18 ± 0.05 mm^3/s) and banded (0.15 ± 0.05 mm^3/s) embryonic chick hearts ($p = 0.32$) (Figure 6c).

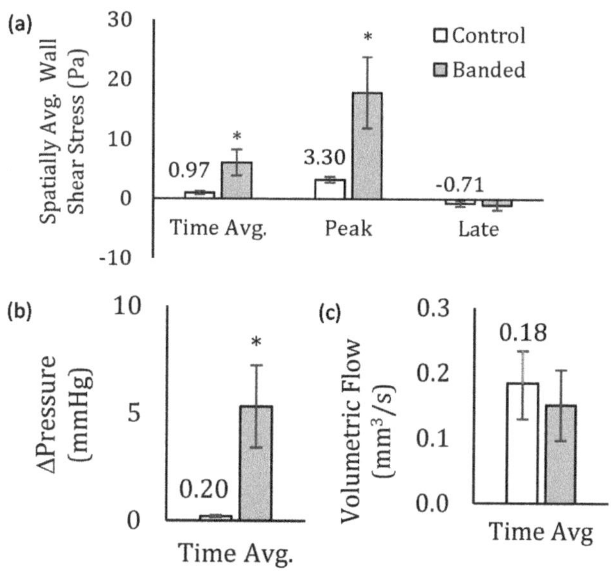

Figure 6. Hemodynamic variables, including (**a**) the spatially-averaged wall shear stress at the time-averaged flow condition, during peak flow conditions and late in the cardiac cycle during retrograde flow, (**b**) time-averaged pressure gradient and (**c**) the volumetric flow rate. * $p < 0.05$.

3.4. Effect of OFT Banding on Relative Expression of Genes Involved in Valve Development

Real-time PCR was carried out to investigate the effects of constricting the OFT on the expression of a selected panel of genes that are critical to valve development (Table 2). Transcript levels of the mechanotransducer *rhoA* were significantly lower in the OFT from banded hearts relative to OFT of control hearts ($p = 0.02$). No significant differences were observed in the mRNA expression of shear-responsive *klf2* between OFT of banded and control hearts ($p = 0.12$).

The OFT of banded hearts exhibited significantly decreased mRNA levels of *collagen1α1* ($p = 0.01$) and increased transcript levels of *periostin* ($p = 0.01$) compared to OFT tissue of the control hearts. Though there was a downregulated trend in the expression of *tenascin C* ($p = 0.08$) in OFT from banded hearts, there were no significant differences in the mRNA levels of *elastin* ($p = 0.19$) and *vinculin* ($p = 0.12$) in the OFT of banded *vs.* control hearts.

The expression of *TGFβRIII* mRNA and that of *TGFβ3* were significantly upregulated ($p = 0.004$ and $p = 0.02$, respectively) in OFT of banded *vs.* control hearts; however, there were no differences in the expression levels of *TGFβ2* ($p = 0.25$) in OFT tissue from hearts in these two groups. Moreover, no significant differences were observed in the transcript levels of *snai2* ($p = 0.14$) and *has2* ($p = 0.1$), while mRNA expression of *mmp2* was significantly upregulated ($p = 0.03$) in the OFT from banded hearts compared to OFT tissue from controls. Though the mRNA expression levels of *CDH11* were significantly downregulated ($p = 0.02$) in OFT of banded hearts, there were no significant changes in transcript levels of *filamin A* ($p = 0.34$) between OFT of banded *vs.* control hearts.

Table 2. Differential expression of genes critical to valve development, upon OFT banding, in OFT tissue of banded and control hearts. * $p < 0.05$.

Gene	OFT from Control Hearts	OFT from Banded Hearts	*p*-Value
Shear-/Flow-Responsive			
rhoA	1.00 ± 0.08	0.88 ± 0.04	0.02 *
klf2	1.00 ± 0.24	0.83 ± 0.07	0.12
ECM			
collagen1a1	1.00 ± 0.23	0.60 ± 0.06	0.01 *
periostin	1.00 ± 0.36	2.15 ± 0.38	0.01 *
tenascinC	1.00 ± 0.20	0.80 ± 0.12	0.08
elastin	1.00 ± 0.32	0.83 ± 0.12	0.19
vinculin	1.00 ± 0.07	1.07 ± 0.06	0.12
EMT/Cell Migration			
TGFβRIII	1.00 ± 0.12	1.28 ± 0.05	0.004 *
TGFβ2	1.00 ± 0.18	0.92 ± 0.10	0.25
TGFβ3	1.00 ± 0.20	1.34 ± 0.13	0.02 *
snai2	1.00 ± 0.47	0.72 ± 0.09	0.14
has2	1.00 ± 0.04	0.95 ± 0.05	0.10
mmp2	1.00 ± 0.05	1.54 ± 0.27	0.03 *
CDH11	1.00 ± 0.12	0.77 ± 0.09	0.02 *
filamin A	1.00 ± 0.23	0.97 ± 0.09	0.34

4. Discussion

Valvular disease is the most common type of CHD. Disease conditions due to abnormal cardiac valve structure and function, including stenosis and regurgitation, may occur congenitally, but may be symptomatic only in adulthood. Consequently, replacement of diseased heart valves is the second most common heart surgery in the U.S., with a majority of the replaced aortic valves exhibiting congenital abnormalities [18]. This underscores the importance for understanding the mechanisms underlining the development of cardiac valves.

The fact that hemodynamics strongly influences heart valve development has been established by several models of altered blood flow, resulting in abnormal valves and defective septa [19–24]. It is well established that EMT is vital in the development of heart valves; however, it is not clear how hemodynamics regulates the EMT process. The present study aims to understand the role of blood as a physical factor in the developmental process of OFT valves at the embryonic stage.

Hemodynamics in the chicken embryonic heart were altered by banding the OFT at the OVJ. This constriction led to a significant "jet effect" at the OVJ, as revealed by ultrasound-mediated flow velocity measurements and prolonged increased levels of wall shear stress. Despite the increased cardiac afterload, the volumetric flowrate and heart rate were similar between controls and banded hearts. This result is indicative of adequate distal tissue perfusion and little change to systemic cardiovascular physiology. A subsequent lumen narrowing was also experienced in the distal portions of the OFT and confirmed by AMIRA 3D reconstructions. This distal lumen narrowing is consistent with the findings of other researchers [25], who hypothesized that this effect may be due to paracrine factors released at the banding site. Regardless, at a consistent volumetric flow, the narrowed lumen led to an increase in spatially-averaged wall shear stresses and a concatenate increase in the differential pressure. Flow-induced wall shear stresses are a result of the viscous properties of flowing blood, thereby creating physical signals that are sensed directly by the epithelial cell-lined lumen. The present work focuses on the effects of alteration in shear stresses; however, pressure and the physical constraints imposed by the banding model could play a pivotal role in the EMT process and the differentiation, morphology and gene expression effects observed herein. The role of these loads and the physical constraints are reserved for future work.

The control peak flow velocities measured for the OFT in our study (8.57 ± 1.28 cm/s) compare well to those of prior researchers, including Bharadwaj *et al.* for HH16 (9.2 ± 0.09 cm/s) and Liu *et al.* for HH18 (6.2 ± 0.7 cm/s) [26,27]. Liu *et al.* also reported a retrograde flow velocity of -2.0 ± 2.0 cm/s, and we found this value to be very close at -0.72 ± 0.77 cm/s. An estimation of time-averaged velocities from the full velocity profile of both of the aforementioned studies is also in the range of our measured value of 2.54 ± 0.68 cm/s. Our banding model, however, has Doppler measured centerline velocities much greater than those presented by Midgett *et al.* [28]. Despite those differences, our results are reasonable when considering proportional changes in cross-sectional area caused by the banding process.

Spatially-averaged wall shear stresses were determined using computational fluid dynamics simulations of 3D reconstructed hearts. CFD, rather than analytical approaches, was employed to enable the implementation of realistic geometries that allow for out-of-plane rotations and changes in cross-section shape. Although analytical solutions provide a good estimate of developed blood flow behavior in a circular cross-section, we observed that actual geometries, especially around the OFT, were non-uniform. The reconstruction and smoothing process can lead to undesired errors in sensitive hemodynamic properties. Despite this, we found time-averaged (0.97 ± 0.26 Pa) and peak (3.30 ± 0.50 Pa) wall shear stress values to be near those found by Bharadwaj *et al.* for the HH16 chick (0.36 Pa and 0.97 Pa, respectively) [26]. Liu *et al.* also showed graphically the peak wall shear stress for the HH18 chick to be somewhere around 6 Pa [27]. Our values fall between these two estimates, and the differences could be attributed to the source tissue location, assumptions on the velocity profile, tissue fixation geometry or from spatially averaging across a larger tissue area. Without more advanced imaging modalities (e.g., micro-CT), we are unable to quantify cushion expansion in real time and require tissue fixed under physiological conditions for our geometric-based CFD analysis. These two factors contribute to error in our shear stress calculations and are acknowledged limitations to this work. Regardless, the results of our CFD study provide a reasonable comparison between control and banded tissues.

Cushion volume and number of cells undergoing EMT were decreased by 39% and 69%, respectively, in the OFT of the banded hearts relative to control hearts. These observations highlight the fact that hemodynamics plays a significant role in the formation of the valve primordia during the initial stages of valve development that occur in HH16–17 embryos, the stage chosen for the OFT banding surgery. These reductions in OFT cushion volume and cell number could potentially lead to the formation of abnormal, hypocellular OFT valves.

As evidenced in the CFD model, there is a significant change in wall shear stress in, and distal to, the banding regions. However, for technical reasons, cushion tissues (including the myocardial sleeve) of the entire OFT were collected, which includes regions directly beneath/surrounding the band, as well as regions post- and pre-constriction. Thus, the gene expression results reported in this study represent changes that occur in the whole OFT tissue rather than at discrete locations. Since CFD simulations predicted spatially-averaged wall shear stresses to be significantly higher in the banded model, we compared the entire tissue gene expression to the entire tissue shear stresses. Our future work will focus on the local effects of shear stresses on markers of gene expression.

Endocardial cells, which line the lumen of the embryonic heart and the adult cardiovascular system, are the first to experience and respond to shear stress by mechanotransduction signaling pathways. When comparing flow (therefore, shear stress) to no flow (no shear), we have previously shown that *rhoA*, a small GTPase involved in regulating the actin cytoskeleton, is upregulated in the presence of flow in *in vitro* cultures of HH25 AV [13] and OFT [14] cushions and is also an important mechanotransducer, in 3D-cultured AV cushion explants [13]. At high levels of shear stress, however, *rhoA* was shown to be downregulated compared to physiological levels [14]. In the present study, we also observed a significant decrease in *rhoA* transcript levels in OFT of banded hearts. This decrease in *rhoA* transcription could potentially lead to inappropriate mechanotransduction and, thus, altered ECM production, leading to abnormally-formed OFT valves. Krüppel-like factor 2 (klf2) is an important shear-responsive transcription factor [29,30], appears to have a role in normal valve development and regulates the EMT process [31]. We did not observe any significant change in the mRNA expression of this gene upon constricting the OFT. This may be a consequence of analyzing the expression of this gene in whole OFT and not just the region where shear stress is altered.

The production/deposition of fibrous ECM proteins is important to maintain valvular integrity in order to allow valves to function efficiently and to prevent the backflow of blood during the cardiac cycle; consequently, aberrant expression and deposition of valve ECM proteins is associated with abnormalities in valve development and pathological states [18]. Collagen is the most abundant fibrous ECM protein in the mature valve, with mutations in collagen1α1 leading to, among other conditions, aortic valve insufficiency that requires valve replacement [18]. Tenascin C is a matricellular protein that is highly expressed during development and is associated with endocardial cushion tissue EMT. Elastin is found in the ventricularis, the aspect of the OFT valves that faces blood flow. It has been shown, in humans, that elastin content increases in the outflow valves from the fetal stage to adult [32]. In our study, we found a decreased expression of *collagen1α1* at the mRNA level and a downregulated trend in mRNA expression of *tenascinC* in OFT from banded hearts relative to that from controls. We have previously shown that in the presence of flow and, therefore, shear stress, transcript levels of *collagen1α1* and *tenascin C* are decreased in *in vitro* 3D-cultured HH25 OFT cushions compared to no flow controls [14]. Yet, when compared to physiological levels of shear stress, there were no observable differences when shear stresses were elevated to pathologically high levels (e.g., those generated from OVJ banding) [14]. The reduction in *collagen1α1* may be attributed to the change in shear stress through the banded OFT. However, it appears that spatially-averaged shear stress does not significantly influence expression of *elastin* and *vinculin*, at least at the mRNA level, at this embryonic stage. Importantly, it should be pointed out that the presence of flow did decrease mRNA expression of *elastin* in 3D-cultured OFT cushions from HH25 hearts and that pathologically high levels of shear stress also increased mRNA expression [14]. These differences are also likely attributable to the stage-dependent influence of hemodynamics on the transcription of this gene. In the present study, we observed an increase in transcripts of *periostin* in the high shear stress model, which are in agreement with our *in vitro* 3D OFT explant experiments [14], where transcript levels of *periostin* were upregulated in OFT cushion tissue. Periostin is a product of TGFβ3 signaling and has been shown to regulate chick AV valve maturation [33].

In the current study, we investigated the expression of a representative panel of genes important for EMT. The type III TGFβ receptor (TGFβRIII) is the ligand-presenting receptor and plays an important role in cushion EMT [34,35]. We observed a significant increase in gene expression of *TGFβRIII* and *TGFβ3* in the OFT tissue of banded hearts. However, there was no significant difference in expression levels of *TGFβ2* between OFT of the banded and control hearts. Snai2 is an important transcription factor of TGFβ signaling that induces EMT by decreasing the expression of adhesion molecules, including E-cadherin [3]. Even though we did not observe any alteration in gene expression of *Snai2* in OFT tissue from the banded hearts, there was a significant decrease in the number of cells undergoing EMT and, thus, invading the cushion tissue. This may be due to the effect of altered hemodynamics on a Snai2-independent EMT process. Thus, there seems to be activation of only the upstream events of TGFβ signaling in OFT tissue by the change in hemodynamics in the heart. The increase in *TGFβ3* levels could partially contribute to the enhanced expression of *periostin* in OFT tissue of the banded heart. Cadherin-11 (CDH11) is a type II classical cadherin that is found in the endothelium and mesenchyme of embryonic cushion tissue and may play a migratory role in populating the cardiac jelly [36]. OFT banding led to a significant downregulation in the expression of *CDH11* in OFT tissue. This indicates that changing cardiac hemodynamics in the embryonic heart could potentially affect the migration of endothelial cells, an important process of valve formation. Lastly, we found a significant increase in the expression of matrix metalloproteinase 2 (*mmp2*) in the OFT of banded hearts. MMP2 is required for degradation of the ECM and cell migration. However, it should be noted that mmp2 has to be proteolytically activated [37], which was not investigated in our study. Thus, we can only conclude that altered intracardiac hemodynamics seems to influence the expression of this gene at the mRNA level. These gene expression studies support the central theme that altered hemodynamics regulate critical valve gene expression. Moreover, using this new *ex ovo* model, we can continue to examine the role of hemodynamics and begin to correlate changes with corresponding cellular responses *in vivo*. Something to this point could not previously be achieved.

5. Conclusion

In summary, altered hemodynamics led to changes in OFT cushion volume, the number of invading mesenchymal cells in the OFT cushions and the expression of genes involved in ECM development, EMT signaling and cell migration. The present study, thus, contributes to the field of valvulogenesis and highlights the importance of normal hemodynamics in proper valve development.

Acknowledgements

The authors thank Bob Price, of the Instrumentation Resource Facility (IRF), University of South Carolina (USC), Columbia, and also the IRF staff, Anna Harper and Lorain Junor, for technical assistance, as well as Susan Lessner for technical assistance on three-dimensional software models. This study was funded in part by a University of South Carolina Research Development Fund grant (JP and VM), FirstString Research Inc. (JP) and NIH IDeA Networks of Biomedical Research Excellence (INBRE) grant for South Carolina P20GM103499 (JE).

Author Contributions

JDP was responsible for the construction and design of the experiments and assisted in writing and editing the manuscript. JE was responsible for interpreting the hemodynamic data and creating the corresponding models. RG was responsible for editing the manuscript and designing the experiments. VM was responsible for acquiring much of the data and helping in manuscript preparation.

Conflicts of Interest

The authors declare no conflict of interest.

References

1. Neeb, Z.; Lajiness, J.; Bolanis, E.; Conway, S. Cardiac outflow tract anomalies. *Wiley Interdiscip Rev. Dev. Biol.* **2013**, *2*, 499–530.
2. Hinton, R.; Yutzey, K. Heart valve structure and function in development and disease. *Annu Rev. Physiol.* **2011**, *73*, 29–46.
3. Von Gise, A.; Pu, W. Endocardial and epicardial epithelial to mesenchymal transitions in heart development and disease. *Circ. Res.* **2012**, *110*, 1628–1645.
4. Person, A.; Klewer, S.; Runyan, R. Cell biology of cardiac cushion development. *Int. Rev. Cytol.* **2005**, *243*, 287–335.
5. De Vlaming, A.; Sauls, K.; Hajdu, Z.; Visconti, R.; Mehesz, A.; Levine, R.; Slaugenhaupt, S.; Hagège, A.; Chester, A.; Markwald, R.; *et al.* Atrioventricular valve development: New perspectives on an old theme. *Differentiation* **2012**, *84*, 103–116.
6. Nakaya, Y.; Sheng, G. EMT in developmental morphogenesis. *Cancer Lett.* **2013**, *341*, 9–15.
7. Bernanke, D.; Markwald, R. Migratory behavior of cardiac cushion tissue cells in a collagen-lattice culture system. *Dev. Biol.* **1982**, *91*, 235–245.
8. Runyan, R.; Markwald, R. Invasion of mesenchyme into three-dimensional collagen gels: A regional and temporal analysis of interaction in embryonic heart tissue. *Dev. Biol.* **1983**, *95*, 108–114.
9. Mjaatvedt, C.; Lepera, R.; Markwald, R. Myocardial specificity for initiating endothelial-mesenchymal cell transition in embryonic chick heart correlates with a particulate distribution of fibronectin. *Dev. Biol.* **1987**, *119*, 59–67.
10. Culver, J.C.; Dickinson, M.E. The effects of hemodynamic force on embryonic development. *Microcirculation* **2010**, *17*, 164–178.

11. Butcher, J.; McQuinn, T.; Sedmera, D.; Turner, D.; Markwald, R. Transitions in early embryonic atrioventricular valvular function correspond with changes in cushion biomechanics that are predictable by tissue composition. *Circ. Res.* **2007**, *100*, 1503–1511.
12. Hove, J.; Köster, R.; Forouhar, A.; Acevedo-Bolton, G.; Fraser, S.; Gharib, M. Intracardiac fluid forces are an essential epigenetic factor for embryonic cardiogenesis. *Nature* **2003**, *421*, 172–177.
13. Tan, H.; Biechler, S.; Junor, L.; Yost, M.; Dean, D.; Li, J.; Potts, J.; Goodwin, R. Fluid flow forces and rhoa regulate fibrous development of the atrioventricular valves. *Dev. Biol.* **2013**, *374*, 345–356.
14. Biechler, S.; Junor, L.; Evans, A.; Eberth, J.; Price, R.; Potts, J.; Yost, M.; Goodwin, R. The impact of flow-induced forces on the morphogenesis of the outflow tract. *Front. Physiol.* **2014**, *5*, doi:10.3389/fphys.2014.00225.
15. Schneider, C.; Rasband, W.; Eliceiri, K. NIH image to ImageJ: 25 years of image analysis. *Nat. Methods* **2012**, *9*, 671–675.
16. McDonald, D. *Blood Flow in Arteries*; 2nd ed.; Edward Arnold: London, UK, 1974.
17. Pfaffl, M. A new mathematical model for relative quantification in real-time RT-PCR. *Nucleic Acids Res.* **2001**, *29*, e45.
18. Combs, M.; Yutzey, K. Heart valve development: Regulatory networks in development and disease. *Circ. Res.* **2009**, *105*, 408–421.
19. Hu, N.; Clark, E. Hemodynamics of the stage 12 to stage 29 chick embryo. *Circ. Res.* **1989**, *65*, 1665–1670.
20. Hogers, B.; DeRuiter, M.; Gittenberger-de Groot, A.; Poelmann, R. Unilateral vitelline vein ligation alters intracardiac blood flow patterns and morphogenesis in the chick embryo. *Circ. Res.* **1997**, *80*, 473–481.
21. Hogers, B.; DeRuiter, M.; Gittenberger-de Groot, A.; Poelmann, R. Extraembryonic venous obstructions lead to cardiovascular malformations and can be embryolethal. *Cardiovasc. Res.* **1999**, *41*, 87–99.
22. Reckova, M.; Rosengarten, C.; de Almeida, A.; Stanley, C.; Wessels, A.; Gourdie, R.; Thompson, R.; Sedmera, D. Hemodynamics is a key epigenetic factor in development of the cardiac conduction system. *Circ. Res.* **2003**, *93*, 77–85.
23. Stekelenburg-de Vos, S.; Ursem, N.; Hop, W.; Wladimiroff, J.; Gittenberger-de Groot, A.; Poelmann, R. Acutely altered hemodynamics following venous obstruction in the early chick embryo. *J. Exp. Biol.* **2003**, *206*, 1051–1057.
24. Lucitti, J.; Tobita, K.; Keller, B. Arterial hemodynamics and mechanical properties after circulatory intervention in the chick embryo. *J. Exp. Biol.* **2005**, *208*, 1877–1885.
25. Shi, L.; Goenezen, S.; Haller, S.; Hinds, M.; Thornburg, K.; Rugonyi, S. Alterations in pulse wave propagation reflect the degree of outflow tract banding in hh18 chicken embryos. *Am. J. Physiol. Heart Circ. Physiol.* **2013**, *305*, H386–H396.
26. Bharadwaj, K.; Spitz, C.; Shekhar, A.; Yalcin, H.; Butcher, J. Computational fluid dynamics of developing avian outflow tract heart valves. *Ann. Biomed. Eng.* **2012**, *40*, 2212–2227.
27. Liu, A.; Nickerson, A.; Troyer, A.; Yin, X.; Cary, R.; Thornburg, K.; Wang, R.; Rugonyi, S. Quantifying blood flow and wall shear stresses in the outflow tract of chick embryonic hearts. *Comput. Struct.* **2011**, *89*, 855–867.

28. Midgett, M.; Goenezen, S.; Rugonyi, S. Blood flow dynamics reflect degree of outflow tract banding in hamburger-hamilton stage 18 chicken embryos. *J. R. Soc. Interface* **2014**, *11*, doi:10.1098/rsif.2014.0643.
29. Groenendijk, B.; Van der Heiden, K.; Hierck, B.; Poelmann, R. The role of shear stress on ET-1, KLF2, and NOS-3 expression in the developing cardiovascular system of chicken embryos in a venous ligation model. *Physiology (Bethesda)* **2007**, *22*, 380–389.
30. Huddleson, J.; Ahmad, N.; Srinivasan, S.; Lingrel, J. Induction of KLF2 by fluid shear stress requires a novel promoter element activated by a phosphatidylinositol 3-kinase-dependent chromatin-remodeling pathway. *J. Biol. Chem.* **2005**, *280*, 23371–23379.
31. Chiplunkar, A.; Lung, T.; Alhashem, Y.; Koppenhaver, B.; Salloum, F.; Kukreja, R.; Haar, J.; Lloyd, J. Krüppel-like factor 2 is required for normal mouse cardiac development. *PLoS ONE* **2013**, *8*, e54891.
32. Aikawa, E.; Whittaker, P.; Farber, M.; Mendelson, K.; Padera, R.; Aikawa, M.; Schoen, F. Human semilunar cardiac valve remodeling by activated cells from fetus to adult: Implications for postnatal adaptation, pathology, and tissue engineering. *Circulation* **2006**, *113*, 1344–1352.
33. Norris, R.; Potts, J.; Yost, M.; Junor, L.; Brooks, T.; Tan, H.; Hoffman, S.; Hart, M.; Kern, M.; Damon, B.; *et al.* Periostin promotes a fibroblastic lineage pathway in atrioventricular valve progenitor cells. *Dev. Dyn.* **2009**, *238*, 1052–1063.
34. Garside, V.; Chang, A.; Karsan, A.; Hoodless, P. Co-ordinating notch, BMP, and TGF-β signaling during heart valve development. *Cell. Mol. Life Sci.* **2013**, *70*, 2899–2917.
35. Brown, C.; Boyer, A.; Runyan, R.; Barnett, J. Requirement of type III TGF-β receptor for endocardial cell transformation in the heart. *Science* **1999**, *283*, 2080–2082.
36. Zhou, J.; Bowen, C.; Lu, G.; Knapp, C., III; Recknagel, A.; Norris, R.; Butcher, J. Cadherin-11 expression patterns in heart valves associate with key functions during embryonic cushion formation, valve maturation and calcification. *Cells Tissues Organs* **2013**, *198*, 300–310.
37. Alexander, S.; Jackson, K.; Bushnell, K.; McGuire, P. Spatial and temporal expression of the 72-KDA type IV collagenase (MMP-2) correlates with development and differentiation of valves in the embryonic avian heart. *Dev. Dyn.* **1997**, *209*, 261–268.

8

Advanced Electrocardiography Identifies Left Ventricular Systolic Dysfunction in Non-Ischemic Cardiomyopathy and Tracks Serial Change over Time

Kerryanne Johnson [1,*], Stacey Neilson [1], Andrew To [1], Nezar Amir [1], Andrew Cave [1], Tony Scott [1], Martin Orr [1,2], Mia Parata [1], Victoria Day [1] and Patrick Gladding [1,3,4]

1 North Shore hospital, Waitemata District Health Board, Takapuna, 0620 Auckland, New Zealand; E-Mails: Stacey.Neilson@waitematadhb.govt.nz (S.N.); Andrew.To@waitematadhb.govt.nz (A.T.); Nezar.Amir@waitematadhb.govt.nz (N.A.); Andrew.Cave@waitematadhb.govt.nz (A.C.); Tony.Scott@waitematadhb.govt.nz (T.S.); Martin.Orr@waitematadhb.govt.nz (M.O.); Mia.Parata@waitematadhb.govt.nz (M.P.); Victoria.Day@waitematadhb.govt.nz (V.D.); Patrick.Gladding@waitematadhb.govt.nz (P.G.)

2 Clinical Informatics Systems Group, North Shore Hospital, Waitemata District Health Board, Takapuna, 0620 Auckland, New Zealand

3 Theranostics Laboratory, North Shore Hospital, Waitemata District Health Board, Takapuna, 0620 Auckland, New Zealand

4 Auckland Bioengineering Institute, University of Auckland, 0620 Auckland, New Zealand

* Author to whom correspondence should be addressed; E-Mail: kerryannejohnson@hotmail.com

Academic Editor: Andy Wessels

Abstract: Electrocardiogram (ECG)-based detection of left ventricular systolic dysfunction (LVSD) has poor specificity and positive predictive value, even when including major ECG abnormalities, such as left bundle branch block (LBBB) within the criteria for diagnosis. Although machine-read ECG algorithms do not provide information on LVSD, advanced ECG (A-ECG), using multiparameter scores, has superior diagnostic utility to strictly conventional ECG for identifying various cardiac pathologies, including LVSD. Methods: We evaluated the diagnostic utility of A-ECG in a case-control study of

40 patients with LVSD (LV ejection fraction < 50% by echocardiography), due to non-ischemic cardiomyopathy (NICM), and 39 other patients without LVSD. Diagnostic sensitivity and specificity for LVSD were determined after applying a previously validated probabilistic A-ECG score for LVSD to stored standard (10 s) clinical 12L ECGs. In 25 of the NICM patients who had serial ECGs and echocardiograms, changes in the A-ECG score *versus* in echocardiographic LV ejection fraction were also studied to determine the level of agreement between the two tests. Results: Analyses by A-ECG had a sensitivity of 95% for LVSD (93% if excluding $N = 11$ patients with LBBB) and specificity of 95%. In the 29 NICM patients without LBBB who had serial ECGs, sensitivity improved to 97% when all ECGs were considered. By comparison, human readers in a busy clinical environment had a sensitivity of 90% and specificity of 63%. A-ECG score trajectories demonstrated improvement, deterioration or no change in LVSD, which agreed with echocardiography, in 76% of cases ($n = 25$). Conclusion: A-ECG scoring detects LVSD due to NICM with high sensitivity and specificity. Serial A-ECG score trajectories also represent a method for inexpensively demonstrating changes in LVSD. A-ECG scoring may be of particular value in areas where echocardiography is unavailable, or as a gatekeeper for echocardiography.

Keywords: left ventricular systolic dysfunction; advanced ECG; non-ischemic cardiomyopathy; echocardiography

1. Introduction

Since the advent of the electrocardiogram (ECG) over a century ago, its utility as a cost-effective and accessible diagnostic tool has been proven repeatedly. Through the application of rules and recognition of certain patterns, expert readers of ECGs can infer a wide variety of cardiac diagnoses. For these reasons the ECG has become a standard of care in the investigation of patients with suspected left ventricular systolic dysfunction (LVSD), and is a particularly valuable tool in primary healthcare [1].

Due to the abundance of patients presenting with dyspnoea, but relative inaccessibility of echocardiography and delays in laboratory testing, the ECG represents one of the most cost-effective point-of-care diagnostic instruments available in the community. Its utility however is limited by the experience of its users and quality of machine-read algorithms, which are often dismissed due to their perceived poor diagnostic quality. However modern advances in digital recording, signal processing, and machine learning have significantly improved accuracy of diagnostic ECG algorithms.

Advanced ECG (A-ECG) analysis utilises a number of these processes, but also typically derives from standard 12L ECG recordings results from additional techniques such as "3-dimensional" (spatial/spatiotemporal) ECG [2–5]; detailed studies of waveform complexity by singular value decomposition (SVD) [4,6–8] and, when longer recordings are available, also high-frequency QRS ECG [9]; and beat-to-beat QT variability (QTV) [10–13] and R-wave to R-wave variability (RRV) [14,15]. By combining the most applicable results from these advanced techniques into scores that rely on large underlying ECG databases and advanced statistics [16], diagnostic yield is increased substantially [17]. In addition as these databases grow, with additional cases and clinical feedback, iterative learning is facilitated and a virtuous circle completed.

In this retrospective case-controlled study, we applied a previously validated A-ECG score for LVSD [17] to the stored digital 12L ECG recordings of patients with a clinical diagnosis of non-ischemic cardiomyopathy (NICM), and to corresponding recordings from randomly selected matched patients who had normal echocardiograms. We used the electronically stored echocardiographic and other clinical information to evaluate the diagnostic accuracy of A-ECG for NICM.

2. Methods

2.1. Patient Selection

A local review of the study protocol by the North Shore Knowledge Centre (Auckland, New Zealand) classified this report as an observational review of electronic clinical records and therefore exempt from Ethics review (Ethical Guidelines for Observational Studies 2012. Health and Disability Ethics Committees of New Zealand) [18].

Patients who had undergone an echocardiogram with a referral stating "non-ischemic cardiomyopathy" or "NICM" were identified using a SQL server search of an Excelera (Philips Healthcare, Best, The Netherlands) database. Their data were included in the study if ≥2 serial echocardiograms had been performed. Controls were identified by choosing other patients from within the same database who had had clinical echocardiograms read as "normal". Corresponding digital 12-lead ECGs were taken from Epiphany's Cardio Server ECG management software (Version 3.2.3.1, Epiphany Healthcare, Midlothian, VA, USA), de-identified, and converted to an analysable, binary format by using an Octave script, then sent to Advanced ECG Services (Nicollier-Schlegel SARL, Trélex, Switzerland, https://aecg.ch) for A-ECG analyses.

2.2. A-ECG Analysis

Because the de-identified 12-lead ECGs were standard clinical ECGs containing only 10-s worth of information, A-ECG analyses were limited to only those parameters that can be accurately assessed from 10-s recordings. Analyzed parameters included those derived from signal averaging of all QRS and T complexes within the 10-s recordings by using software originally assembled at NASA [8,17] to generate results for: (1) several spatial (derived 3-dimensional) ECG parameters, including the spatial mean and peaks QRS-T angles, the spatial ventricular gradient, and various spatial waveform azimuths, elevations, and time-voltages [17], all derived by using the Frank-lead reconstruction technique of Kors *et al.* [19]; (2) parameters of QRS and T-waveform complexity derived by SVD that can be reproducibly obtained from 10-s ECGs, for example the principal component analysis (PCA) ratio ([8] and the dipolar voltage equivalents [4,17]) of the QRS and T waveforms; and (3) the most applicable parameters from the conventional scalar 12-lead ECG. The majority of these parameters and their related detailed methods have been described in previous publications [8,17,19,20]. To specifically judge the presence *versus* absence of LVSD by A-ECG, and then to also qualitatively follow the status of LVSD by A-ECG over time, we utilized a previously validated A-ECG score for LVSD that was originally constructed on the basis of multivariate logistic regression of A-ECG data from a larger data set of previous patients with known LVSD [17].

Results for this 5-component score are also derivable from the standard ~10-s 12-lead ECG recordings utilized in the present study. The score specifically incorporates results from a patient's spatial mean QRS-T angle, derived Frank Z-lead integral, total (12-lead) QRS voltage, and SVD-derived QRS-wave nondipolar and T-wave dipolar voltages [17]. The exact coefficients utilized in the score can also be found within Supplemental Table 2 of [17].

2.3. Human Reader Sub-Study

A sub-study was also conducted wherein four human readers were also asked to provide a diagnosis for a random sample of 22 conventional 12L ECGs taken from all the ECGs in this study. 10 of these ECGs were from patients with NICM, and 12 were from control patients without NICM. Two respondents were cardiologists and two were general practitioners. The number of ECGs was reduced to limit the impact of time on clinicians with other clinical duties. For all 22 ECGs, the respondents were posed a single hypothetical patient with nonspecific breathlessness and instructed to provide a diagnosis of normal *versus* abnormal ECG. Moreover, for any ECG considered abnormal, they were asked to further segregate it into a most likely diagnostic category from amongst the following four choices: (a) coronary artery disease; (b) left ventricular hypertrophy or hypertrophic cardiomyopathy; (c) ischemic or non-ischemic cardiomyopathy (*i.e.*, LV ejection fraction < 50%); or (d) Long QT syndrome (LQTS) or other channelopathy.

2.4. Echocardiography

Echocardiograms were performed as part of clinical care on a GE Vivid 7 ultrasound machine. All echocardiograms were performed by an experienced trainee sonographer under cardiologist (ASE level III) supervision. The dates and data for each study were entered into a database and compared over serial assessment and with serial ECGs. Simpson biplanes estimates of ejection fraction were performed on all studies.

2.5. Statistics

Diagnostic sensitivity and specificity for LVSD (LV ejection fraction <50%) were determined after applying the aforementioned validated A-ECG score for LVSD [17] and the human reader results to the analyzed 12L ECGs. Cochran's Q test was used for determining differences in accuracy between cardiologists, general practitioners and automated A-ECG in correctly identifying patients with *versus* without LVSD. For patients who had serial echocardiograms (LV ejection fractions) and corresponding serial A-ECG scores, the respective serial results were also characterized as improved, worsened or unchanged (i.e., when directional change was less than ±10%), thus allowing for qualitative comparison between directional changes in LV ejection fraction and the A-ECG score. Because the A-ECG score for LVSD was originally designed to determine, in a simple binary fashion, whether or not LVSD (defined as LV ejection fraction < 50%) was present, and not to attempt to track LV ejection fraction quantitatively [17], we performed a quantitative correlation between the two continuous parameters for academic purposes only. Finally, we also obtained A-ECG-related linear discriminant analysis (LDA) plots for purely descriptive purposes.

3. Results

3.1. Cases

Forty patients with LVSD due to clinically specified non-ischemic cardiomyopathy (NICM) were identified through the database search along with 39 controls without LVSD. Baseline patient characteristics are shown in Tables 1 and 2.

Table 1. Patient characteristics.

	Cases (n = 41)	Controls (n = 38)	p-Value
Age (mean/SD)	57 (14)	44(19)	0.76
Type 2 DM (%)	9 (22)	2 (5)	0.06
HTN (%)	18 (44)	9 (24)	0.1
Current Smoker (%)	7 (2)	6 (16)	0.07
Ex-smoker (%)	15 (37)	9 (24)	0.3
IHD (%)	2 (5)	2 (5)	0.6
Dyslipidaemia (%)	12 (29)	7 (18)	0.37
PVD (%)	1 (2)	-	0.81
CVA/TIA (%)	4 (10)	-	0.14
AF (%)	12 (29)	1 (3)	0.005
Alcohol excess (%)	3(7)	-	0.29
Mental Health Dx (%)	3 (7)	3 (8)	0.8
Substance abuse (%)	2 (5)	-	0.49
Gout (%)	6 (15)	3 (8)	0.54
CKD (%)	2 (5)	2 (5)	0.6
Obesity (%)	21 (51)	11 (29)	0.08

DM: Diabetes, IHD: Ischemic heart disease, PVD: Peripheral vascular disease, CVA/TIA: Cerebrovascular accident/Transient ischemic attack, AF: Atrial fibrillation, Alcohol excess ≥ 21 standard drinks/week in a male or >14 in a female. CKD: Chronic kidney disease, Obesity = Body Mass Index > 30.

Nineteen patients underwent cardiac MRI for investigation of their cardiomyopathy. NICM was confirmed in 18 of these patients with only one patient also having myocardial scar consistent with the presence of coronary artery disease.

Twenty six patients underwent a coronary angiogram. Six of these were found to have moderate (≤50%–69%) to severe coronary artery disease (≥70%), eight had no disease and the remaining 12 had trivial to mild disease. Three of the six patients with moderate to severe coronary disease had undergone a cardiac MRI showing NICM, and the remaining three had a clinical diagnosis of NICM. Only one patient within the cohort was ultimately considered to have a mixed non-ischemic and ischemic cardiomyopathy based on information that became available, only after study completion.

Table 2. Patient medication and left ventricular (LV) ejection fraction at each echocardiogram date.

	Echo 1 ($n = 41$)		Echo 2 ($n = 41$)		Echo 3 ($n = 21$)		Controls ($n = 38$)	
Ejection Fraction (mean/SD)	25% (9)		31% * (11)		38% ¥ (13)		55%–60%	
	Drug Rx	**Max dose**	**Drug Rx**	**Max dose**	**Drug Rx**	**Max dose**	**Drug Rx**	**Max dose**
Betablocker (%)	15 (37)	2 (5)	39 (95)	14 (34)	17 (81)	12 (57)	8 (21)	1 (3)
ACEI (%)	17 (41)	7 (7)	30 (73)	12 (29)	13 (62)	7 (33)	6 (16)	2 (5)
ARB (%)	4 (10)	2 (5)	10 (24)	2 (5)	5 (24)	3 (14)	2 (5)	2 (5)
CCHB (%)	5 (12)	1 (2)	2 (5)	-	3 (14)	-	6 (16)	2 (5)
Spironolactone (%)	9 (22)	7 (7)	24 (59)	19 (46)	11 (52)	7 (33)	-	-
Digoxin (%)	2 (5)	-	4 (10)	-	4 (19)	-	-	-
Loop Diuretic (%)	9 (22)	-	27 (66)	-	11 (52)	-	-	-
Thiazide diuretic (%)	2 (5)	2 (5)	1 (2)	1 (2)	-	-	1 (3)	1 (3)
Statin (%)	10 (24)	2 (5)	18 (44)	1 (2)	6 (29)	1 (5)	9 (24)	1 (3)
Aspirin (%)	13 (32)	12 (29)	12 (29)	12 (29)	1 (5)	1 (5)	7 (18)	7 (18)
Warfarin (%)	3 (7)	-	12 (29)	-	7 (33)	-	-	-
Dabigatran (%)	-	-	2 (5)	-	1 (5)	-	-	-
Dipyridamole (%)	1 (2)	1 (2)	1 (2)	1 (2)	-	-	-	-
Amiodarone (%)	1 (2)	-	3 (7)	-	-	-	-	-
Clopidogrel (%)	-	-	1 (2)	-	-	-	1 (3)	-
ISMN (%)	-	-	-	-	-	-	1 (3)	-

t test comparison between Echo1 and Echo 2, * $p = 0.004$; and Echo 2 and Echo 3. ¥ $p = 0.01$.

The baseline characteristics for the control (non-NICM) group, including administered medications, are also shown in Tables 1 and 2. The median number of days between the ECG and echocardiogram in controls was 81 days (range 1 to 758).

The maximum or target dose has been defined as follows: BB: Carvedilol 25 mg bd, Metoprolol 190 mg. Bisoprolol 10 mg. ACEI: Accupril 20mg bd, Lisonopril 20 mg Enalopril 20 mg. ARB: Losartan 50 mg, Candesartan 32 mg. Diuretics: Spironolactone 25 mg, Bendrofluazide 2.5 mg, Frusemide NA. CCHB: Diltiazem 360 mg, Amlodipine 10 mg, Felodipine 10 mg. Anti-arrhythmics: Digoxin NA, Amiodarone NA. Statins: Simvastatin 80 mg, Atorvastatin 80 mg. Anticoagulant/platelets: Aspirin 100 mg, Dipyridamole 25 mg bd, Clopidogrel 75 mg, Warfarin NA. Where the thiazide diuretic is in the form of a combination with ACEI it is assumed to be at maximum/target dose

The patients' ECGs were obtained both before and after echocardiography. The median number of days between the first echocardiogram and ECG was 6 (range 0 to 114). The median number of days between the first and second echocardiogram was 321 (range 58 to 1287). The median number of days between the second echocardiogram and second ECG was 14 (range 0 to 147).

3.2. A-ECG

Eleven of the patients with NICM had LBBB such that their ECGs could not be fully analysed for A-ECG. In the remaining patients ($N = 68$ total: 29 patients with NICM and 39 controls), A-ECG had a sensitivity of 93% for LVSD (95% if including the $N = 11$ patients with LBBB) and specificity of 95%. In the 29 NICM patients without LBBB who had serial ECGs, sensitivity of A-ECG also improved to 97% when all serial ECGs were considered. Trajectories in the A-ECG score for LVSD demonstrated improvement, deterioration or no change in LVSD, which agreed with changes in echocardiographic LV ejection fraction, in 76% of cases ($n = 25$). The quantitative correlation between the results of the A-ECG score for LVSD and the echocardiographic LVEF was $r = 0.32$ ($p = 0.01$). The correlation between the change in the A-ECG score for LVSD and the change in the LV ejection fraction between the first and second echocardiograms and A-ECGs (i.e., in patients who had serial results for both) was $r = 0.35$ ($p = 0.01$) (Figure 1). Fourteen patients had atrial fibrillation, a condition that did not preclude A-ECG scoring unless an LBBB was concomitantly present.

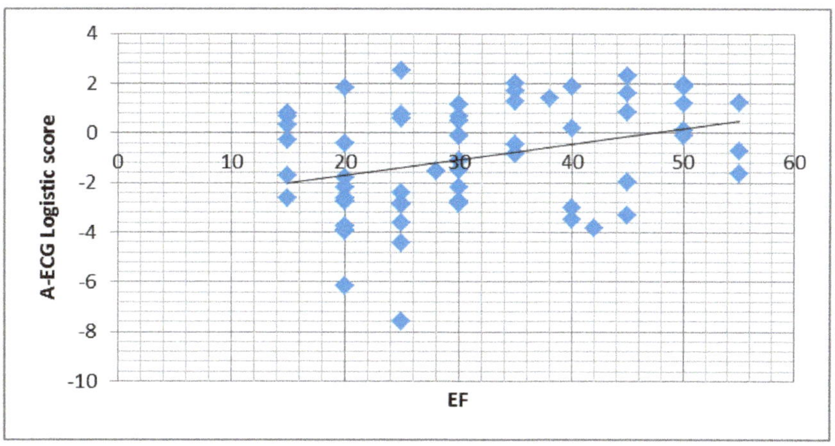

Figure 1. *Cont.*

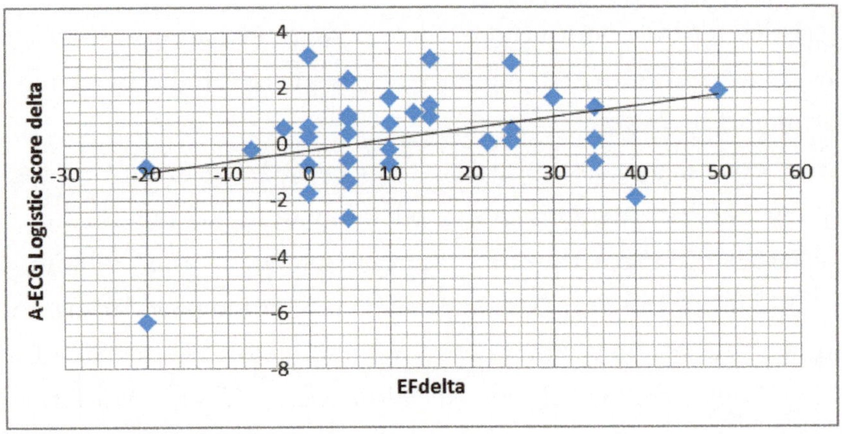

Figure 1. (Top): Baseline ejection fraction (EF) *versus* baseline A-ECG logistic score for left ventricular systolic dysfunction (LVSD), in all serial NICM patient ECGs; and (Bottom) Change in EF *versus* change in A-ECG logistic score.

3.3. Human Reader Sub-Study

The human readers' sensitivity and specificity for correctly designating, on the subset of 22 conventional 12L ECG tracings, the presence *versus* absence of LVSD through calls of "abnormal ECG", and also for correctly designating the appropriate (*i.e.*, ultimately clinically proven) diagnostic category, are listed in Table 3. For both types of diagnosis, the performance of the cardiologists tended to be better than that of the general practitioners, although this difference was not statistically significant (Cochran's Q = 1, df = 3, $p = 0.8$). However, the performance of the A-ECG score for LVSD was statistically significantly better than that of the clinical readers (Cochran's Q 12.8, df = 4, $p = 0.01$).

Table 3. Diagnostic accuracy of cardiologists and general practitioners assessing for LVSD.

Multiple Diagnoses	**Cardiologists**	**General Practitioners**
Sensitivity	25%	15%
Specificity	71%	42%
Binary Diagnosis (Normal/Abnormal)	**Cardiologists**	**General Practitioners**
Sensitivity	90%	85%
Specificity	63%	58%

Average sensitivity and specificity for two readers reporting on a random sample of 22 ECGs from the overall cohort.

3.4. Controls

Of the 39 controls, 18 had abnormalities reported by A-ECG that were not related to LVSD. Two of these had interventricular conduction delays (QRS > 120 ms) such that their ECGs could not be fully analysed for A-ECG. A linear discriminant analysis (LDA) depicting the control population's A-ECG results in 2D and 3D space is shown in Figure 2. In the LDA, the probability of the presence of a given disease state is grossly demonstrated by the relative proximity of the patient's given study number to a given disease state (larger circles), the latter being derived from a pre-existing database of A-ECG information from thousands of earlier patients with known, imaging-proven cardiac health or disease. Seven of the patients in the control group had A-ECG-related LDA results reporting a high probability of coronary artery disease. Of these, 6 patients had one or more cardiovascular risk factors. The 7th patient had late gadolinium enhancement on cardiac MRI and a diagnosis of myocarditis. The most abnormal A-ECG from this subgroup suggested a previous inferior myocardial infarction, which was confirmed by observation of regional wall motion abnormalities on echocardiography and by prior history.

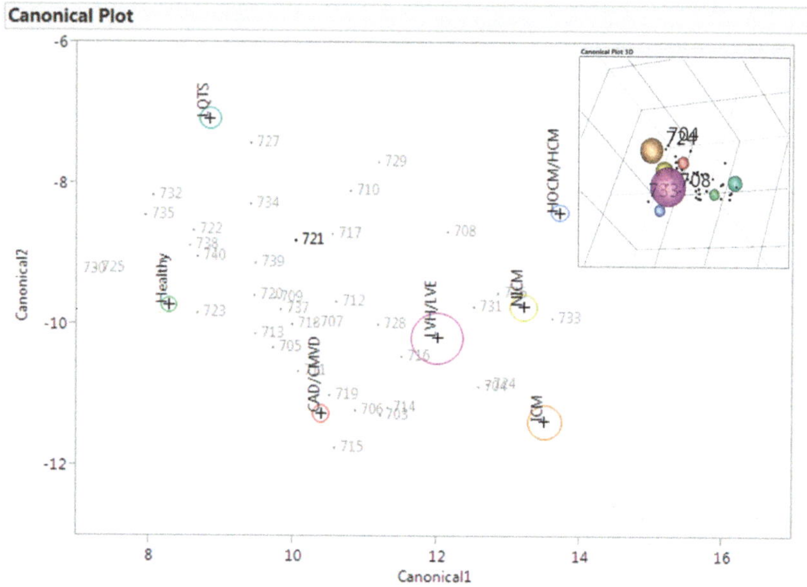

Figure 2. 2D and 3D Linear Discriminant Analysis plot of control ECGs. Each individual control (non-NICM) patient's A-ECG result as denoted by a number plotted within a 2-dimensional (2D) linear discriminant space. Probability of the presence of a given disease state is grossly demonstrated by the relative proximity of the patient's given number to a given disease state (larger circles), the latter being derived from a pre-existing database of A-ECG information from thousands of earlier patients with known, imaging-proven cardiac health or disease. Note however that because this is a 2D representation of a 3D space (right upper inset), a patient's number may sometimes have the appearance of proximity to a disease circle in the x and y planes shown, but in the z plane the distance may actually be closer to some other sphere. CAD/CMVD = Coronary Artery Disease and/or Coronary Microvascular Disease Population; LVH/LVE = Left Ventricular Hypertrophy or Enlargement population; HOCM/HCM = Hypertrophic Cardiomyopathy population; NICM = Non-Ischemic Cardiomyopathy population; ICM = Ischemic Cardiomyopathy population; and LQTS = Long QT Syndrome (LQTS) population, respectively.

The A-ECG LDA suggested a high probability of LV hypertrophy or enlargement in 5 other controls without NICM. One of these controls had a previous repair of a ventricular septal defect but no evidence of LV hypertrophy on echocardiography. Another had suspected Marfan's syndrome with slender body habitus and a history of ablation of a Wolf-Parkinson-White pre-excitation pathway. The remaining three patients had hypertension.

Two of the controls without NICM had A-ECG patterns consistent with the Long QT syndrome, despite having QTc intervals within the normal range. Both of these patients had a history of recurrent syncope. One of these patients was non contactable while the other was recalled to clinic for possible genetic and other testing. Of all the patients in this cohort, 7 (18%) had conditions wherein genetic information might have aided diagnosis.

4. Discussion

In this retrospective case-control study, we prospectively further validated, in a group of patients with *versus* without NICM, the diagnostic utility of a previously published A-ECG score for LVSD [17]. In our patients, the A-ECG score had a sensitivity of 93% for LVSD (95% if including $N = 11$ patients with LBBB) and specificity of 95%. Thus screening by A-ECG would have accurately identified nearly all patients with existing LVSD due to NICM, distinguishing them from patients with normal LV ejection fraction and allowing the identification by ECG of those who needed more extensive cardiac investigations. Secondarily, we also demonstrated the same A-ECG's scores qualitative ability to serially track changes in LVEF over time, based on the 76% correspondence between its results, when classified as improved, worsened or unchanged, with corresponding results from serial echocardiography.

Although the value of the ECG in the diagnosis of structural heart disease, such as ischemic heart disease, is well established, its utility in diagnosing LVSD is less so. The ability of the ECG to predict the presence of LVSD has been evaluated in a number of studies involving ECGs read both by humans and machine [1,21–23]. However with both types of readings the prediction of LVSD was ultimately allowed by indirect means, e.g., the presence of atrial fibrillation, or previous myocardial infarction or major nonspecific ECG abnormalities such as axis deviation or left bundle branch block (LBBB). Hence although the presence of a human-read major ECG abnormality can have high sensitivity for LVSD (90%–94%), the specificity is poor (58%–61%) [1,23]. In relation to our own sub-study of human-read ECGs, it is worth noting that most previous studies have asked readers to sort ECGs into normal or abnormal categories, using abnormality as a surrogate for LVSD. So although the sensitivity for the presence of LVSD appears high for human readers, this only applies to the detection of ECG abnormalities in the breathless patient, and hence *prediction* of LVSD presence, rather than its diagnosis. In this case-control study, we further validated not only A-ECG scoring's equivalent sensitivity for LVSD (NICM) compared to human reading of conventional ECGs, but also its superior specificity. Furthermore A-ECG results as applied to discriminant analyses provided a spectrum of further diagnoses for each individual ECG, which could not be matched in sensitivity or specificity by human readers who did not have further clinical information.

Two factors are noteworthy in this respect. First, the sensitivity of a human read ECG is highly influenced by experience, with reported sensitivity of 87% for less experienced readers [1]. By comparison A-ECG provides consistency unmatched by a human reader, who may also have external pressures of time, workload and fatigue. Second, LBBB is included as a major ECG abnormality in many of the human read ECG pathways to triage echocardiography [23]. By including patients with LBBB in the present cohort, the sensitivity of A-ECG in the diagnosis of LVSD would increase to 95%. And even when excluding patients with LBBB, sensitivity would also further increase to 97% if/when all serial ECGs were scored by A-ECG.

Whilst many ECG parameters, such as the QRS duration [24], are known to alter with left ventricular dilation and dysfunction, modest changes in these continuous parameters are not easily perceptible to human readers. Computerised ECG scores have been described since the 1970s and

1980s and initially showed, in small populations of patients with ischemic cardiomyopathy, remarkable sensitivity (93%) and specificity (88%) for LVSD as well as strong correlations with LVEF (r = 0.8 to 0.9) [21,22]. However, the performance of these older, strictly conventional ECG scores was notably diminished during subsequent attempts at validation with further (larger *N*) cases of ischemic cardiomyopathy [25], such that they were never translated into clinical practice [26]. In addition, these scores focused only on detecting LVSD in the context of ischemic cardiomyopathy, emphasising changes in Q and R wave amplitudes to estimate the extent of infarction and thereby an ejection fraction. As such, they also never demonstrated any effectiveness for detecting nonischemic cardiomyopathy, in contradistinction to the effectiveness of A-ECG scoring in this study. Finally, although there was a modest, statistically significant correlation between the results (and changes in) the A-ECG score for LVSD in this study and those in echocardiographic LV ejection fraction, we agree with the general notion that clinically, one should not attempt to use ECG measures as linear surrogates for purely anatomical phenomena like echocardiographically estimated LV ejection fraction (as in our study) or mass (as noted by Bacharova) [27].

ECG, by its very nature, measures cardiac electrical phenomena and thus estimates changes in cardiac electrical status, not mechanical status. And while clinically speaking, changes in cardiac electrical and mechanical function often accompany and correlate with one another, they are not the same thing, nor is it necessarily helpful to consider them the same thing. For example, a degree of "left ventricular electrical remodelling" that can be ascertained from a change in an electrical phenomenon (such as a change in the spatial QRS-T angle, one of the components of the 5-parameter A-ECG score for LVSD evaluated in this study) [17] may actually have more prognostic importance than one ascertained from a mechanical phenomenon, especially at relatively equivalent levels of mechanical heart failure [28]. In addition, A-ECG combined with additional clinical information, such as genomic, proteomic and metabolomic biomarkers, might lead to a new appreciation of heart failure and its intermediate pathophenotypes. Notably 18% of our control patients also had conditions wherein genetic information would have aided diagnosis.

Although ECGs are often repeated over serial time points, the ability to assess, in detail, changes in one person's conventional ECG in a single visualisation generally requires not only computerisation and dedicated software, but also the serial use of a single manufacturer's ECG platform. In a previous study [20], we demonstrated that analysis of A-ECG results by linear discriminant analyses can also allow for visualisation of changes in one person's A-ECG condition over time in a fashion that is independent of the ECG manufacturer or platform. For population studies, including the present one, the same visualization technique can also have utility in direct comparison of ECG results between individuals, the identification of diseases or patterns of potential concern in groups of individuals, and in identifying isolated conditions in single patients. In this study, although the control patients were identified as having normal echocardiograms, it was evident from the A-ECG discriminant analysis, and also often verified clinically, that a number of these patients nonetheless had significant cardiac pathology, some of which had not been detected during their visits through tertiary care centres. This appeared to be particularly apparent for suspected hereditary conditions, such as the Long QT syndrome, though this diagnosis is yet to be confirmed in the aforementioned patients.

In single patients A-ECG also demonstrated an ability to identify trajectories towards greater health or disease based on a comparison of A-ECG-related results with those from echocardiography.

Previous studies have shown that standard ECG parameters alter, in the short term, with diuresis in patients with heart failure [29]. In the Framingham heart study, ECG evidence of LV hypertrophy was shown to not only correlate with blood pressure but also changed with time [30]. The ECG changes were also predictive of subsequent cardiovascular events. The ability of the A-ECG to more objectively track changes than strictly conventional ECG may have utility in management decisions, such as helping to determine when further imaging or tailored treatment is appropriate. Given the cost-effectiveness and improved access of ECG compared with cardiac imaging, this improved upstream accuracy may lead to improved downstream decision making, reducing the costs of unnecessary investigations. In addition the distributed application of digital A-ECG lends itself well to telemedicine initiatives with greater community and primary care presence. In relation to this, whilst the A-ECG score that was further validated in this study clearly requires the derivation of several sophisticated ECG parameters, this does not necessarily imply that for its clinical application, the logic and signal processing behind the score must be directly programmed into the computer software or firmware of the various ECG machine manufacturers. For example it is already possible for any clinician to obtain such score results for his patients today, currently within hours, but in the future presumably within minutes, simply by uploading the patient's raw digital ECG data file(s) to a secure central server site (see e.g., https://aecg.ch).

5. Conclusions

We have demonstrated that A-ECG scoring, a novel method of analysis of standard 12L ECG, has high sensitivity and specificity for detecting mechanical LVSD in a cohort with NICM, exceeding that described in previous studies. The A-ECG method also identified directional changes in mechanical LVSD over time which agreed with serial echocardiography findings in 76% of cases. In addition visualisations of multivariate A-ECG results by means of discriminant analyses were useful for identifying patients in the control group with other cardiac disease, notably those with possible hereditary conditions consistent with patient symptomatology. The high sensitivity and specificity of A-ECG, as well as its breadth of diagnostic ability, might make it an ideal population screening tool and method for triaging patients for noninvasive imaging. This may particularly be the case when used in conjunction with disruptive low cost imaging methods, such as pocket echocardiography [31]. Fully prospective application of this technology should be trialled in the clinical setting with human supervision to assess its utility and cost-effectiveness as both a diagnostic and screening tool.

Limitations

The number of patients in this study was limited and the patient and control groups were not well matched for age, for the presence of atrial fibrillation and LBBB, and for medication use (drugs like digitals and amiodarone certainly also affecting the ECG). As ECGs were analysed retrospectively as part of clinical care they often occurred at time intervals distant to the echocardiogram. It is possible therefore that there would have been a change in ejection fraction over that time, partially accounting for the variability seen in Figure 1. Patients with ischemic cardiomyopathy were excluded and therefore the results may not be applicable to these patients. The reason for excluding them however was to evaluate the effectiveness of A-ECG in population of NICM patients without surrogate indicators of probable LVSD, such as widespread Q waves, *etc*. Although no scar was visible on most MRIs, only 26 patients underwent a coronary angiogram, such that potential contributions to LVSD by ischemia could not be fully excluded in all patients. Due to workload pressures and funding constraints, some ECGs were also not assessed by the human readers. However in relation to this, it should be noted that A-ECG is not currently applicable as a screening method for patients with IVCD or LBBB, an echocardiogram usually being immediately indicated for such patients based on their conventional ECG findings alone. A-ECG is also not intended to be a substitute for echocardiography, which provides a wealth of additional information such as chamber size, valvular function, *etc*, but is rather more suitable as an augmentation to traditional methods for sequential diagnostic testing, in the assessment of undifferentiated patients [31].

Acknowledgments

We thank Hamish Hart and Jonathan Christiansen for reviewing the project.

Author Contributions

P.G, M.O. and T.S. conceived and designed the research project; M.P and V.D collected data. A.C, M.O, K.J and P.G collected and analyzed the data; S.N performed the echocardiograms; A.T. and N.A. read the echocardiograms; K.J and P.G. wrote the paper.

Conflicts of Interest

The authors declare no conflict of interest.

References

1. Goudie, B.M.; Jarvis, R.I.; Donnan, P.T.; Sullivan, F.M.; Pringle, S.D.; Jeyaseelan, S.; Struthers, A.D. Screening for left ventricular systolic dysfunction using GP-reported ECGs. *Br. J. Gen. Pract.* **2007**, *57*, 191–195.
2. Kardys, I.; Kors, J.A.; van der Meer, I.M.; Hofman, A.; van der Kuip, D.A.; Witteman, J.C. Spatial QRS-T angle predicts cardiac death in a general population. *Eur. Heart J.* **2003**, *24*, 1357–1364.
3. Fayn, J.; Rubel, P.; Pahlm, O.; Wagner, G.S. Improvement of the detection of myocardial ischemia thanks to information technologies. *Int. J. cardiol.* **2007**, *120*, 172–180.
4. Rautaharju, P.M.; Kooperberg, C.; Larson, J.C.; LaCroix, A. Electrocardiographic predictors of incident congestive heart failure and all-cause mortality in postmenopausal women, the Women's Health Initiative. *Circulation* **2006**, *113*, 481–489.
5. Yamazaki, T.; Froelicher, V.F.; Myers, J.; Chun, S., Wang, P. Spatial QRS-T angle predicts cardiac death in a clinical population. *Heart rhythm* **2005**, *2*, 73–78.
6. Okin, P.M.; Malik, M.; Hnatkova, K.; Lee, E.T.; Galloway, J.M.; Best, L.G.; Howard, B.V.; Devereux, R.B. Repolarization abnormality for prediction of all-cause and cardiovascular mortality in American Indians: the Strong Heart Study. *J. Cardiovasc. Electrophysiol.* **2005**, *16*, 945–951.

7. Zabel, M.; Malik, M.; Hnatkova, K.; Papademetriou, V.; Pittaras, A.; Fletcher, R.D.; Franz, M.R. Analysis of T-wave morphology from the 12-lead electrocardiogram for prediction of long-term prognosis in male US veterans. *Circulation* **2002**, *105*, 1066–1070.
8. Batdorf, B.H.; Feiveson, A.H.; Schlegel, T.T. The effect of signal averaging on the reproducibility and reliability of measures of T-wave morphology. *J. Electrocardiol.* **2006**, *39*, 266–270.
9. Schlegel, T.T.; Kulecz, W.B.; DePalma, J.L.; Feiveson, A.H.; Wilson, J.S.; Rahman, M.A.; Bungo, M.W. Real-time 12-lead high-frequency QRS electrocardiography for enhanced detection of myocardial ischemia and coronary artery disease. *Mayo. Clin. Proc.* **2004**, *79*, 339–350.
10. Berger, R.D.; Kasper, E.K.; Baughman, K.L.; Marban, E.; Calkins, H.; Tomaselli, G.F. Beat-to-beat QT interval variability: Novel evidence for repolarization lability in ischemic and nonischemic dilated cardiomyopathy. *Circulation* **1997**, *96*, 1557–1565.
11. Piccirillo, G.; Magri, D.; Matera, S.; Magnanti, M.; Torrini, A.; Pasquazzi, E.; Schifano, E.; Velitti, S.; Marigliano, V.; Quaglione, R.; *et al.* QT variability strongly predicts sudden cardiac death in asymptomatic subjects with mild or moderate left ventricular systolic dysfunction: A prospective study. *Eur. Heart. J.* **2007**, *28*, 1344–1350.
12. Vrtovec, B.; Sinkovec, M.; Starc, V.; Radovancevic, B.; Schlegel, T.T. Coronary artery disease alters ventricular repolarization dynamics in type 2 diabetes. *Pacing. Clin. Electrophysiol.* **2005**, *28* (Suppl 1), S178–S181.
13. Starc, V.; Schlegel, T.T. Real-time multichannel system for beat-to-beat QT interval variability. *J. Electrocardiol.* **2006**, *39*, 358–367.
14. Marek, M.J.; Thomas, B.A.; Camm, J.; Kleiger, R.E.; Malliani, A.; Moss, A.J.; Schwartz, P.J. Heart rate variability. Standards of measurement, physiological interpretation, and clinical use. Task Force of the European Society of Cardiology and the North American Society of Pacing and Electrophysiology. *Eur. Heart J.* **1996**, *17*, 354–381.
15. Goldberger, A.L.; Amaral, L.A.; Hausdorff, J.M.; Ivanov, P.; Peng, C.K.; Stanley, H.E. Fractal dynamics in physiology: Alterations with disease and aging. *Proc. Natl. Acad. Sci. USA* **2002**, *99* (Suppl 1), 2466–2472.
16. Jain, A.K.; Duin, R.P.W.; Jianchang, M. Statistical pattern recognition: A review. *IEEE Trans. Pattern Anal. Mach. Intell.* **2000**, *22*, 4–37.
17. Schlegel, T.T.; Kulecz, W.B.; Feiveson, A.H.; Greco, E.C.; DePalma, J.L.; Starc, V.; Vrtovec, B.; Rahman, M.A.; Bungo, M.W.; Hayat, M.J.; *et al.* Accuracy of advanced versus strictly conventional 12-lead ECG for detection and screening of coronary artery disease, left ventricular hypertrophy and left ventricular systolic dysfunction. *BMC Cardiovasc. Disord.* **2010**, *10*, doi:10.1186/1471-2261-10-28.
18. Committee, N.E.A. Streamlined ethical guidelines for health and disability research. http://neac.health.govt.nz/streamlined-ethical-guidelines-health-and-disability-research (accessed on 12 May 2015).
19. Kors, J.A.; van Herpen, G.; Sittig, A.C.; van Bemmel, J.H. Reconstruction of the Frank vectorcardiogram from standard electrocardiographic leads: diagnostic comparison of different methods. *Eur. Heart J.* **1990**, *11*, 1083–1092.

20. Gladding, P.; Cave, A.; Zareian, M.; Smith, K.; Hussan, J.; Hunter, P.; Erogbogbo, F.; Aguilar, Z.; Martin, D.; Chan, E.; *et al*. Open Access Integrated Therapeutic and Diagnostic Platforms for Personalized Cardiovascular Medicine. *J. Pers. Med.* **2013**, *3*, 203–237.
21. Palmeri, S.T.; Harrison, D.G.; Cobb, F.R.; Morris, K.G.; Harrell, F.E.; Ideker, R.E.; Selvester, R.H.; Wagner, G.S. A QRS scoring system for assessing left ventricular function after myocardial infarction. *N. Engl. J. Med.* **1982**, *306*, 4–9.
22. Gottwik, M.G.; Parisi, A.F.; Askenazi, J.; McCaughan, D. Computerized orthogonal electrocardiogram: relation of QRS forces to left ventricular ejection fraction. *Am. J. Cardiol.* **1978**, *41*, 9–13.
23. Davie, A.P.; Francis, C.M.; Love, M.P.; Caruana, L.; Starkey, I.R.; Shaw, T.R.; Sutherland, G.R.; McMurray, J.J. Value of the electrocardiogram in identifying heart failure due to left ventricular systolic dysfunction. *BMJ* **1996**, *312*, doi:10.1136/bmj.312.7025.222.
24. Velavan, P.; Khan, N.K.; Rigby, A.S.; Goode, K.; Komajda, M.; Follath, F.; Swedberg, K.; Madeira, H.; Clark, A.L.; Cleland, J.G. Relation between severity of left ventricular systolic dysfunction and repolarisation abnormalities on the surface ECG: A report from the Euro heart failure survey. *Heart* **2006**, *92*, 255–256.
25. Fioretti, P.; Brower, R.W.; Lazzeroni, E.; Simoons, M.L.; Wijns, W.; Reiber, J.H.; Bos, R.J.; Hugenholtz, P.G. Limitations of a QRS scoring system to assess left ventricular function and prognosis at hospital discharge after myocardial infarction. *Br. Heart J.* 1985, *53*, 248–252.
26. Young, S.G.; Abouantoun, S.; Savvides, M.; Madsen, E.B.; Froelicher, V. Limitations of electrocardiographic scoring systems for estimation of left ventricular function. *J. Am. Coll. Cardiol.* **1983**, *1*, 1479–1488.
27. Bacharova, L. Electrocardiography-left ventricular mass discrepancies in left ventricular hypertrophy: Electrocardiography imperfection or beyond perfection? *J. Electrocardiol.* **2009**, *42*, 593–596.
28. Borleffs, C.J.W.; Scherptong, R.W.C.; Man, S.C.; van Welsenes, G.H.; Bax, J.J.; van Erven, L.; Swenne, C.A.; Schalij, M.J. Predicting Ventricular Arrhythmias in Patients With Ischemic Heart Disease: Clinical Application of the ECG-Derived QRS-T Angle. *Circulation* **2009**, *2*, 548–554.
29. Madias, J.E.; Song, J.; White, C.M.; Kalus, J.S.; Kluger, J. Response of the ECG to short-term diuresis in patients with heart failure. *Ann. Noninvasive Electrocardiol.* **2005**, *10*, 288–296.
30. Levy, D.; Salomon, M.; D'Agostino, R.B.; Belanger, A.J.; Kannel, W.B. Prognostic implications of baseline electrocardiographic features and their serial changes in subjects with left ventricular hypertrophy. *Circulation* **1994**, *90*, 1786–1793.
31. Kitada, R.; Fukuda, S.; Watanabe, H.; Oe, H.; Abe, Y.; Yoshiyama, M.; Song, J.M.; Sitges, M.; Shiota, T.; Ito, H.; *et al*. Diagnostic accuracy and cost-effectiveness of a pocket-sized transthoracic echocardiographic imaging device. *Clin. Cardiol.* **2013**, *36*, 603–610.

9

Preliminary Evidence for Aortopathy and an X-Linked Parent-of-Origin Effect on Aortic Valve Malformation in a Mouse Model of Turner Syndrome

Robert B. Hinton [1,*], Amy M. Opoka [1], Obah A. Ojarikre [2], Lawrence S. Wilkinson [3,4] and William Davies [3,4]

1 The Heart Institute, Division of Cardiology, Cincinnati Children's Hospital Medical Center, Cincinnati, OH 45208, USA; E-Mail: amy.opoka@cchmc.org
2 Mill Hill Laboratory, Francis Crick Institute, London NW7 1AA, UK; E-Mail: andrew.ojarikre@crick.ac.uk
3 MRC Centre for Neuropsychiatric Genetics and Genomics and Institute of Psychological Medicine and Clinical Neurosciences, School of Medicine, Cardiff University, Cardiff CF24 4HQ, UK; E-Mails: wilkinsonl@cardiff.ac.uk (L.S.W.); daviesw4@cardiff.ac.uk (W.D.)
4 Neuroscience and Mental Health Research Institute, Schools of Medicine and Psychology, Cardiff University, Cardiff CF24 4HQ, UK

* Author to whom correspondence should be addressed; E-Mail: bingrbh@icloud.com

Academic Editor: Andy Wessels

Abstract: Turner syndrome (TS), most frequently caused by X-monosomy (45,X), is characterized in part by cardiovascular abnormalities, including aortopathy and bicuspid aortic valve (BAV). There is a need for animal models that recapitulate the cardiovascular manifestations of TS. Extracellular matrix (ECM) organization and morphometrics of the aortic valve and proximal aorta were examined in adult 39,XO mice (where the parental origin of the single X was paternal (39,X^{P}O) or maternal (39,X^{M}O)) and 40,XX controls. Aortic valve morphology was normal (tricuspid) in all of the 39,X^{P}O and 40,XX mice studied, but abnormal (bicuspid or quadricuspid) in 15% of 39,X^{M}O mice. Smooth muscle cell orientation in the ascending aorta was abnormal in all 39,X^{P}O and 39,X^{M}O mice examined, but smooth muscle actin was decreased in 39,X^{M}O mice only. Aortic dilation was present with reduced penetrance in 39,XO mice. The 39,XO mouse demonstrates aortopathy and an X-linked parent-of-origin effect on aortic valve malformation, and the candidate gene *FAM9B* is polymorphically expressed in control and diseased human aortic valves. The 39,XO mouse model may be valuable for examining the mechanisms underlying the cardiovascular findings in TS, and suggest there are important genetic modifiers on the X chromosome that modulate risk for nonsyndromic BAV and aortopathy.

Keywords: cardiovascular malformation; valves; heritability; disease models; genomic imprinting; *Xlr3b*; *FAM9B*; 39,XO

1. Introduction

Turner syndrome (TS), most frequently caused by X-monosomy (45,X), is characterized by diverse developmental, endocrine and cardiovascular abnormalities, and affects approximately 1 in 2500 live born females [1]. Cardiovascular malformations (CVM) are present in 75% of TS fetuses and 20%–45% of live born infants, with bicuspid aortic valve (BAV), typically resulting from fusion of the right and left coronary cusps, being the most commonly observed malformation (20%–30% of TS cases) [2,3]. Aortic coarctation and thoracic aortic aneurysm also occur [4].

Two distinct genetic mechanisms may contribute to the phenotype of individuals with a 45,X constitution: first, haploinsufficiency for one or more of products of genes that escape X-inactivation (~15%–20% of the X-linked genetic complement [5]). Second, phenotypic variability within 45,X individuals may be due to the parental origin of the single X chromosome; in ~70% of TS cases, the X chromosome is inherited from the mother ($45,X^M$) whereas in the remainder it is inherited from the father ($45,X^P$). X-linked parent-of-origin effects (POE), *i.e.* where the appearance of $45,X^M$ and $45X^P$ subjects differs significantly, have been described on diverse phenotypes including: brain morphology and cognitive function, neck webbing, sensorineural hearing loss, renal and ocular abnormalities [6–9]. Some limited evidence exists for increased rates of non-syndromic CVMs (including aortic valve malformation and aortopathy) in $45,X^M$ subjects relative to $45,X^P$ subjects [6,10], somewhat consistent with increased rates of aortic valve malformation in males ($46,X^MY$) relative to females ($46,X^PX^M$) [11]. However, other studies have shown no difference in CVMs, including specifically BAV, between $45,X^M$ and $45,X^P$ individuals [2,12,13]. X-linked POE could be explained by the presence of X-linked imprinted genes (*i.e.*, genes that are solely, or predominantly, expressed from either the paternally or maternally inherited allele) [14]; to date, no X-linked imprinted genes have been identified in man. Alternatively, such POE might be explained by the presence of cryptic mosaicism (notably the presence of Y-linked sequences in $45,X^M$ individuals only) [15].

The 39,XO mouse model, where the parental origin of the X chromosome can be varied ($39,X^PO$ or $39,X^MO$) partially recapitulates several aspects of the Turner syndrome phenotype, including X-linked POE on cognition [16]; as a consequence of how they are generated, these mice cannot possess cryptic X or Y-linked sequences [17]. Here, we studied the cardiovascular system of 39,XO mice for the first time. We hypothesized that $39,X^MO$ mice would exhibit higher rates of aortopathy and aortic valve malformation than $39,X^PO$ (and 40,XX female) mice.

2. Methods and Materials

40,XX, 39,X^PO and 39,X^MO mice were bred on an MF1 outbred albino strain background and karyotyped *post mortem* as described previously [16]. Mice aged 6 weeks to 12 months were used. We used an outbred background because: (a) 39,XO mouse physiology has previously been extensively characterized on this background; and (b) humans are not inbred, hence the data obtained in our model may have greater translational relevance. Adult hearts were dissected, fixed in 4% paraformaldehyde, dehydrated in ethanol and stored in 70% ethanol at −20 °C before histological processing. Importantly, cardiovascular morphology was analyzed blind to karyotype. Briefly, short axis serial sections showing the aortic valve *en face* were examined to determine aortic valve morphology based on the number and location of cusp attachments, which was classified as unicuspid, bicuspid, tricuspid (normal), or quadricuspid according to established definitions [18]. Morphometrics were performed using sections obtained in the long axis to examine aortic valve tissue (annulus area, cusp length, and hinge thickness), aorta tissue (medial thickness in the aortic root and ascending aorta), and the caliber of the aortic lumen at different levels (aortic valve annulus, aortic root, sinotubular junction and ascending aorta dimensions), analogous to clinical measures, as previously described [19]. By early adulthood the bodyweights of 40,XX and 39,XO mice do not differ significantly [16], therefore there is no need to normalize aorta measurements for body size as is done in TS subjects due to short stature [20,21]. Extracellular matrix (ECM) organization of both the aortic valve and the ascending aorta was assessed using Movat's pentachrome stain [22]. The aorta was studied further by examining the presence of alpha smooth muscle actin (SMA) and phospho-histone H3 (a marker of proliferation) using immunohistochemistry. Smooth muscle cell orientation was assessed by measuring the angle of the plane of the cell relative to the adjacent elastic fiber; an angle greater than 60 degree was considered abnormal. Our model allowed us to assess the effects of X-monosomy (40,XX *vs.* 39,XO), and X-linked POE (39,X^PO *vs.* 39,X^MO) on the measures described. Morphometric data were analyzed by One Way ANOVA with a between-group factor of KARYOTYPE. Data regarding frequency of aortic valve malformations were analyzed by a one-tailed Freeman Halton extension of Fisher's Exact Test. Human *FAM9B* expression was examined in human aortic valve control and disease samples by reverse transcriptase polymerase chain reaction using the following primers: 5′-CGCCTCTAGCTTCC CAGGACAA-3′ and 5′-GGCTTCTTGGTATTAGCCCCCGT-3′. *FAM9B* cDNA was used as the positive control (Thermo Fisher MGC cDNA, MHS6278-211690668).

3. Results and Discussion

3.1. Aortic Valve

The overall prevalence of aortic valve malformation in 39,XO mice was 4/45 (8%). While aortic valve morphology was normal (tricuspid) in all of the 39,X^PO (n = 18) and 40,XX (n = 21) mice studied, four mice (15%) from the 39,X^MO group (n = 27) exhibited valve abnormalities (p = 0.03); three 39,X^MO mice displayed BAV and one a quadricuspid aortic valve (Figure 1D–G). Two of the BAVs seen in the 39,X^MO group had fusion of the right and left coronary cusps, and one had fusion of the right and non-coronary cusps, consistent with the frequency identified in human studies [2]. There was no gross evidence of raphe or partial fusion. The aortic valve findings appear highly specific in that ECM trilaminar organization and valve morphometrics were equivalent in 40,XX, $39,X^PO$ and $39,X^{M}O$ mice (One Way ANOVA effect of KARYOTYPE on hinge thickness: $F_{[2,23]} = 1.58$, $p = 0.23$, cusp thickness: $F_{[2,23]} = 0.21$, $p = 0.81$, cusp length: $F_{[2,23]} = 0.51$, $p = 0.61$ and on annulus area: $F_{[2,23]} = 1.19$, $p = 0.32$, Table 1, Figure 1). While our current data provide intriguing initial support for an X-linked parent-of-origin effect on aortic valve malformation, we cannot completely discount the possibility that such abnormalities are seen in both $39,X^PO$ and $39,X^{M}O$ groups; this will require testing in further larger-scale studies.

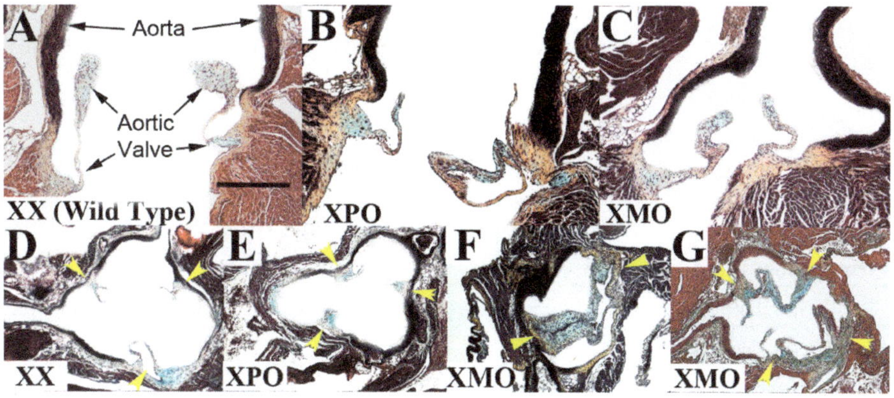

Figure 1. Aortic valve morphology is abnormal in $39,X^{M}O$ mice only. Aortic valves and proximal aortas are shown in the long axis view in adult 40,XX wild type controls (**A**) $39,X^PO$ (**B**) and $39,X^{M}O$ (**C**) mice. Trilaminar extracellular matrix (ECM) organization in both aortic valve and aorta tissue is preserved in 39, XO mice (**B,C**). Normal aortic valve morphology is seen in the short axis view in 40,XX (**D**) and $39,X^PO$ mice (**E**), *i.e.*, a tricuspid pattern with three commissures (yellow arrowheads); however, $39,X^{M}O$ mice demonstrate a variety of malformation patterns, including bicuspid aortic valve (BAV), as evidenced by two commissures (**F**), and quadricuspid aortic valve, which shows four commissures (**G**). Panels shown at 20× magnification; scale bar 250 µm.

Table 1. Aortic Valve and Aorta Morphometrics in a Mouse Model of Turner Syndrome.

	Valve Annulus Area (μm^2)	**Valve Hinge Thickness** (µm)	**Valve Cusp Length** (µm)	**Aortic Root Thickness** (µm)	**Ascending Aorta Thickness** (µm)
XX ($n = 8$)	5563 ± 1628	47 ± 14	279 ± 57	58 ± 8	111 ± 16
X^PO ($n = 6$)	4738 ± 1639	50 ± 6	325 ± 101	63 ± 4	103 ± 5
$X^{M}O$ ($n = 12$)	7180 ± 1328	59 ± 19	318 ± 112	57 ± 7	104 ± 14

Mean ± Standard Deviation.

3.2. Ascending Aorta

There were no significant differences across 40,XX ($n = 5$), $39,X^PO$ ($n = 5$) and $39,X^{M}O$ ($n = 9$) groups with regard to aortic root dimensions ($F_{[2,16]} = 3.14$, $p = 0.07$), aortic dimensions ($F_{[2,14]} = 2.38$, $p = 0.13$), or aortic valve annulus size ($F_{[2,16]} = 2.08$, $p = 0.16$), but there appeared to be a trend whereby all aortic measurements were greater in 39,XO mice than 40,XX mice with $39,X^{M}O$ mice showing the greatest deviation from 40,XX subjects; a proportion of 39,XO mice showed aorta measures greater than two standard deviations from the 40,XX mean (Table 2). Interestingly, while elastic fiber architecture, including gross lamellae number and medial thickness, was ostensibly normal across all three experimental groups, smooth muscle cell orientation in the ascending aorta was abnormal in all 39,X^PO and 39,X^MO mice examined when compared with 40,XX mice, demonstrating misaligned cells arranged in a plane orthogonal to the lamellae rather than the normal parallel plane; the average proportion of cells misaligned in 40,XX ($n = 5$), 39,X^PO ($n = 5$) and 39,X^MO ($n = 9$) was 12.5%, 72.7% and 82.6%, respectively ($x^2_{[2]} = 165.43$, $p < 0.0001$, Figure 2A–C). The cell density and proliferation index were not different between genotypes (data not shown). Interestingly, SMA staining was decreased in 39,X^MO mice only (Figure 2D–F). To our knowledge, this intriguing phenotype has not previously been reported in individuals with TS and warrants further investigation in this population.

Table 2. Aorta Dimensions by Pathology in a Mouse Model of Turner Syndrome.

	Valve Annulus Dimension (μm)	Aortic Root Dimension (μm)	Sinotubular Junction Dimension (μm)	Ascending Aorta Dimension (μm)
XX ($n = 5$)	486 ± 40	735 ± 52	502 ± 54	517 ± 41
X^PO ($n = 5$)	500 ± 36 (0/5, 0%)	778 ± 65 (1/5, 20%)	531 ± 62 (1/5, 20%)	559 ± 25 (1/5, 20%)
X^MO ($n = 9$)	537 ± 50 (3/9, 33%)	826 ± 63 (5/9, 56%)	540 ± 59 (3/9, 33%)	566 ± 44 (2/7, 29%)

Mean ± Standard Deviation; parentheses reflect proportion of mice > 2 SDs from the XX mean.

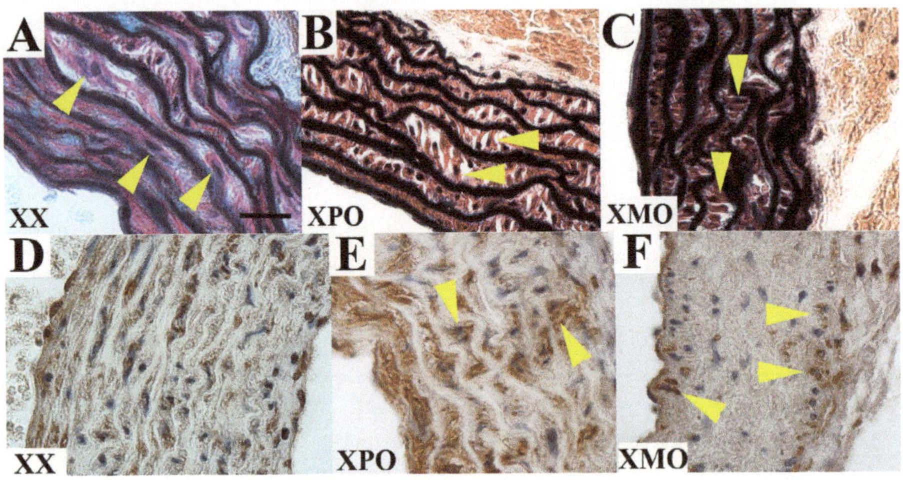

Figure 2. Aorta smooth muscle cell orientation is abnormal in both 39,X^MO and 39,X^PO mice, but content is decreased in 39,X^MO mice only. High magnification of the ascending aorta in adult 40,XX wild type controls (**A**) 39,X^PO (**B**) and 39,X^MO (**C**) mice demonstrate intact elastic fiber architecture and subtle smooth muscle cell misalignment abnormalities in both 39,X^PO and 39,X^MO mice. Note the plane of the smooth muscle cells in the 39, XO mice (yellow arrowheads) is orthogonal to the plane of elastic fibers, when compared with the normal parallel orientation of the cells (yellow arrowheads in panel H). SMA staining shows normal diffuse expression in 40,XX (**D**) aortas, as well as 39,X^PO (**E**) aortas despite the cell orientation abnormality, but significantly decreased expression in 39,X^MO mice (**F**). Panels are shown at 100×; scale bar 25 μm.

3.3. Discussion

Here we have demonstrated preliminary evidence for aortic valve malformation and aortopathy in the 39,XO mouse. Our aortic data from mutant mice suggest abnormalities in smooth muscle cell adhesion to the elastic fiber, similar to previous studies in a mouse model of aortopathy [23], but not overt elastic fiber pathology, and a propensity for latent dilation of the proximal aorta, particularly in 39,X^MO subjects. Aortic dilation in 39,XO mice is consistent with observations in TS individuals with aortic valve pathology [24]; unfortunately as our aortic valve and aortic size measurements were assessed from short and long axis sections respectively, we could not determine the frequency of both defects being present in the same individual mice. Further *in vivo* work in large cohorts of older 39,XO animals, as well as replication in other inbred strains, will be required to identify mechanisms underlying the aberrant smooth muscle orientation observation, to verify any dilated aorta phenotype, and to more accurately ascertain its prevalence, age of onset, potential POEs and relevance to pathophysiology. While the variable ages used in this study do not impact the evaluation of a congenital defect like BAV, they do confound the determination of TAA since the manifestation of this disease is typically sometime after birth. In addition, a more comprehensive assessment of cardiac structure in these mice is warranted to evaluate for subtle but clinically significant CVM associated with TS, such as partial anomalous pulmonary venous return. The finding of a quadricuspid aortic valve suggests there is a related spectrum of aortic valve malformation ranging from unicuspid to quadricuspid, a concept that has been forwarded previously [25]. While there was no conspicuous evidence of more severe CVM, such as hypoplastic left heart syndrome (HLHS), it is important to note that 39,XO mice, unlike TS patients, do not appear to show significant *in utero* mortality, an observation that may represent a significant limitation of the model but also suggests this mouse may be a good model for individuals with TS who survive to birth, including those who may be XX, XO mosaics. Lymphatic abnormalities resulting in hydrops are widely regarded as the primary cause of fetal loss in TS. Studies have sought to establish that "flow-related" CVMs, ranging from BAV to HLHS are caused by the hygroma in TS, but CVM occurs without lymphatic abnormality, fetal loss occurs in the absence of CVM, and severe CVM, including HLHS, is viable in TS [26,27], suggesting that CVM is neither necessary nor sufficient for fetal loss in TS. The lack of fetal loss in mice may be attributable to the fact that far fewer X-linked genes escape X-inactivation in the mouse than in humans (hence the loss of an X chromosome is less deleterious).

Our aortic valve malformation data indicate an overall prevalence of ~8% in 39,XO mice (consistent with increased rates in TS) with 39,X^MO mice being selectively affected. While this putative X-linked POE on aortic valve morphology cannot be explained by cryptic mosaicism, it could theoretically result from the fact that the 39,X^MO mice are generated from a separate cross to 40,XX and 39,X^PO mice; the fact that the 39,X^MO mice were born to wild type 40,XX mothers, and raised in identical conditions to the other two experimental groups strongly argues against this possibility. The most parsimonious explanation for this finding is that there are one or more X-linked imprinted genes that influence aortic valve development in mice; the expression/function of these genes might be affected by modifier genes and/or the environment, hence why not all 39,X^MO mice exhibited aortic valve abnormalities. To date, the only X-linked gene known to be imprinted in the mouse heart is *Xlr3b*, the expression of which is approximately 12-fold greater in 39,X^MO than 39,X^PO mice during late embryogenesis [16]. The function(s) of *Xlr3b* are currently unknown, but roles in chromatin metabolism and in response to toxic insults have been suggested [14,28]. Therefore, *Xlr3b* represents a potentially important genetic candidate for predisposing to developmental aortic valve abnormalities in mice, and further work on the role of this protein within the mammalian heart is warranted. It will also be worthwhile comparing gene expression in 39,X^PO and 39,X^MO heart tissue to identify novel underlying X-linked imprinted gene candidates.

In terms of relevance to Turner syndrome, our data indicate two possibilities: (i) there is an X-linked POE on aortic valve morphology in mice but not in humans due to species' different physiology; or (ii) there is an X-linked POE in both species, in the same direction, and of a similar magnitude. It is possible that, in some studies, an X-linked POE in humans could have been obscured by the presence of mosaicism (*i.e.*, 46,XX and 45,X^MO cells in some individuals), by the relatively low frequency of abnormalities in the 45,X^M group, and/or by using scanning techniques to examine cardiac morphology rather than *post mortem* histology. An obvious candidate gene for any X-linked POE on aortic valve development in humans is *FAM9B*, the closest orthologue of *Xlr3b* [16]. *FAM9B* is located on the short arm of the X chromosome at Xp22.32 within a region recently shown to be important in aortic valve and aorta development [29]. In an additional analysis, we have shown that *FAM9B* is polymorphically expressed in human aortic valves (Figure 3). In this small sample, there was no clear relationship between *FAM9B* expression status and gender (male or female), aortic valve morphology (tricuspid or bicuspid), or the presence of aortic valve disease (AVD) (pediatric or adult). Whether *FAM9B* is imprinted in human heart tissue, why it is polymorphically expressed in the aortic valve, and how it influences cardiac biology remains to be investigated.

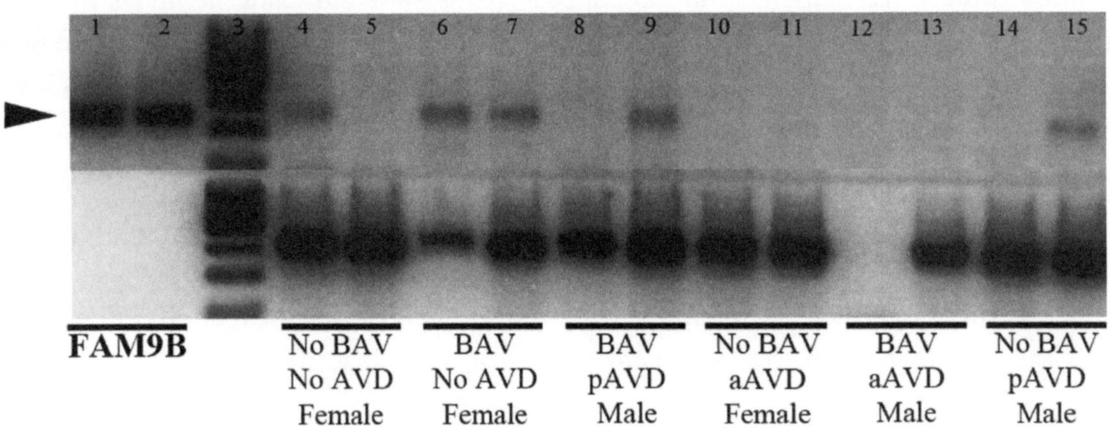

Figure 3. *FAM9B* is polymorphically expressed in human aortic valve tissue. *FAM9B* is expressed in control (No BAV, No AVD) human aortic valve tissue; however, there is no clear relationship between *FAM9B* expression (black arrowhead at ~275 bp) status, when compared with positive control expression from a human *FAM9B* cDNA clone (left columns), and aortic valve morphology (tricuspid or bicuspid), the presence of aortic valve disease (pediatric or adult), or gender (male or female). Samples were run simultaneously two per group (black bars), except BAV aAVD Male due to a technical failure (lane 12), and beta-actin (ACTB) was used as the housekeeping gene. BAV bicuspid aortic valve; AVD aortic valve disease; p: pediatric; a: adult; loading control (lane 3).

4. Conclusions

In summary, our findings suggest the 39,XO mouse as a much-needed animal model for examination of the biological mechanisms underlying the cardiovascular findings in Turner syndrome, and indicate that there may be important genetic modifiers on the X chromosome in nonsyndromic BAV, aortic valve disease and aortopathy. Specifically, our work suggests *FAM9B* as a potential novel X-linked genetic modulator of CVM risk.

Acknowledgments

The work was supported by a Research Councils United Kingdom Fellowship to W.D., a Cardiff University LINK Award to L.S.W., and by core Medical Research Council (MRC) funding (U117532009) to O.A.O. We would like to thank the animal technicians at MRC National Institute of Medical Research and Cardiff University for their expert animal husbandry.

Author Contributions

Study conception and design: R.B.H., W.D.; Acquisition of data: R.B.H., A.M.O., O.A.O., W.D.; Analysis and interpretation of data: R.B.H., L.S.W., W.D.; Drafting of manuscript: R.B.H., W.D.; Critical revision and final approval of manuscript: R.B.H., A.M.O., O.A.O., L.S.W., W.D.

Conflicts of Interest

The authors declare no conflict of interest.

References

1. Sybert, V.P.; McCauley, E. Turner's syndrome. *N. Engl. J. Med.* **2004**, *351*, 1227–1238.
2. Sachdev, V.; Matura, L.A.; Sidenko, S.; Ho, V.B.; Arai, A.E.; Rosing, D.R.; Bondy, C.A. Aortic valve disease in Turner syndrome. *J. Am. Coll. Cardiol.* **2008**, *51*, 1904–1909.
3. Sybert, V.P. Cardiovascular malformations and complications in Turner syndrome. *Pediatrics* **1998**, *101*, E11.
4. Lin, A.E.; Lippe, B.; Rosenfeld, R.G. Further delineation of aortic dilation, dissection, and rupture in patients with Turner syndrome. *Pediatrics* **1998**, *102*, e12.
5. Carrel, L.; Willard, H.F. X-inactivation profile reveals extensive variability in X-linked gene expression in females. *Nature* **2005**, *434*, 400–404.
6. Chu, C.E.; Donaldson, M.D.; Kelnar, C.J.; Smail, P.J.; Greene, S.A.; Paterson, W.F.; Connor, J.M. Possible role of imprinting in the Turner phenotype. *J. Med. Genet.* **1994**, *31*, 840–842.
7. Lepage, J.F.; Hong, D.S.; Mazaika, P.K.; Raman, M.; Sheau, K.; Marzelli, M.J.; Hallmayer, J.; Reiss, A.L. Genomic imprinting effects of the X chromosome on brain morphology. *J. Neurosci.* **2013**, *33*, 8567–8574.
8. Sagi, L.; Zuckerman-Levin, N.; Gawlik, A.; Ghizzoni, L.; Buyukgebiz, A.; Rakover, Y.; Bistritzer, T.; Admoni, O.; Vottero, A.; Baruch, O.; *et al.* Clinical significance of the parental origin of the X chromosome in turner syndrome. *J. Clin. Endocrinol. Metab.* **2007**, *92*, 846–852.

9. Skuse, D.H.; James, R.S.; Bishop, D.V.; Coppin, B.; Dalton, P.; Aamodt-Leeper, G.; Bacarese-Hamilton, M.; Creswell, C.; McGurk, R.; Jacobs, P.A. Evidence from Turner's syndrome of an imprinted X-linked locus affecting cognitive function. *Nature* **1997**, *387*, 705–708.
10. Abd-Elmoniem, K.Z.; Bakalov, V.K.; Matta, J.R.; Muldoon, N.; Hanover, J.A.; Bondy, C.A.; Gharib, A.M. X Chromosome Parental Origin and Aortic Stiffness in Turner Syndrome. *Clin. Endocrinol.* **2014**, *81*, 467–470.
11. Davies, M.J.; Treasure, T.; Richardson, P.D. The pathogenesis of spontaneous arterial dissection. *Heart* **1996**, *75*, 434–435.
12. Bondy, C.A.; Matura, L.A.; Wooten, N.; Troendle, J.; Zinn, A.R.; Bakalov, V.K. The physical phenotype of girls and women with Turner syndrome is not X-imprinted. *Hum. Genet.* **2007**, *121*, 469–474.
13. Ko, J.M.; Kim, J.M.; Kim, G.H.; Lee, B.H.; Yoo, H.W. Influence of parental origin of the X chromosome on physical phenotypes and GH responsiveness of patients with Turner syndrome. *Clin. Endocrinol.* **2010**, *73*, 66–71.
14. Davies, W.; Isles, A.R.; Burgoyne, P.S.; Wilkinson, L.S. X-linked imprinting: Effects on brain and behaviour. *Bioessays* **2006**, *28*, 35–44.
15. Henn, W.; Zang, K.D. Mosaicism in Turner's syndrome. *Nature* **1997**, *390*, 569, doi:10.1038/37514.
16. Davies, W.; Isles, A.; Smith, R.; Karunadasa, D.; Burrmann, D.; Humby, T.; Ojarikre, O.; Biggin, C.; Skuse, D.; Burgoyne, P.; *et al. Xlr3b* is a new imprinted candidate for X-linked parent-of-origin effects on cognitive function in mice. *Nat. Genet.* **2005**, *37*, 625–629.
17. Lynn, P.M.; Davies, W. The 39,XO mouse as a model for the neurobiology of Turner syndrome and sex-biased neuropsychiatric disorders. *Behav. Brain Res.* **2007**, *179*, 173–182.
18. Hinton, R.B. Bicuspid aortic valve and thoracic aortic aneurysm: Three patient populations, two disease phenotypes, and one shared genotype. *Cardiol. Res. Pract.* **2012**, *2012*, 926975, doi:10.1155/2012/926975.
19. Hinton, R.B.; Alfieri, C.M.; Witt, S.A.; Glascock, B.J.; Khoury, P.R.; Benson, D.W.; Yutzey, K.E. Mouse heart valve structure and function: Echocardiographic and morphometric analyses from the fetus through the aged adult. *Am. J. Physiol. Heart Circ. Physiol.* **2008**, *294*, H2480–H2488.
20. Matura, L.A.; Ho, V.B.; Rosing, D.R.; Bondy, C.A. Aortic dilatation and dissection in Turner syndrome. *Circulation* **2007**, *116*, 1663–1670.
21. Carlson, M.; Airhart, N.; Lopez, L.; Silberbach, M. Moderate aortic enlargement and bicuspid aortic valve are associated with aortic dissection in Turner syndrome: Report of the international turner syndrome aortic dissection registry. *Circulation* **2012**, *126*, 2220–2226.
22. Hinton, R.B.; Lincoln, J.; Deutsch, G.H.; Osinska, H.; Manning, P.B.; Benson, D.W.; Yutzey, K.E. Extracellular matrix remodeling and organization in developing and diseased aortic valves. *Circ. Res.* **2006**, *98*, 1431–1438.
23. Bunton, T.E.; Biery, N.J.; Myers, L.; Gayraud, B.; Ramirez, F.; Dietz, H.C. Phenotypic alteration of vascular smooth muscle cells precedes elastolysis in a mouse model of Marfan syndrome. *Circ. Res.* **2001**, *88*, 37–43.
24. Olivieri, L.J.; Baba, R.Y.; Arai, A.E.; Bandettini, W.P.; Rosing, D.R.; Bakalov, V.; Sachdev, V.; Bondy, C.A. Spectrum of aortic valve abnormalities associated with aortic dilation across age groups in Turner syndrome. *Circ. Cardiovasc. Imaging* **2013**, *6*, 1018–1023.

25. Ward, C. Clinical significance of the bicuspid aortic valve. *Heart* **2000**, *83*, 81–85.
26. Lacro, R.V.; Jones, K.L.; Benirschke, K. Coarctation of the aorta in Turner syndrome: A pathologic study of fetuses with nuchal cystic hygromas, hydrops fetalis, and female genitalia. *Pediatrics* **1988**, *81*, 445–451.
27. Iyer, N.P.; Tucker, D.F.; Roberts, S.H.; Moselhi, M.; Morgan, M.; Matthes, J.W. Outcome of fetuses with Turner syndrome: A 10-year congenital anomaly register based study. *J. Matern. Fetal Neonatal Med.* **2012**, *25*, 68–73.
28. Davies, W. Genomic imprinting on the X chromosome: Implications for brain and behavioral phenotypes. *Ann. N.Y. Acad. Sci.* **2010**, *1204*, E14–E19.
29. Bondy, C.A.; Bakalov, V.K.; Cheng, C.; Olivieri, L.; Rosing, D.R.; Arai, A.E. Bicuspid aortic valve and aortic coarctation are linked to deletion of the X chromosome short arm in Turner syndrome. *J. Med. Genet.* **2013**, *50*, 662–665.

10

Imaging of Mitral Valve Prolapse: What Can We Learn from Imaging about the Mechanism of the Disease?

Ronen Durst * and Dan Gilon

Heart Institute, Ein Kerem Campus, Hadassah Hebrew University Medical Center, POB 12000, 92110 Jerusalem, Israel; E-Mail: dangi@ekmd.huji.ac.il

* Author to whom correspondence should be addressed; E-Mail: durst@hadassah.org.il

Academic Editors: Russell Norris and Cheryl L. Maslen

Abstract: Mitral valve prolapse (MVP) is the most common mitral valve disorder affecting 2%–3% of the general population. Two histological forms for the disease exist: Myxomatous degeneration and fibroelastic disease. Pathological evidence suggests the disease is not confined solely to the valve tissue, and accumulation of proteoglycans and fibrotic tissue can be seen in the adjacent myocardium of MVP patients. MVP is diagnosed by demonstrating valve tissue passing the annular line into the left atrium during systole. In this review we will discuss the advantages and limitations of various imaging modalities in their MVP diagnosis ability as well as the potential for demonstrating extra associated valvular pathologies.

Keywords: mitral valve prolapse; imaging; myxomatous degeneration; fibroelastic deficiency

---

1. History of MVP Diagnosis

MVP is a common cardiovascular disorder, originally described in the 1960s and is considered today the most common cause of mitral regurgitation [1–3]. Barlow and Bosman described a constellation of clinical findings consisting of non-ejection systolic clicks and a late systolic murmur, T-wave abnormalities, and systolic aneurysmal billowing of the posterior mitral leaflet into the left atrium on left ventriculography [4]. MVP is defined by the abnormal relationship of the mitral leaflets to their surrounding structures as diagnosed by imaging. In early studies, MVP prevalence was considered to be between 5% and 15%, with some estimates even as high as 35% [5–10]. These studies relied on auscultation and single-dimensional M-mode echo techniques, which provide only a limited appreciation of cardiac anatomy and produce varying results depending on the orientation of the ultrasound transducer on the chest [11–14]. Despite the improved spatial appreciation and view standardization achieved with two-dimensional echocardiography, similarly high diagnostic rates could still be obtained based on the assumption that the mitral annulus is planar, and that leaflet displacement relative to the annulus in any view is abnormal [15–17]. Three-dimensional echocardiographic pioneering studies by Levine and colleagues have shown that the mitral annulus is not a flat plane but rather has a saddle-like shape with high points positioned anteriorly and posteriorly and low points medially and laterally (Figure 1) [16–19]. Recognition of the saddle shape has significantly increased the specificity of diagnostic criteria without loss of sensitivity. Commonly today, a displacement of 2 mm or above of the leaflet above the annular plane in parasternal long axis view is considered diagnostic (Figure 2A) [4,20]. The three-dimensional understanding of the mitral valve shape and the new more accurate MVP diagnostic criteria have reduced the prevalence of the disease in various series to 2%–3% of the general population [3,14]. Strengthening the accuracy of this criterion is the fact that it has been used in genetic studies to successfully clone MVP segregating allelic loci [21,22]. The definition of MVP is based on demonstrating the anatomical relation between mitral valve leaflet excursion into the left atrium relative to the annulus. Often, pathologies are found in other valve as well. Sometimes the tricuspid valve demonstrates prolapsing segments and leakage, although criteria for defining tricuspid valve prolapse are currently lacking. In some instances, aortic valve pathologies in families segregating MVP were reported [23–25]. This relation can be demonstrated by non-invasive imaging. Imaging can also provide an insight into the pathology associated with valve structure as well as potential myocardial abnormalities. The purpose of this paper is to review the advantages and limitations of the various imaging modalities in diagnosing MVP and related pathologies.

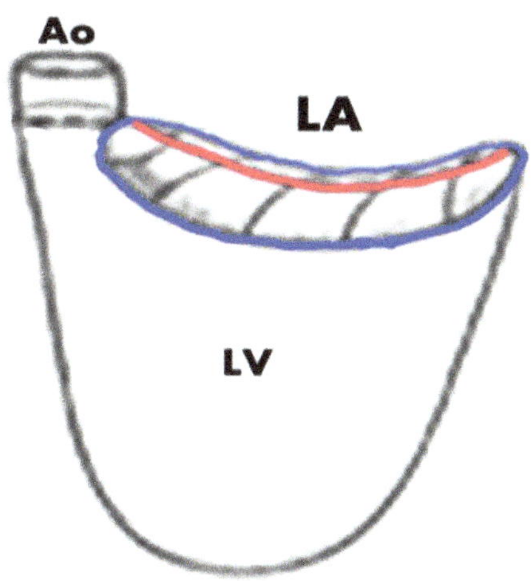

Figure 1. Scheme of the mitral valve anatomy with the saddle shaped annulus (**blue**) and the plane of the valve as seen in para-sternal long axis view on echo (**pale red**) showing the two high points of the annulus. Ao = aorta, LV = left ventricle, LA = left atrium.

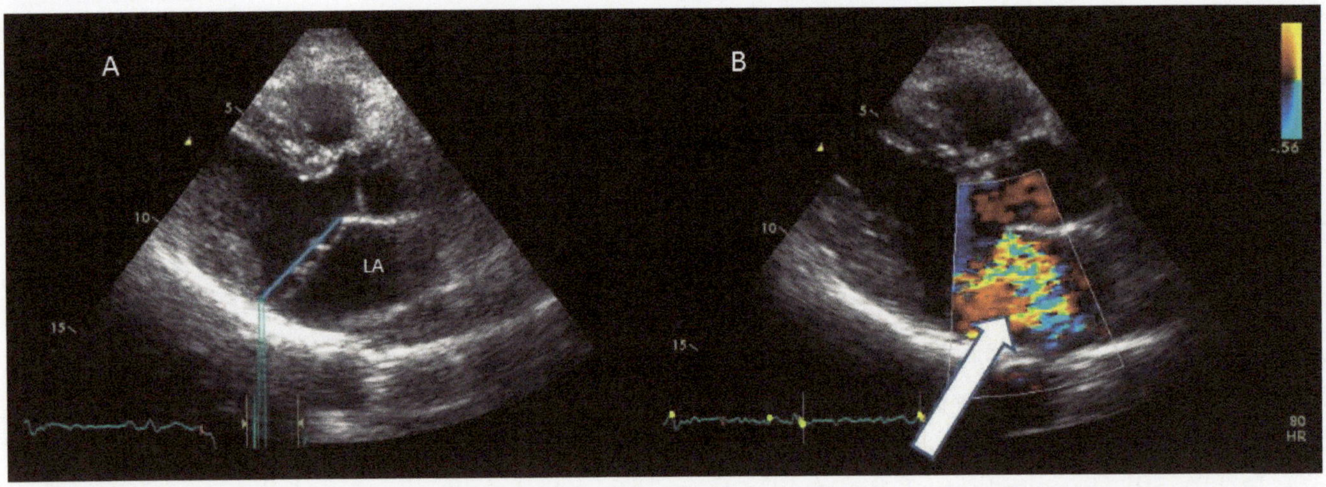

Figure 2. A parasternal long axis view of a prolapsing valve. Panel **A** shows the prolapsing valve relative to the annular line (**blue line**). Panel **B** shows color Doppler through the prolapsing valve demonstrating a severe jet of regurgitation (**arrow**). LA = left atrium.

2. Echocardiography

Degenerative processes resulting in regurgitation of the mitral valve have two main phenotypes: Diffuse myxomatous degeneration (or "Barlow disease"), which may present as a genetic disorder, and a markedly different fibroelastic deficiency (FED) [1,26], which might be caused by an accelerated aging process. Barlow disease is characterized by excess connective tissue, with redundant, thickened and yellowish leaflets, marked annulus dilatation, elongated and thin (sometimes ruptured) or thick (frequently calcified) chordae, disrupted collagen and elastic layers, and with excess of acid mucopolyssacharides. Patients with MVP usually present young or at middle aged after a long history of murmur and/or mitral regurgitation (Figure 2B). Familial clustering of MVP has recently been described in the Framingham heart study [27,28]. Myxomatous degeneration is sometimes associated with connective tissure disorders, such as Marfan's disease, Loeys–Dietz syndrome, Ehlers–Danlos syndrome and Stickler syndrome. It may also be non-syndromic [4]. FED is characterized by decreased connective tissue, deficient in collagen, elastin and proteoglycans; thin, smooth and translucent leaflets without excess tissue and only moderate annulus dilatation; and thin, slightly elongated chordae. Patients frequently present at an older age with chordal rupture and flail after a rather shorter clinical history. While most of the leaflet is thin, localized myxomatous degeneration and thickening occur within the flail scallop, mainly of the posterior leaflet [28–30].

Pathological processes in MVP are not limited to the valves only. Pathological studies of MVP patients with sudden death or death from other causes have shown proteoglycan depositions similar to the deposition within the leaflet also in the myocardial tissue, fibrous endocardial plaque depositions, and non-specific interstitial fibrosis [31–35]. These depositions are thought to play a role in the increased tendency of MVP patients for cardiac arrhythmia, sudden death and chest pain [35,36]. Few studies tried to define echocardiographic criteria to differentiate FED from myxomatous degeneration. Because FED patients tend to be of older age, FED is more often associated with other marks of degenerative valve disease such as annular calcification, aortic sclerosis and pupillary muscle calcification [37,38]. In contrast, myxomatous valves usually show billowing of the body of one or both leaflets with prolapse of the margin of either or both leaflets adjacent to the annular ring. The valve is typically large, with elongated and redundant billowing leaflets; leaflets are bulky and thickened. Leaflet thickness often exceeds 3 mm. Another common feature is displacement of the insertion of the posterior leaflet away from the ventricular crest and toward the atrium, creating an out-pouching at the leaflet base [38]. While these features may help clinicians differentiate FED from myxomatous degeneration, studies are needed to define the sensitivity and specificity of echocardiography in discriminating between the two. This is particularly important because FED tends to have a favorable surgical outcome, whereas myxomatous degeneration is probably more likely to have a genetic etiology. First degree relatives of patients with myxomatous mitral valve disease should be screened by echocardiography.

Echocardiography can be used to assess pathologies in other valves. Echocardiographic definition for tricuspid valve prolapse is still lacking. With the advent of three-dimensional imaging, authors have suggested that 3D images are more suitable for defining the prolapsing segment of the tricuspid valve as well as better define the regurgitant orifice area [39].

Echocardiography is the most widely used imaging tool for evaluating cardiac function. For clinicians, left ventricular chamber size as well as function, and regurgitation severity are important for clinical decision making.

3. Magnetic Resonance Imaging (MRI)

In recent years cardiac MRI has emerged as a practical, non-invasive tool for cardiac imaging. MRI has several advantages over echocardiography. These include the ability for tissue characterization, unlimited imaging planes, it does not depend on an acoustic window, and it is less invasive then transesophageal echocardiography [40]. Han *et al.* were the first to provide a practical road map for MVP evaluation by MRI [41]. Understanding the saddle shape of mitral valve, Han *et al.* chose a stack of cine SSFP images in the LVOT view spanning the entire mitral valve to evaluate MVP (Figure 3). These imaging planes do not only parallel parasternal long axis and apical long axis of echo in showing the two mitral annulus high points in the a single image, but also enables definition of the prolapsing segments (scallop) [42]. With this approach, the sensitivity and specificity of MVP detection was as high as 100% compared to echocardiography. MRI was also proven to be accurate in evaluating the mitral valve annular dimensions, which may be important whenever a mitral valve prosthesis implantation or repair is planned [43]. While these results are very promising, several topics need to be considered: First, the views used in this study are not routine in every cardiac MRI study [44]. Therefore, the sensitivity specificity reported might only be applied to studies planned a priori for MVP evaluation in which all the relevant image planes have been obtained. Second, one of the key characteristics of myxomatous changes occurring in many patients with MVP is valve thickening. MRI, due to insufficient spatial resolution and volume averaging effect, failed to demonstrate valve thickening.

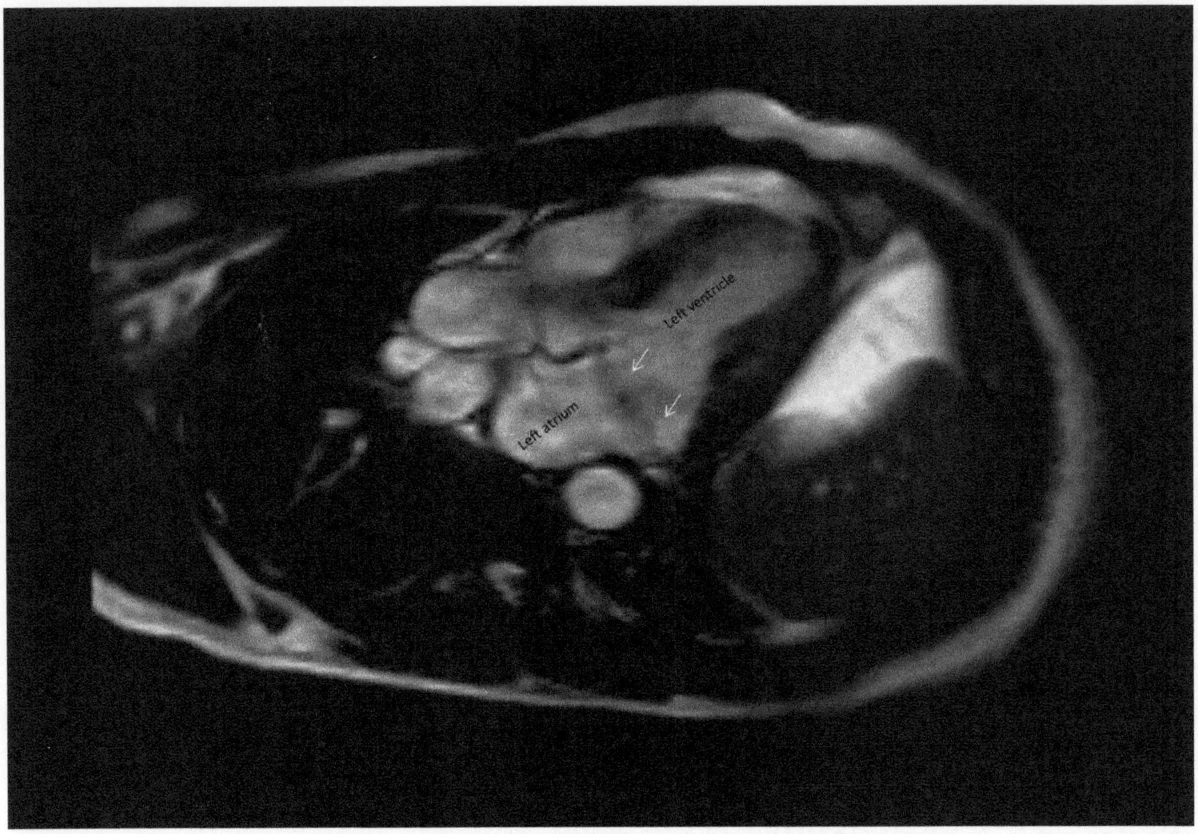

Figure 3. A steady state free precession image on parasternal long axis view of the mitral valve. Note the atrial displacement of both leaflets (arrows).

MRI, like echocardiography, can provide information on the severity of regurgitation. MRI can provide an estimate of the volume of regurgitation and its relation with the overall left ventricular ejection fraction [43]. On the technical level, the volume of mitral regurgitation is quantified indirectly by subtracting the forward flow over the aorta, measured directly with phase-contrast sequence from the left ventricular ejected volume as measured volumetrically. The mitral regurgitant volume is the calculated difference between the LV stroke volume, and the aortic forward stroke volume [45].

One of the major advantages of MRI is the ability for tissue characterization. Several studies were able to demonstrate pathological delayed enhancement in the papillary muscle and other regions of the myocardium [41,46,47]. One study demonstrated increased extracellular space by T1 mapping [47]. These delayed enhancement patterns and increased extracellular space may represent fibrosis or proteoglycan depositions or fibrosis. Indeed, myocardial histological analysis of patients demonstrated diffuse fibrosis [47]. The clinical significance of delayed enhancement in MVP patients is unclear. However, in the future, these myocardial changes may prove to correlate with MVP complications such as sudden death or heart failure and therefore may be useful for clinical decision processes and for prognostication.

MRI can provide high-resolution volumetric images of the left ventricle as well as provide quantitative assessment of regurgitant volume. These are important for clinical decision-making and are an added value of MR imaging.

4. Computed Tomography (CT)

Computed tomography (CT) of the heart has emerged in recent years as valuable tool for noninvasive imaging of the heart. It provides high-resolution volumetric datasets that can be post-processed to provide views suitable for MVP diagnosis. After acquisition, images in planes demonstrating both superior aspect of the saddle shaped annulus of the mitral valve are generated. The relation between valve leaflets and annulus can be studied, and the degree of leaflet displacement can be measured [48]. An important advantage of CT over echocardiography is that it allows for the visualization of adjacent anatomic structures, such as the coronary sinus and coronary arteries, which cannot be easily demonstrated by other imaging modalities. Several studies compared the diagnostic accuracy of CT with that of echocardiography and intraoperative findings. They found sensitivity and specificity of 84%–96% and 93%–100%, respectively, compared with echo and had excellent agreement with operative findings in defining the culprit scallop of the valve [48–51]. Other studies failed to demonstrate high correlation with operative findings in demonstrating the prolapsing segment [52]. Additional advantages of CT include the ability to demonstrate thicker valve leaflets compared with controls and the ability to map flailing segments. However, there is no study showing that CT can discriminate between myxomatous degeneration and FED. Also, CT cannot help in tissue characterization and, unlike MRI, it cannot demonstrate myocardial pathology. CT has several other disadvantages compared to the other imaging modalities. CT utilizes ionizing radiation. Radiation exposure ranged in one study from 9–11 mSv [48]. Because systolic images are needed for MVP demonstration (in contrast with coronary angriogrphy where radiation exposure can be limited in many cases to diastole only), radiation reduction techniques cannot be used. While CT is suitable to evaluate left ventricular volume very accurately, it cannot be used to estimate the severity of regurgitation. Thus, although MVP imaging with CT is possible, it should not be used as the preferred imaging modality, unless other clinical information, such as coronary evaluation, which can be provided by CT is needed.

5. Nuclear Imaging

Patients with MVP often complain of palpitations and chest discomfort. These symptoms have led to a notion of increased prevalence of anxiety disorders in MVP patients. This has been referred to as "mitral valve prolapse syndrome" [53]. The association between MVP and anxiety disorders is currently doubted [54]. Several studies of thallium myocardial perfusion scans on MVP patients demonstrated evidence for ischemia in these patients. These studies suggested a possible explanation for the increased prevalence of chest pain and palpitations. The results were conflicting. While some studies showed evidence for ischemia in patients with normal coronaries, particularly at the insertion point of the pupillary muscle, others showed no evidence for it [54–57]. These changes were considered to be related to either ischemia of small vessels or fibrosis in the hypo perfused areas [56]. Because of inconsistent findings in these various studies, it is difficult to conclude whether ischemic changes truly exist in MVP patients and what is their clinical significance. Nuclear imaging is routinely used for quantification of chamber size and function, because they are important for clinical evaluation of the patients.

6. Conclusions

MVP is diagnosed by imaging modalities by demonstrating valve leaflets ascending into the left atrium passing over the two high points of the saddle shaped annulus into the left atrium during systole. Echocardiography has a central role in diagnosis of MVP and is used as the main tool for this purpose. High special resolution imaging modalities such as MRI and CT can also demonstrate the anatomical relation between the mitral valve annular line and leaflet excursion needed for appropriate diagnosis. The now well-established criteria for definition of MVP based on proper understanding of the mitral valve three-dimensional anatomy and shape has allowed better definition of the disease culminating in finding gene and biological pathways leading to myxomatous degeneration and prolapse. Pathological findings in MVP are not confined to the valve tissue only. Some imaging modalities, such as MRI and, to a lesser, extent nuclear imaging, have demonstrated pathologies in muscle tissue of MVP patients. The pathological correlates of these findings, however, as well as their clinical significance are currently uncertain.

Acknowledgments

This work was supported by the European Union international reintegration program-PIRG08-2010-276984-MVP gen.

Conflicts of Interest

The authors declare no conflict of interest.

References

1. Barlow, J.B.; Bosman, C.K. Aneurysmal protrusion of the posterior leaflet of the mitral valve. An auscultatory-electrocardiographic syndrome. *Am. Heart J.* **1966**, *71*, 166–178.
2. Devereux, R.B.; Brown, W.T.; Kramer-Fox, R.; Sachs, I. Inheritance of mitral valve prolapse: Effect of age and sex on gene expression. *Ann. Intern. Med.* 1982, **97**, 826–832.
3. Freed, L.A.; Levy, D.; Levine, R.A.; Larson, M.G.; Evans, J.C.; Fuller, D.L.; Lehman, B.; Benjamin, E.J. Prevalence and clinical outcome of mitral-valve prolapse. *N. Engl. J. Med.* **1999**, *341*, 1–7.
4. Nishimura, R.A.; McGoon, M.D. *Perspectives on Mitral-Valve Prolapse. N. Engl. J. Med.* **1999**, *341*, 48–50.
5. Markiewicz, W.; Stoner, J.; London, E.; Hunt, S.A.; Popp, R.L. Mitral valve prolapse in one hundred presumably healthy young females. *Circulation* **1976**, *53*, 464–473.
6. Procacci, P.M.; Savran, S.V.; Schreiter, S.L.; Bryson, A.L. Prevalence of clinical mitral-valve prolapse in 1169 young women. *N. Engl. J. Med.* **1976**, *294*, 1086–1088.
7. Savage, D.D.; Devereux, R.B.; Garrison, R.J.; Castelli, W.P.; Anderson, S.J.; Levy, D.; Thomas, H.E.; Kannel, W.B.; Feinleib, M. Mitral valve prolapse in the general population. 2. Clinical features: The Framingham Study. *Am. Heart J.* **1983**, *106*, 577–581.

8. Savage, D.D.; Devereux, R.B.; Garrison, R.J.; Castelli, W.P.; Anderson, S.J.; Levy, D.; Thomas, H.E.; Kannel, W.B.; Feinleib, M. Mitral valve prolapse in the general population. 1. Epidemiologic features: The Framingham Study. *Am. Heart J.* **1983**, *106*, 571–576.
9. Bryhn, M.; Persson, S. The prevalence of mitral valve prolapse in healthy men and women in Sweden. An echocardiographic study. *Acta Med. Scand.* **1984**, *215*, 157–160.
10. Levy, D.; Savage, D. Prevalence and clinical features of mitral valve prolapse. *Am. Heart J.* **1987**, *113*, 1281–1290.
11. Shah, P.M. Echocardiographic diagnosis of mitral valve prolapse. *J. Am. Soc. Echocardiogr.* **1994**, *7*, 286–293.
12. Markiewicz, W.; London, E.; Popp, R.L. Effect of transducer placement on echocardiographic mitral valve motion. *Am. Heart J.* **1978**, *96*, 555–556.
13. Leatham, A.; Brigden, W. Mild mitral regurgitation and the mitral prolapse fiasco. *Am. Heart J.* **1980**, *99*, 659–664.
14. Gilon, D.; Buonanno, F.S.; Joffe, M.M.; Leavitt, M.; Marshall, J.E.; Kistler, J.P.; Levine, R.A. Lack of evidence of an association between mitral-valve prolapse and stroke in young patients. *N. Engl. J. Med.* **1999**, *341*, 8–13.
15. Warth, D.C.; King, M.E.; Cohen, J.M.; Tesoriero, V.L.; Marcus, E.; Weyman, A.E. Prevalence of mitral valve prolapse in normal children. *J. Am. Coll. Cardiol.* **1985**, *5*, 1173–1177.
16. Levine, R.A.; Triulzi, M.O.; Harrigan, P.; Weyman, A.E. The relationship of mitral annular shape to the diagnosis of mitral valve prolapse. *Circulation* **1987**, *75*, 756–767.
17. Levine, R.A.; Stathogiannis, E.; Newell, J.B.; Harrigan, P.; Weyman, A.E. Reconsideration of echocardiographic standards for mitral valve prolapse: Lack of association between leaflet displacement isolated to the apical four chamber view and independent echocardiographic evidence of abnormality. *J. Am. Coll. Cardiol.* **1988**, *11*, 1010–1019.
18. Levine, R.A.; Handschumacher, M.D.; Sanfilippo, A.J.; Hagege, A.A.; Harrigan, P.; Marshall, J.E.; Weyman, A.E. Three-dimensional echocardiographic reconstruction of the mitral valve, with implications for the diagnosis of mitral valve prolapse. *Circulation* **1989**, *80*, 589–598.
19. Perloff, J.K.; Child, J.S. Mitral valve prolapse. Evolution and refinement of diagnostic techniques. *Circulation* **1989**, *80*, 710–711.
20. Bonow, R.; Carabello, B.; de Leon, A.C., Jr.; Edmunds, L.H., Jr.; Fedderly, B.J.; Freed, M.D.; Gaasch, W.H.; McKay, C.R.; Nishimura, R.A.; O'Gara, P.T. ACC/AHA guidelines for the management of patients with valvular heart disease: A report of the American College of Cardiology/American Heart Association Task Force on practice guidelines (Committee on management of patients with valvular heart disease). *J. Am. Coll. Cardiol.* **1998**, *32*, 1486–1582.
21. Freed, L.A.; Acierno, J.S., Jr.; Dai, D.; Leyne, M.; Marshall, J.E.; Nesta, F.; Levine, R.A.; Slaugenhaupt, S.A. A locus for autosomal dominant mitral valve prolapse on chromosome 11p15.4. *Am. J. Hum. Genet.* **2003**, *72*, 1551–1559.
22. Nesta, F.; Leyne, M.; Yosefy, C.; Simpson, C.; Dai, D.; Marshall, J.E.; Hung, J.; Slaugenhaupt, S.A.; Levine, R.A. New locus for autosomal dominant mitral valve prolapse on chromosome 13: Clinical insights from genetic studies. *Circulation* **2005**, *112*, 2022–2030.
23. Van Son, J.A.; Miles, C.M.; Starr, A. Tricuspid valve prolapse associated with myxomatous degeneration. *Ann. Thorac. Surg.* **1995**, *59*, 1237–1239.

24. Lardeux, A.; Kyndt, F.; Lecointe, S.; Marec, H.L.; Merot, J.; Schott, J.J.; Le Tourneau, T.; Probst, V. Filamin-A-Related Myxomatous Mitral Valve Dystrophy: Genetic, Echocardiographic and Functional Aspects. *J. Cardiovasc. Transl. Res.* **2011**, *4*, 748–756.
25. Weinreich, D.J.; Burke, J.F.; Bharati, S.; Lev, M. Isolated prolapse of the tricuspid valve. *J. Am. Coll. Cardiol.* **1985**, *6*, 475–481.
26. Carpentier, A.; Chauvaud, S.; Fabiani, J.N.; Deloche, A.; Relland, J.; Lessana, A.; D'Allaines, C.; Blondeau, P.; Piwnica, A.; Dubost, C. Reconstructive surgery of mitral valve incompetence: Ten-year appraisal. *J. Thorac. Cardiovasc. Surg.* **1980**, *79*, 338–348.
27. Delling, F.N.; Rong, J.; Larson, M.G.; Lehman, B.; Osypiuk, E.; Stantchev, P.; Slaugenhaupt, S.A.; Benjamin, E.J.; Levine, R.A.; Vasan, R.S. Familial clustering of mitral valve prolapse in the community. *Circulation* **2015**, *131*, 263–268.
28. Fornes, P.; Heudes, D.; Fuzellier, J.F.; Tixier, D.; Bruneval, P.; Carpentier, A. Correlation Between Clinical and Histologic Patterns of Degenerative Mitral Valve Insufficiency: A Histomorphometric Study of 130 Excised Segments. *Cardiovasc. Pathol.* **1999**, *8*, 81–92.
29. Messika-Zeitoun, D.; Topilsky, Y.; Enriquez-Sarano, M. The Role of Echocardiography in the Management of Patients with Myxomatous Disease. *Cardiol. Clin.* **2013**, *31*, 217–229.
30. Matsumaru, I.; Eishi, K.; Hashizume, K.; Kawano, H.; Tsuneto, A.; Hayashi, T. Clinical and pathological features of degenerative mitral valve disease: Billowing mitral leaflet versus fibroelastic deficiency. *Ann. Thorac. Cardiovasc. Surg.* **2014**, *20*, 987–994.
31. Morales, A.R.; Romanelli, R.; Boucek, R.J.; Tate, L.G.; Alvarez, R.T.; Davis, J.T. Myxoid heart disease: An assessment of extravalvular cardiac pathology in severe mitral valve prolapse. *Hum. Pathol.* **1992**, *23*, 129–137.
32. Farb, A.; Tang, A.L.; Atkinson, J.B.; McCarthy, W.F.; Virmani, R. Comparison of cardiac findings in patients with mitral valve prolapse who die suddenly to those who have congestive heart failure from mitral regurgitation and to those with fatal noncardiac conditions. *Am. J. Cardiol.* **1992**, *70*, 234–239.
33. Dollar, A.L.; Roberts, W.C. Morphologic comparison of patients with mitral valve prolapse who died suddenly with patients who died from severe valvular dysfunction or other conditions. *J. Am. Coll. Cardiol.* **1991**, *17*, 921–931.
34. La Vecchia, L.; Ometto, R.; Centofante, P.; Varotto, L.; Bonanno, C.; Bozzola, L.; Bevilacqua, P.; Vincenzi, M. Arrhythmic profile, ventricular function, and histomorphometric findings in patients with idiopathic ventricular tachycardia and mitral valve prolapse: Clinical and prognostic evaluation. *Clin. Cardiol.* **1998**, *21*, 731–735.
35. Burke, A.P.; Farb, A.; Tang, A.; Smialek, J.; Virmani, R. Fibromuscular dysplasia of small coronary arteries and fibrosis in the basilar ventricular septum in mitral valve prolapse. *Am. Heart J.* **1997**, *134*, 282–291.
36. Düren, D.R.; Becker, A.E.; Dunning, A.J. *Long*-term follow-up of idiopathic mitral valve prolapse in 300 patients: A prospective study. *J. Am. Coll. Cardiol.* **1988**, *11*, 42–47.
37. Adawil, S.; Aronson, D.; Halon, D.A.; Aviram, S.; Lewis, B.S.; Shiran, A. Non-myxomatous flail mitral valve: Clinical and echocardiographic characteristics and long-term clinical outcome. *J. Heart Valve Dis.* **2007**, *16*, 336–343.

38. Anyanwu, A.C.; Adams, D.H. Etiologic Classification of Degenerative Mitral Valve Disease: Barlow's Disease and Fibroelastic Deficiency. *Semin. Thorac. Cardiovasc. Surg.* **2007**, *19*, 90–96.
39. Elsayed, M.; Thind, M.; Nanda, N.C. Two- and Three-dimensional Transthoracic Echocardiographic Assessment of Tricuspid Valve Prolapse with Mid-to-Late Systolic Tricuspid Regurgitation. *Echocardiography* **2015**, *32*, 1022–1025.
40. Pennell, D.J. Cardiovascular Magnetic Resonance. *Circulation* **2010**, *121*, 692–705.
41. Han, Y.; Peters, D.C.; Salton, C.J.; Bzymek, D.; Nezafat, R.; Goddu, B.; Kissinger, K.V.; Zimetbaum, P.J.; Manning, W.J.; Yeon, S.B. Cardiovascular magnetic resonance characterization of mitral valve prolapse. *JACC Cardiovasc. Imaging* **2008**, *1*, 294–303.
42. Foster, G.P.; Isselbacher, E.M.; Rose, G.A.; Torchiana, D.F.; Akins, C.W.; Picard, M.H. Accurate Localization of Mitral Regurgitant Defects Using Multiplane Transesophageal Echocardiography. *Ann. Thorac. Surg.* **1998**, *65*, 1025–1031.
43. Christiansen, J.P.; Karamitsos, T.D.; Myerson, S.G. Assessment of Valvular Heart Disease by Cardiovascular Magnetic Resonance Imaging: A Review. *Heart Lung Circ.* **2011**, *20*, 73–82.
44. Boxt, L.M. From the RSNA Refresher Courses: Cardiac MR Imaging: A Guide for the Beginner. *Radiographics* **1999**, *19*, 1009–1025.
45. Chan, K.M.; Wage, R.; Symmonds, K.; Rahman-Haley, S.; Mohiaddin, R.H.; Firmin, D.N.; Pepper, J.R.; Pennell, D.J.; Kilner, P.J. Towards comprehensive assessment of mitral regurgitation using cardiovascular magnetic resonance. *J. Cardiovasc. Magn. Reson.* **2008**, *10*, 61, doi:10.1186/1532-429X-10-61.
46. Van de Heyning, C.M.; Magne, J.; Piérard, L.A.; Bruyère, P.J.; Davin, L.; de Maeyer, C.; Paelinck, B.P.; Vrints, C.J.; Lancellotti, P. Late gadolinium enhancement CMR in primary mitral regurgitation. *Eur. J. Clin. Investig.* **2014**, *44*, 840–847.
47. Edwards, N.C.; Moody, W.E.; Yuan, M.; Weale, P.; Neal, D.; Townend, J.N.; Steeds, R.P. Quantification of Left Ventricular Interstitial Fibrosis in Asymptomatic Chronic Primary Degenerative Mitral Regurgitation. *Circ.: Cardiovasc. Imaging* **2014**, *7*, 946–953.
48. Feuchtner, G.M.; Alkadhi, H.; Karlo, C.; Sarwar, A.; Meier, A.; Dichtl, W.; Leschka, S.; Blankstein, R.; Gruenenfelder, J.; Stolzmann, P.; *et al*. Cardiac CT Angiography for the Diagnosis of Mitral Valve Prolapse: Comparison with Echocardiography. *Radiology* **2010**, *254*, 374–383.
49. Smith, T.; Gurudevan, S.; Cheng, V.; Trento, A.; Derobertis, M.; Thomson, L.; Friedman, J.; Hayes, S.; Siegel, R.J.; Berman, D.S. Assessment of the morphological features of degenerative mitral valve disease using 64-slice multi detector computed tomography. *J. Cardiovasc. Comput. Tomogr.* **2012**, *6*, 415–421.
50. Shah, R.G.; Novaro, G.M.; Blandon, R.J.; Wilkinson, L.; Asher, C.R.; Kirsch, J. Mitral valve prolapse: Evaluation with ECG-gated cardiac CT angiography. *AJR Am. J. Roentgenol.* **2010**, *194*, 579–584.
51. Koo, H.J.; Yang, D.H.; Oh, S.Y.; Kang, J.W.; Kim, D.H.; Song, J.K.; Lee, J.W.; Chung, C.H.; Lim, T.H. Demonstration of Mitral Valve Prolapse with CT for Planning of Mitral Valve Repair. *RadioGraphics* **2014**, *34*, 1537–1552.
52. Ghosh, N.; Al-Shehri, H.; Chan, K.; Mesana, T.; Chan, V.; Chen, L.; Yam, Y.; Chow, B.J. Characterization of mitral valve prolapse with cardiac computed tomography: Comparison to echocardiographic and intraoperative findings. *Int. J. Cardiovasc. Imaging* **2012**, *28*, 855–863.

53. Hancock, E.W.; Cohn, K. The syndrome associated with midsystolic click and late systolic murmur. *Am. J. Med.* **1966**, *41*, 183–196.
54. Alpert, M.A.; Sabeti, M.; Kushner, M.G.; Beitman, B.D.; Russell, J.L.; Thiele, J.R.; Mukerji, V. Frequency of isolated panic attacks and panic disorder in patients with the mitral valve prolapse syndrome. *Am. J. Cardiol.* **1992**, *69*, 1489–1490.
55. Gaffney, F.A.; Wohl, A.J.; Blomqvist, C.G.; Parkey, R.W.; Willerson, J.T. Thallium-201 myocardial perfusion studies in patients with the mitral valve prolapse syndrome. *Am. J. Med.* **1978**, *64*, 21–26.
56. Butman, S.; Chandraratna, P.A.; Milne, N.; Olson, H.; Lyons, K.; Aronow, W.S. Stress myocardial imaging in patients with mitral valve prolapse: Evidence of a perfusion abnormality. *Cathet. Cardiovasc. Diagn.* **1982**, *8*, 243–252.
57. Butman, S.; Chandraratna, P.A.; Milne, N.; Olson, H.; Lyons, K.; Aronow, W.S. Stress myocardial imaging in mitral leaflet prolapse syndrome. *Am. J. Cardiol.* **1978**, *42*, 746–750.

11

Glucose Serum Concentrations and Cardiovascular Disease in Patients on the End Stage of Renal Disease without Diabetes Mellitus

Vaia D. Raikou [1,*] and Despina Kyriaki [2]

[1] Department of Medicine—Propaedaetic, National and Kapodistrian University of Athens, School of Medicine, Athens, 11527, Greece

[2] Department of Nuclear Medicine, General Hospital "LAÏKO", Athens, 11527, Greece; E-Mail: dkyriaki@gmail.com

* Author to whom correspondence should be addressed; E-Mail: vraikou@med.uoa.gr

Academic Editor: Andy Wessels

Abstract: *Background/Aim*: It is still controversial whether tighter glycemic control is associated with better clinical outcomes in patients with kidney failure. We examined the association between glucose serum concentrations and cardiovascular disease in patients on the end stage of renal disease without diabetes mellitus. *Methods*: We studied 76 patients on on-line hemodiafiltration. Cardiovascular disease was defined by the existence of coronary disease (CD). Arterial stiffness was measured as carotid-femoral pulse wave velocity (c-fPWV) and carotid augmentation index (AIx). The concentrations of beta2-microglobulin (β2M) and insulin were measured by radioimmunoassays and insulin resistance by HOMA-IR. We built a logistic-regression analysis to examine the role of glucose on cardiovascular disease after adjustment for the traditional and specific risk factors for dialysis patients. *Results*: Serum glucose was positively correlated with beta2M, insulin and HOMA-IR (r = 0.361, p = 0.002, r = 0.581, p = 0.001 and r = 0.753, p = 0.001 respectively). Logistic-regression analysis did not show significant impact of glucose concentrations on cardiovascular disease after adjustment for traditional and specific risk factors. *Conclusions*: The association between elevated glucose serum concentrations and represented by coronary syndrome cardiovascular disease in patients on the end stage of renal disease without diabetes mellitus was not found significant.

Keywords: glucose; HOMA-IR; cardiovascular disease; hemodiafiltration

1. Introduction

Poor glycemic control is associated with the development of comorbidities such as coronary artery disease and myocardial infarction in the general population [1]. Hyperglycemia has been shown to play a significant role on the development of microangiopathy and endothelial dysfunction [2]. Moreover, glycemia is known to influence the electrolyte balance, the function of potassium and calcium channels and sympathetic activity, all associated to arrhythmogenesis and sudden cardiac death of patients with kidney failure [3]. However, it is not clear whether patients on the end stage of renal disease (ESRD) with or/and without diabetes mellitus benefit from strict glycemic control [4].

In this study, we examined the association between glucose serum concentrations and cardiovascular disease in patients on the end stage of renal disease without diabetes mellitus.

2. Material and Methods

2.1. Subjects

We studied 76 hemodialyzed patients (hemodialysis mean duration =7.3 ± 6.0 years), 47 men and 29 women on mean age 62.2 ± 15 years. The treatment modality which was applied was on-line- predilution hemodiafiltration (on-l HDF). We excluded the patients with multiple intradialytic hypotensive episodes, fibrillation and the patients with interdialytic weight gain of > 5% of total body weight. Also, those with significant infection or malignancy were excluded from our study. The enrolled patients did not have interdialytic peripheral edema, high BP, interdialytic orthostatic hypotension or other characteristics of an inaccurate dry body weight.

The hemodialysis treatment was performed three-times weekly with a dialysis time of 3.5–4 h per session, a filter of 1.5–2 m^2 surface area and a blood flow of 350–400 mL/min. A bicarbonate-based ultrapure buffer dialysis solution was used with a dialysate flow rate of 500–600 mL/min, a calcium concentration of 1.50–1.75 mmol/L, a sodium concentration of 138–145 mmol/L and low molecular weight heparin as anticoagulant therapy. We used high-flux synthetic membrane, defined by an ultrafiltration coefficient > 20 mL/h [5]. Dialysis dose was defined by Kt/V for urea, which was calculated according to the formula of Daugirdas [6]. The patients, who had Kt/V for urea < 1.2, were excluded from the study.

Cardiovascular disease was represented by the presence of coronary disease (CD, n = 25, 32.9%), which might be the underlying disease for heart failure or peripheral arterial disease.

The coronary syndrome was documented by history of myocardial infarction, coronary artery angioplasty or bypass surgery, clinical signs of angina pectoris or electrocardiographic ischaemic findings.

Patients with interdialytic blood pressure ≥ 160/90 (n = 29, 38.2%) were considered hypertensive, as well as the patients who were receiving anti-hypertensive drugs, such as calcium channel blockers, beta-blockers or inhibitors of agiotensin II receptors.

The family history for cardiovascular events or hypertension was positive at a ratio of 64.5% of the studied patients.

In our data, the renal failure was caused by hypertensive nephrosclerosis at a ratio of 33% and by chronic glomerulonephritis at a ratio of 30%.

2.2. Blood Collection

Blood samples were drawn just before the start of the mean weekly dialysis session in a 12 h fasting state from the vascular access. At the end of the treatment, the blood pump speed was reduced to < 80 mL/min and blood samples was obtained at 2 min post-dialysis from the arterial dialysis tubing for the calculation of the adequacy of dialysis by kt/V for urea. The blood samples were centrifuged, and kept at a temperature of −80 °C.

In each subject, three sequences of samples were received for the serum glucose measurements, and their average was used for statistical analysis.

2.3. Laboratory Measurements

Albumin, the ratio of low density lipoproteins (LDL) to high density lipoproteins (HDL) (LDL/HDL) and serum glucose concentrations were measured by biochemical analysis. Hematocrit, hemoglobin and monocytes blood cells values were also measured.

The concentrations of beta2-microglobulin, insulin and intact-parathormone (i-PTH) were measured by radioimmunoassays (Immunotech by Beckman, Prague, Czech Republic, BioSource Europe SA, Nivelles, Belgium and CIS bio international, Gif- sur-Yvette, France respectively).

Insulin resistance was calculated using the homeostasis model assessment of insulin resistance (HOMA-IR) [7].

High sensitivity C-reactive protein (hsCRP) and oxidized LDL (ox-LDL) serum concentrations were measured using enzyme linked immunoabsorbed assays (ELISA, Immundiagnostik AG., Bensheim, Germany) according to manufacturer's specifications.

Normalized protein catabolic rate for dry body mass (nPCR) was calculated from the urea generation rate [8]. Body mass index (BMI) was obtained from height and post-dialysis body weight.

2.4. Hemodynamic Measurements

Predialysis peripheral systolic and diastolic blood pressures (SBP and DBP, respectively) were calculated as the mean of 10 measurements during a treatment month using an automatic sphygmomanometer OMRON M4-I (Co Ltd Kyoto Japan). Mean peripheral pre-dialysis BP (MBP) was calculated as: MBP = DBP + 1/3 (SBP − DBP). Before the mid-week dialysis session, the patients were allowed to rest for at least 10 min prior to their haemodynamic measurements. Arterial stiffness was measured as carotid-femoral pulse wave velocity (c-fPWV) and carotid augmentation index (AIx) using the SphygmoCor system® (AtCor Medical Pty.Ltd, Sydney, Australia) according to manufacturer's specifications. In each subject two sequences of measurements were performed, and their mean was used for statistical analysis. Pulse pressure (PP) was derived. Also, a 12-lead electrocardiographic examination was used to estimate the ischaemic findings.

3. Approval and Consent

The study was approved by the ethics committee of the Hospitals "Laiko, University General Hospital of Athens" and Renal Unit of "Diagnostic and Therapeutic Center of Athens Hygeia SA". Written informed consent was obtained from all subjects.

4. Data Analysis

Data were analyzed using SPSS 15.0 statistical package for Windows (SPSS Inc, Chicago, IL, USA) and expressed as mean ± standard deviation or as median value ± interquartile range for data that showed skewed distributions; differences between mean values were assessed by using paired-t test and Mann-Whitney U test and expressed as mean ± standard deviation or as mean rank. Correlations between variables were defined by Pearson and Spearman coefficient and p values less than 0.05 were considered significant. ROC curve analysis was used for the determination of glucose cut off point related to coronary disease. x^2 analysis was used for the correlation between categorical variables.We performed a logistic-regression analysis to investigate serum glucose concentrations as possible independent factor for cardiovascular disease after adjustment for the traditional and specific cardiovascular risk factors for dialysis patients, such as age, hypertension, BMI, dyslipidemia, anemia, inflammation, oxidative status, mineral bone disease, dialysis adequacy defined by Kt/V for urea and family history for cardiovascular disease.

5. Results

We divided our patients in two groups according to found by ROC curve glucose cut off point related to coronary disease value equal to 114.5 mg/dL (greater, n = 18 or lower, n = 58 than 114.5 mg/dL). Characteristics and differences between two groups of patients are listed in Table 1. We observed that the patients with higher glucose concentrations (n = 18) had significantly increased insulin, HOMA-IR, hsCRP, PP values and beta2M serum concentrations than the patients with lower serum glucose values ($p < 0.05$) (Figure 1).

Table 1. Characteristics and differences between groups of patients according to glucose cut off point related to coronary disease (on-line hemodiafiltration, $n = 76$, *: $p < 0.05$).

Characteristic	Patients with Glucose Serum Concentrations Less than 114.5 mg/dL (n = 58, Mean ± SD or Mean Rank)	Patients with Glucose Serum Concentrations More than 114.5 mg/dL (n = 18, Mean ± SD or Mean Rank)
Age (years)	60.8 ± 14.5	67.6 ± 15.5
Dialysis duration (years)	37.8	36.4
BMI (Kg/m^2)	24.2 ± 2.9	25.3 ± 3.1
Urine (mL/day)	226.2 ± 150.6	166.6 ± 115.4

Table 1. *Cont.*

Characteristic	Patients with Glucose Serum Concentrations Less than 114.5 mg/dL ($n = 58$, Mean ± SD or Mean Rank)	Patients with Glucose Serum Concentrations More than 114.5 mg/dL ($n = 18$, Mean ± SD or Mean Rank)
KTVurea	38.22	34.88
nPCR (g/Kg/day)	2.3 ± 0.4	2.5 ± 0.6
Glucose (mg/dL)	85.5 ± 13.7	132.7 ± 26.2 *
SBP (mmHg)	130.0 ± 20.7	138.3 ± 19.7
DBP (mmHg)	80.8 ± 10.2	84.3 ± 7.7
MBP (mmHg)	97.2 ± 12.9	102.3 ± 11.3
c-fPWV(m/s)	11.1 ± 1.8	12.08 ± 1.7
Augmentation index (AIx)	24.1 ± 2.3	24.4 ± 1.7
Pulse Pressure (PP, mmHg)	55.4 ± 17.7	66.7 ± 20.8 *
ABPI	1.12 ± 0.4	1.12 ± 0.5
Hemoglobulin	11.8 ± 1.3	12.01 ± 1.3
Monocytes (K/μL)	0.49 ± 0.2	0.50 ± 0.2
insulin (μU/mL)	32.7	54.7 *
HOMA-IR (mmol/L)	31.4	59.4 *
hsCRP (mg/L)	7.3 ± 6.03	10.6 ± 4.6 *
beta2-microglobulin (mg/L)	34.1	49.5 *
i-PTH (pg/mL)	38.2	34.6
Albumin (gr/dL)	37.9	36.09
LDL/HDL	2.3 ± 0.9	2.2 ± 0.7
ox-LDL (ng/mL)	35.2	45.8

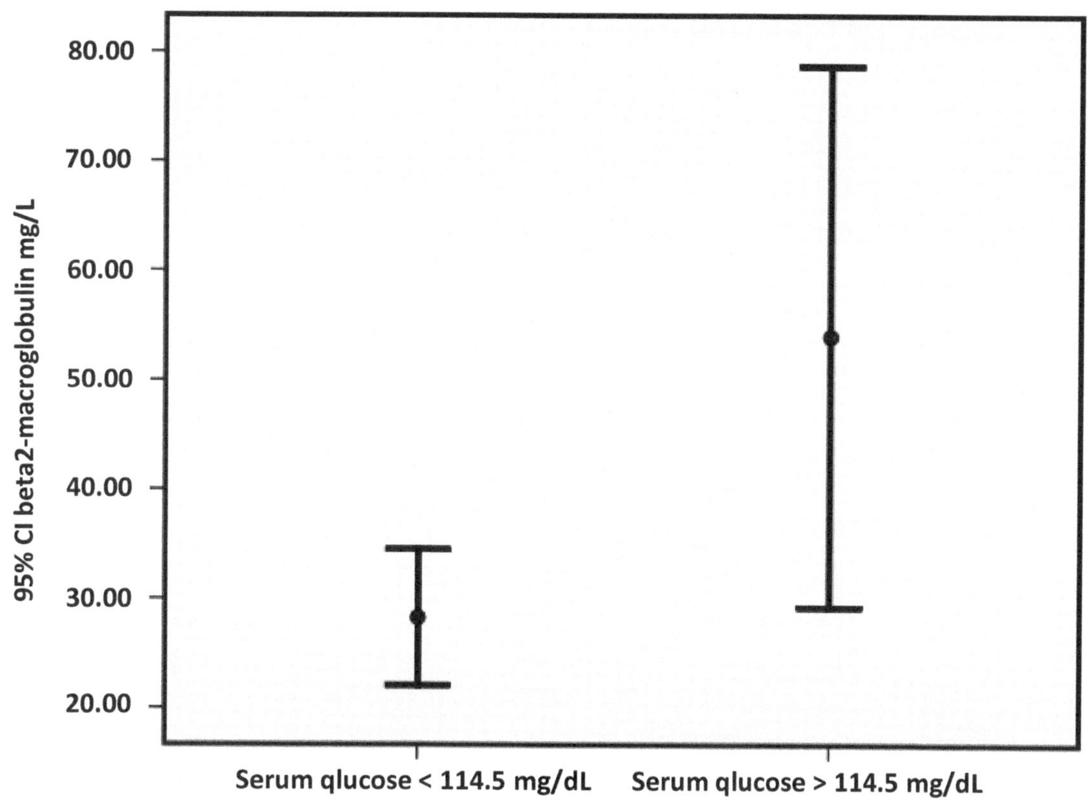

Figure 1. Beta2-microglobulin serum concentrations in patients on hemodiafiltration with glucose serum concentrations less and more than 114.5 mg/dL ($p = 0.04$).

Correlations

In total patients serum glucose was positively correlated with beta2M, insulin, HOMA-IR (Figure 2) and monocytes (r = 0.361, p = 0.002, r = 0.581, p = 0.001, r = 0.753, p = 0.001 and r = 0.272, p = 0.02, respectively). Also, HOMA-IR was significantly associated with both BMI and age (r = 0.303, p = 0.008 and r = 0.317, p = 0.005, respectively), although no significant association between glucose serum concentrations and neither BMI nor age could be found.

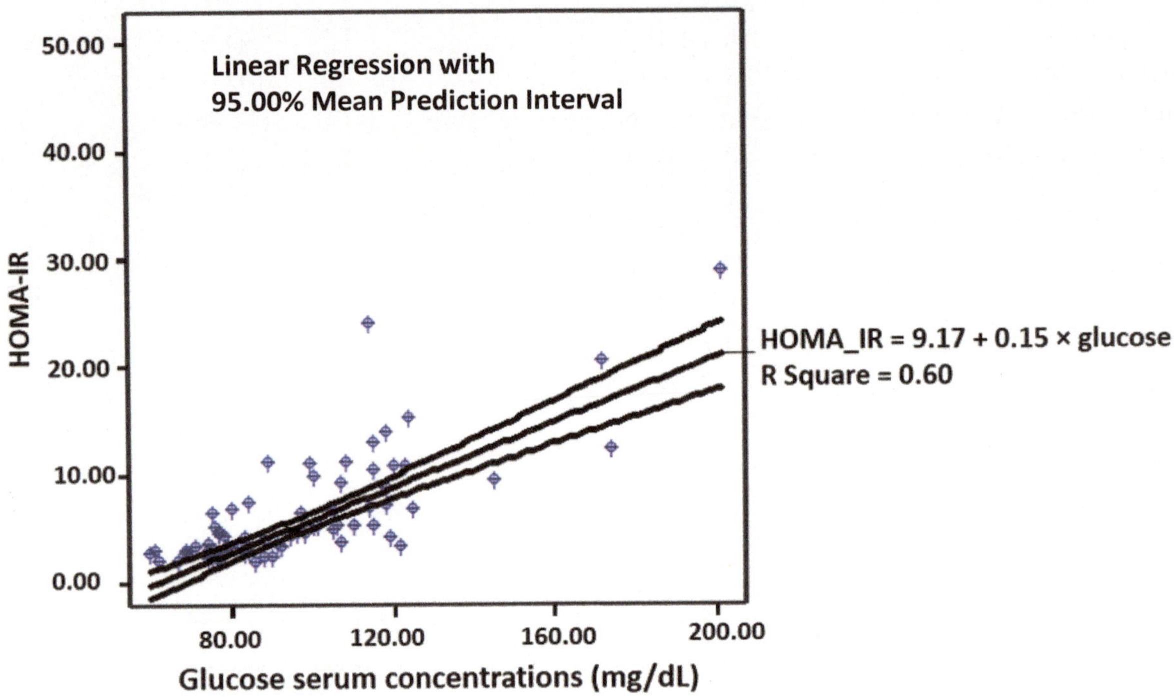

Figure 2. Correlation between glucose serum concentrations and insulin resistance defined by HOMA-IR (n = 76, r = 0.753, p = 0.001).

Table 2. Correlation between glucose serum concentrations and coronary disease in patients on hemodiafiltration after adjustment for risk factors.

Factors	B	S.E.	Sig.	Exp (B)
Glucose	−0.001	0.013	0.937	0.999
age	0.064	0.03	0.042	1.066
hypertension	1.042	0.75	0.169	2.836
BMI	−0.263	0.13	0.044	0.769
LDL/HDL	−1.288	0.55	0.020	0.276
Hb	0.605	0.32	0.060	1.832
hsCRP	0.092	0.06	0.164	1.097
oxLDL	0.011	0.005	0.025	1.011
i-PTH	0.004	0.002	0.025	1.004
Kt/Vurea	−5.816	2.9	0.044	0.003
Family history	0.099	0.824	0.905	1.104

The association of higher or lower serum glucose values with the presence of coronary disease was not found statistically significant by x^2 analysis (p = NS). Also, the built logistic-regression analysis did not show significant impact of serum glucose concentrations on CD, after adjustment for the traditional and specific risk factors for these patients. However, the age, dyslipidemia, BMI, oxidative status defined by oxLDL, i-PTH and dialysis adequacy determined by kt/V for urea showed significant risk factors (Table 2).

6. Discussion

It has been reported that hyperglycemia induced generation of the inflammatory cytokines, oxidative stress and advanced glycation end products (AGEs). These toxins are profibrotic and directly involved in the pathogenesis of the vascular complications [9]. However, the link between intensive glycemic control and cardiovascular events is complex and still debated [10]. Some observational studies indicated the importance of good glycemic control, defined by serum glucose and hemoglobin A(1c), for cardiovascular disease in dialysis patients with diabetes mellitus (DM) [11].

Controversially, in several studies, no association between HbA1c, and neither patient survival nor cardiovascular disease could be shown in dialysis patients with DM [12]. Previous study of 1484 dialysis patients with or without DM showed that higher casual glucose and HbA1c levels were not associated with mortality in maintenance hemodialysis patients [13]. In agreement, we did not find a significant association between high glucose serum concentrations and coronary disease in our data, which included patients on hemodiafiltration without DM adjusting to traditional and specific for these patients' factors.

In this study, we did not measure HbA1c concentrations, as it is known some inaccuracy of the HbA1c measurement in reflecting glucose levels in patients with chronic kidney disease. Studies suggest that glycated albumin is superior to HbA1c in estimating glucose control in dialysis patients [14].

Moreover, in the present study, we did not observe a significant difference for c-fPWV or AIx values in patients with higher glucose levels comparatively to the patients with lower glucose concentrations. c-fPWV and AIx values are used to assess arterial stiffness, which defines cardiovascular disease, and it has been reported that PWV varies during dialysis due to alterations in hydration status [15]. A previous study has reported that volume overload plays an important role in the development of arterial stiffness in HD patients [16]. Also, inflammation, mineral bone disease, hyperlipidemia and anemia have already been reported as specific cardiovascular risk factors for dialyzed patients, due partly to the relationship with arterial stiffness [17].

However, we observed significantly increased PP in patients with higher glucose than in patients with lower glucose levels. PP is influenced by both, arterial stiffness and hydration status, because blood pressure is mainly volume-dependent in these patients. This was related to PP extracellular volume, which might be extended in this group of patients comparatively to the patients with lower glucose concentrations, in whom the liquid balance may be achieved more effectively through dialysis treatment. This may explain the increased PP in the group of patients with higher glucose in comparison to the patients with lower glucose, rather than PP being associated with arterial stiffness.

On the other hand, in this study, the patients with higher glucose concentrations presented elevated insulin values, insulin resistance defined by HOMA-IR, significantly higher hsCRP and beta2M serum concentrations than the patients with lower glucose concentrations. Also, glucose was positively associated with beta2M, insulin, HOMA-IR and circulating monocytes.

It has been reported that hyperglycemia promotes inflammation by the excess generation of inflammatory cytokines and reactive free radicals, causing oxidative stress, which is associated with increased circulating inflammatory cells, elevated insulin resistance and the production of AGEs [2]. In the mean time, during hyperglycemia the generation of elevated AGEs modifies beta2M, which is accumulated in the circulation of dialysis patients [18]. AGE-modified beta2M (AGE-beta2M) may directly stimulate chemotaxis of monocytes and synthesis of cytokines from macrophages (interleukin-1β, TNF-α, and interleukin-6) [19]. Additionally, metabolic acidosis, which is a common condition particularly in end-stage renal disease patients [20] and which also promotes inflammation releasing cytokines [21], may be the connective pathophysiological mechanism between hyperglycemia, increased insulin resistance and increased accumulation of beta2M [22].

7. Conclusions

In this study, the association between elevated glucose serum concentrations and coronary syndrome cardiovascular disease in patients at the end stage of renal disease without diabetes mellitus was not found significant, despite that hyperglycemia was associated with extended extracellular volume and it promoted inflammatory procedure.

Acknowledgments

Financial disclosure: None

Author Contributions

Vaia D. Raikou: the idea of manuscript, the design, the hemodynamic measurements, the statistical analysis and the main writing of the paper. Despina Kyriaki: the collection of blood samples and the total laboratory mearurments.

Conflicts of Interest

The authors declare no conflict of interest.

References

1. Gaede, P.; Vedel, P.; Larsen, N.; Jensen, G.V.; Parving, H.H.; Pedersen, O. Multifactorial intervention and cardiovascular disease in patients with type 2 diabetes. *N. Engl. J. Med.* **2003**, *348*, 383–393.
2. Fang, Z.Y.; Prins, J.B.; Marwick, T.H. Diabetic cardiomyopathy: Evidence, mechanisms, and therapeutic implications. *Endocr. Rev.* **2004**, *25*, 543–567.
3. Ritz, E.; Wanner, C. The challenge of sudden death in dialysis patients. *Clin. J. Am. Soc. Nephrol.* **2008**, *3*, 920–929.
4. Ansari, A.; Thomas, S.; Goldsmith, D. Assessing glycemic control in patients with diabetes and end-stage renal failure. *Am. J. Kidney Dis.* **2003**, *41*, 523–531.

5. Chauveau, P.; Nguyen, H.; Combe, C.; Chêne, G.; Azar, R.; Cano, N.; Canaud, B.; Fouque, D.; Laville, M.; Leverve, X.; *et al*. French Study Group for Nutrition in Dialysis. Dialyzer membrane permeability and survival in hemodialysis patients. *Am. J. Kidney Dis.* **2005**, *45*, 565–571.
6. Daugirdas, J.T. Second generation logarithmic estimates of single-pool variable volume Kt/V: An analysis of error. *J. Am. Soc. Nephrol.* **1993**, *4*, 1205–1213.
7. Silva, E.A.; Flexa, F.; Zanella, M.T. Impact of abdominal fat and insulin resistance on arterial hypertension in non-obese women. *Arq. Bras. Endocrinol. Metabol.* **2009**, *53*, 340–343.
8. Daugirdas, J.T. Simplified equations for monitoring Kt/V, PCRn, eKt/V, and ePCRn. *Adv. Ren. Replace Ther.* **1995**, *2*, 295–304.
9. Johansen, J.S.; Harris, A.K.; Rychly, D.J.; Ergul, A. Oxidative stress and the use of antioxidants in diabetes: Linking basic science to clinical practice. *Cardiovasc. Diabetol.* **2005**, *4*, doi:10.1186/1475-2840-4-5.
10. Ray, K.K.; Seshasai, S.R.; Wijesuriya, S.; Sivakumaran, R.; Nethercott, S.; Preiss, D.; Erqou, S.; Sattar, N. Effect of intensive control of glucose on cardiovascular outcomes and death in patients with diabetes mellitus: A metaanalysis of randomised controlled trials. *Lancet* **2009**, *373*, 1765–1772.
11. Drechsler, C.; Krane, V.; Ritz, E.; Marz, W.; Wanner, C. Glycemic control and cardiovascular events in diabetic hemodialysis patients. *Circulation* **2009**, *120*, 2421–2428.
12. Shima, K.; Komatsu, M.; Kawahara, K.; Minaguchi, J.; Kawashima, S. Stringent glycaemic control prolongs survival in diabetic patients with end-stage renal disease on haemodialysis. *Nephrology (Carlton)* **2010**, *15*, 632–638.
13. Shurraw, S.; Majumdar, S.R.; Thadhani, R.; Wiebe, N.; Tonelli, M.; Alberta Kidney Disease Network. Glycemic control and the risk of death in 1484 patients receiving maintenance hemodialysis. *Am. J. Kidney Dis.* **2010**, *55*, 875–884.
14. Freedman, B.I.; Shenoy, R.N.; Planer, J.A.; Clay, K.D.; Shihabi, Z.K.; Burkart, J.M.; Cardona, C.Y.; Andries, L.; Peacock, T.P.; Sabio, H.; *et al*. Comparison of glycated albumin and hemoglobin A1c concentrations in diabetic subjects on peritoneal and hemodialysis. *Perit Dial. Int.* **2010**, *30*, 72–79.
15. Di Iorio, B.; Nazzaro, P.; Cucciniello, E.; Bellizzi, V. Influence of haemodialysis on variability of pulse wave velocity in chronic haemodialysis patients. *Nephrol. Dial. Transplant.* **2010**, *25*, 1579–1583.
16. Zheng, D.; Cheng, L.T.; Zhuang, Z.; Gu, Y.; Tang, L.J.; Wang, T. Correlation between pulse wave velocity and fluid distribution in hemodialysis patients. *Blood Purif.* **2009**, *27*, 248–252.
17. Ritz, E.; Wanner, C. Lipid abnormalities and cardiovascular risk in renal disease. *J. Am. Soc. Nephrol.* **2008**, *19*, 1065–1070.
18. Tzoulaki, I.; Murray, G.D.; Lee, A.J.; Rumley, A.; Lowe, G.D. Fowkes, F.G. C-reactive protein, interleukin-6, and soluble adhesion molecules as predictors of progressive peripheral atherosclerosis in the general population: Edinburgh Artery Study. *Circulation* **2005**, *112*, 976–983.
19. Miyata, T.; Inagi, R.; Iida, Y.; Sato, M.; Yamada, N.; Oda, O.; Maeda, K.; Seo, H. Involvement of β2-microgbobulin modified with advanced glycation end products in the pathogenesis of hemodialysis-associated amyboidosis. *J. Clin. Invest.* **1994**, *93*, 521–528.
20. Kalantar-Zadeh, K.; Mehrotra, R.; Fouque, D.; Kopple, J.D. Metabolic acidosis and malnutrition-inflammation complex syndrome in chronic renal failure. *Semin. Dial.* **2004**, *17*, 455–465.

21. London, G.M.; Drueke, T.B. Atherosclerosis and arteriosclerosis in chronic renal failure. *Kidney Int.* **1997**, *51*, 1678–1695.
22. Sonikian, M.; Gogusev, J.; Zingraff, J.; Loric, S.; Quednau, B.; Bessou, G.; Siffert, W.; Drüeke, T.B.; Reusch, H.P.; Luft, F.C. Potential effect of metabolic acidosis on beta2-microglobulin generation: *In vivo* and *in vitro* studies. *J. Am. Soc. Nephrol.* **1996**, *7*, 350–356.

12

Embryonic Development of the Bicuspid Aortic Valve

Peter S. Martin [1], Benjamin Kloesel [1], Russell A. Norris [2], Mark Lindsay [3], David Milan [3] and Simon C. Body [1,*]

[1] Department of Anesthesiology, Perioperative and Pain Medicine, Brigham and Women's Hospital, Harvard Medical School, 75 Francis St., Th724, Boston, MA 02115, USA; E-Mails: peter.martin001@umb.edu (P.S.M.); b.kloesel@gmx.net (B.K.)

[2] Department of Regenerative Medicine and Cell Biology, Children's Research Institute, Medical University of South Carolina, 173 Ashley St, Charleston, SC 29403, USA; E-Mail: norrisra@musc.edu

[3] Cardiovascular Research Center, Richard B. Simches Research Center, Massachusetts General Hospital, 185 Cambridge Street, Boston, MA 02114, USA; E-Mails: lindsay.mark@mgh.harvard.edu (M.L.); dmilan@mgh.harvard.edu (D.M.)

* Author to whom correspondence should be addressed: E-Mail: sbody@partners.org

Academic Editor: Cheryl L. Maslen

Abstract: Bicuspid aortic valve (BAV) is the most common congenital valvular heart defect with an overall frequency of 0.5%–1.2%. BAVs result from abnormal aortic cusp formation during valvulogenesis, whereby adjacent cusps fuse into a single large cusp resulting in two, instead of the normal three, aortic cusps. Individuals with BAV are at increased risk for ascending aortic disease, aortic stenosis and coarctation of the aorta. The frequent occurrence of BAV and its anatomically discrete but frequent co-existing diseases leads us to suspect a common cellular origin. Although autosomal-dominant transmission of BAV has been observed in a few pedigrees, notably involving the gene *NOTCH1*, no single-gene model clearly explains BAV inheritance, implying a complex genetic model involving interacting genes. Several sequencing studies in patients with BAV have identified rare and uncommon mutations in genes of cardiac embryogenesis. But the extensive cell-cell signaling and multiple cellular origins involved in cardiac embryogenesis preclude simplistic explanations of this disease. In this review, we examine the series of events from cellular and transcriptional embryogenesis of the heart, to development of the aortic valve.

Keywords: bicuspid aortic valve; heart development; congenital heart disease; aortic valve; aortic stenosis; aortic incompetence

1. Introduction

Congenital heart disease (CHD) is the most frequently occurring birth defect among liveborn humans. Bicuspid aortic valve (BAV) in particular is the most common congenital valvular heart defect, having an overall frequency of 0.5%–1.2% and occurring more frequently in males and white individuals. BAVs result from abnormal aortic cusp formation during valvulogenesis, whereby adjacent cusps fuse into a single large cusp resulting in two, instead of the normal three, aortic cusps [1]. BAV is a strong risk factor for accelerated aortic valve disease, principally aortic stenosis, and ascending aortic aneurysm [2,3].

BAV occurs in several genetic syndromes, including Turner syndrome, and is associated with coarctation of the aorta, hypoplastic left heart syndrome, Holt-Oram syndrome, ventricular noncompaction and adult-onset aortopathy [1]. In addition, BAV occasionally demonstrates complex inheritance in large families without evidence of syndromic features, other congenital heart defects or a family history of CHD. Yet, some 10% of BAV patients have first-degree relatives with the condition or associated non-valvular abnormalities such as aortic coarctation, thoracic aortic aneurysms, mitral valve disease or ventricular septal defects [4].

Over the past few decades, much progress has been made in understanding the embryological development of the heart, including the contributions of various cell populations and the molecular biology of its very complex spatial and temporal anatomical development. Advances in the identification of transcription factors, signaling molecules and structural genes for heart development have assisted the discovery of genes causing CHD. Culprit genes have been identified using genomewide association studies (GWAS) or candidate gene sequencing [5–7], which have elucidated the etiology of some congenital heart defects, notably atrial and ventricular septal defects [8–11] and Tetralogy of Fallot [12–14]. However, the underlying pathology of most structural outflow tract (OFT) defects remains unknown because of the complexity of transcriptional and signaling mechanisms in the developing embryo and the numerous cell types involved in tract development. Thus far, for any single structural defect, numerous genes have been implicated, each in only a small percentage of patients. Similarly, there has been limited progress in defining the molecular etiology of BAV. Although autosomal-dominant transmission of this condition has been observed in some three-generation pedigrees, notably involving the gene *NOTCH1* [15,16], no single-gene model clearly explains BAV inheritance. Likewise, evidence for specific loci for a genetic etiology of sporadic BAV (wherein no first- or second-generation relatives with BAV can be identified) is limited.

In this review, we describe normal development of the aortic valve; the key cellular players; the specifics of cell-cell communication and migration; and pathways possibly involved in BAV development.

2. Progenitor Development of the Vertebrate Heart

The vertebrate heart has remarkable evolutionary conservation and structural similarity that includes divided pulmonary and systemic circulations, a conduction system and valves to create coordinated unidirectional flow at high pressure. These diverse structural and functional features of the vertebrate heart reflect its origination from cardiac neural crest (CNC) cells, which contribute to portions of the OFT and septum; the mesenchyme that comprises the first heart field (FHF) and second heart field (SHF); the endothelium, which provides growth factor signals and precursor cells for formation of the cardiac valves; and the proepicardium, which provides precursors for the coronary vasculature and mural valve leaflets [17,18]. Spatial and temporal integration of these various cell types is required for proper cardiac specification and anatomical morphology during embryogenesis.

2.1. Gastrulation in the Early Embryo

We start at gastrulation as specification of cardiac progenitor cells occurs by this time. After formation of the hollow sphere of cells known as the *blastocyst*, the three germ layers of the embryo (the ectoderm, mesoderm, and endoderm) are formed by development of the primitive streak (along the anterior-posterior axis) and gastrulation—the process of conversion of the spherical blastocyst to the complex and differentiated *gastrula* that forms the organs at about days 15–16 of human embryogenesis (Figure 1). Gastrulation requires cell polarity, axis specification and cell-type specification to establish a three-dimensional map of the embryo.

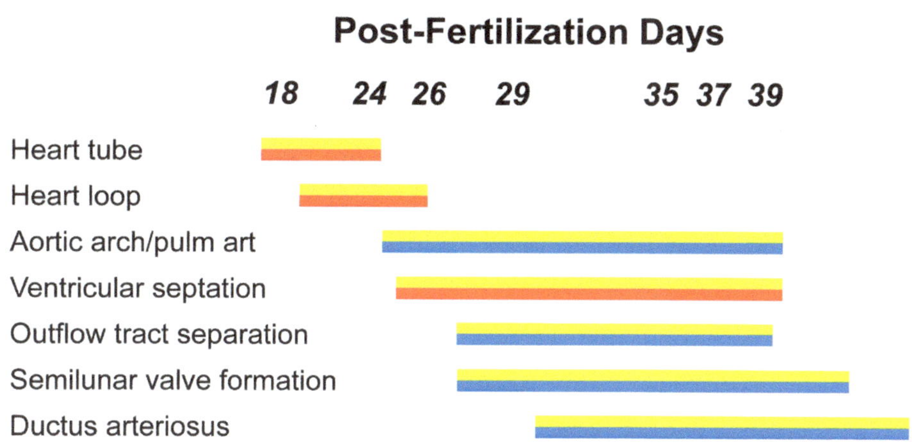

Figure 1. Timeline of outflow tract and semilunar valve development post-fertilization. The colors represent contributions to cardiac development from different cell populations. These contributions are from the first heart field (red), second heart field (yellow) and cardiac neural crest (blue). Modified from [19].

Embryonic progenitor cells derive from the epiblast on either side of the primitive streak. The process of forming three germ layers from the blastocyst requires epiblast migration and epithelial to mesenchymal transition (EMT) to form the mesoderm and endoderm. Finally, cell lineages of the heart, pharyngeal arches and vasculature begin to be defined. EMT is a process by which epithelial cells lose their cell polarity and cell-cell adhesion, and gain migratory and invasive properties to become mesenchymal stem cells, which are multipotent stromal cells that can differentiate into a variety of cell types. After undergoing EMT, mesodermal cells move cranio-laterally before converging medially while forming the lateral plate mesoderm (LPM) and other mesodermal derivatives. The LPM splits into the dorsal somatic and ventral splanchnic mesoderm. The dorsal somatic mesoderm gives rise to the body wall and other derivatives, while the ventral splanchnic mesoderm gives rise to all heart components mentioned earlier as well as other derivatives.

EMT is primarily mediated by transforming growth factor-β (TGF-β) signaling as well as Wnt (wingless-related MMTV integration sites), fibroblast growth factor (FGF) and the bone morphogenic pathway (BMP), amongst others. Expression of cardiac-specific transcription factors, such as the *GATA*, *MEF2*, *NK2*, *TBX* and *HAND* gene families, control cardiac cell fate and the morphogenesis of cardiac structures. Adjacent endodermal cells that are not destined to become cardiac precursors express many of these transcription factors and are paracrine controllers of development. Thus, complexity of the vertebrate heart results from spatial and temporal selectivity of a diverse range of regulatory proteins and regulatory elements on specific cell populations. This specificity in gene regulation probably underlies the restriction of many cardiac defects to specific anatomical regions of the heart [5].

2.2. Cardiac Mesoderm (FHF and SHF)

Mesodermal progenitor cells derived from the LPM arise from the cranial third of the primitive streak during early gastrulation. These mesodermal cells migrate in a cranial-lateral direction to become localized on either side of the primitive streak and undergo EMT to mesodermal cells, then proliferate and migrate in a semicircular fashion. Later, they coalesce in the midline to form the cardiac crescent.

The cellular fate of these cardiac mesodermal cells is initially uncommitted, but after migration, they become specified to differentiate into the cardiogenic mesoderm of the FHF and SHF at about day 18 of human embryogenesis (Figure 2). The FHF is formed from the cells that are first to differentiate from the cardiac crescent and are marked by the transcription factor *Hcn4*. The FHF gives rise to the early heart tube and, later, to much of the left ventricle, portions of both atria and some of the right ventricle [20].

The SHF is composed of undifferentiated progenitor cells from the medial splanchnic mesoderm adjacent to the pharyngeal endoderm. Many transcription factors have been implicated in the development of the SHF, including Mef2c, Tbx1, Islet-1 (Isl1), Hand2, Fgf8 and Fgf10 [20]. Once the rudimentary heart tube is created, cells from the SHF contribute to the OFT, giving rise to the smooth muscle of the aortic root, and join with more distal smooth muscle of the ascending aorta derived from neural crest cells. The SHF is also the source of the majority of the myocardium of the right ventricle, components of the interventricular septum, a small part of the left ventricle and the atria [21,22]. Specifically, the SHF cells reach the heart tube at both the arterial pole (anterior SHF) and venous pole (posterior SHF). At the arterial pole, the anterior SHF-derived mesoderm supplies the myocardium of the right ventricle up to the right side of the ventricular septum. The SHF also contributes to the semilunar valves and the walls of the great arteries. Progenitors of SHF cells are marked by the transcription factor *Isl1* [23].

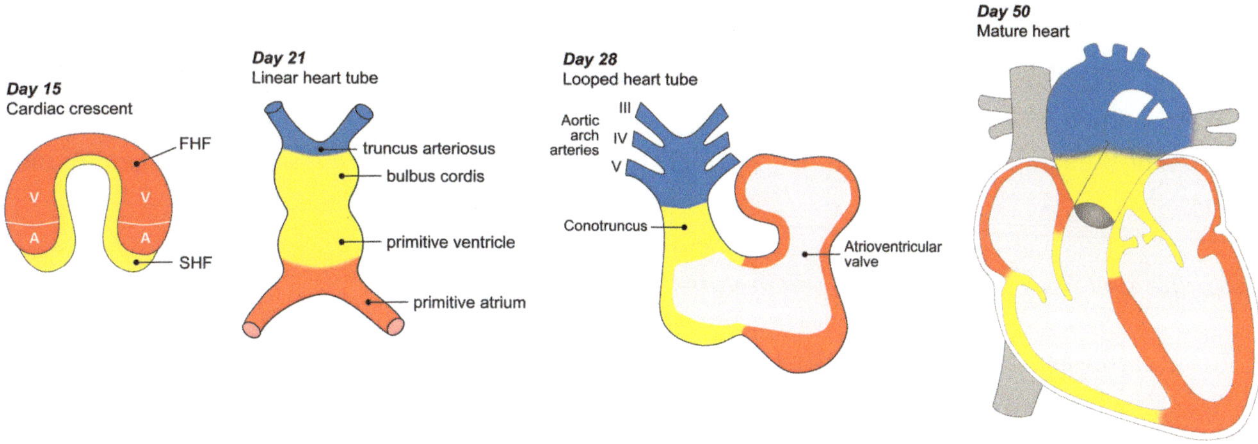

Figure 2. Stages of human cardiac development with color-coding of contributing cell populations, seen from a ventral view. These contributions are from the first heart field (red), second heart field (yellow) and cardiac neural crest (blue). By day 15 post-fertilization, the cardiac crescent is specified to form specific segments of the linear heart tube, which is patterned along the anteroposterior axis to form the looped and mature heart. Cardiac neural crest cells populate the aortic arch arteries (III, IV, and VI) and aortic sac (AS) that together contribute to specific segments of the mature aortic arch. Mesenchymal cells form the cardiac valves from the conotruncal (CT) and atrioventricular valve (AVV) segments. Abbreviations: A, atrium; V, ventricle; RV, right ventricle; LV, left ventricle; RA, right atrium; LA, left atrium; PA, pulmonary artery; Ao, aorta; DA, ductus arteriosus. Modified from [24].

2.3. Cardiac Neural Crest Cells

Neural crest cells form a wide variety of cells types, including nervous tissue, melanocytes, cartilage, bone, connective tissue and smooth muscle. CNC cells are a population of multipotent neural crest cells that originate from the dorsal neural tube at the interface of the ectoderm and neural ectoderm during embryogenesis. They migrate bilaterally into the ectoderm and endoderm of the pharyngeal arches as each arch develops and proliferate with the pharyngeal arteries to form the smooth muscle layer of the carotid artery (3rd pharyngeal arch), upper limb arteries and aortic arch (4th pharyngeal arch), and pulmonary arteries (6th pharyngeal arch).

A subpopulation of CNC cells continues caudal migration to the anterior domain of the SHF to form the OFT [25] at about day 22 in the human, where they contribute to the aorta, main pulmonary artery, and aortic-pulmonary septum via the truncal cushions [26]; valve formation via the endocardial cushions; and perhaps separation of the ventricular myocardium from the aorta and pulmonary artery [26]. The CNC cells at the base of the OFT lie in the medial walls of the arterial trunks, continuous proximally with the remnant of the aorto-pulmonary septum [27]. The 4th and 6th pharyngeal arches are connected to the proximal OFT by the aortic "sac"—a non-muscular intra-pericardial connection that becomes the ascending aorta by septation of these arches; rotation of the OFT enables connection of the septated arches to their respective ventricles [28]. Thus, septation of the elongated spiraling OFT occurs with fusion of the single aorto-pulmonary septum and enlarged endocardial cushions after significant CNC cell colonization of the truncal cushions.

CNC cells also provide signals that shape the developing heart. For example, they pattern the aortic arch, ventricular and atrial septae, and OFT [29]. Similar to requirements for the EMT process, Wnt, FGF and BMP are necessary for CNC cell migration and programming. Disruption of the endothelin, semaphorin, Wnt/β-catenin-Pitx2, Notch, TGF- β, BMP and Hedgehog pathways results in septal and OFT defects.

2.4. Myocardial and Endocardial Cell Contributions

The fate of cardiogenic mesoderm cells is shaped by their communication with the notochord and the pharyngeal endoderm of the embryo. The endocardium in particular plays a crucial role in several steps of the development of the early heart, including cell specification and guiding cell migration. It is thought that mammalian endocardial and myocardial cells are derived from EMT of a common multipotent progenitor within the cardiac mesoderm [30,31]. The endocardium plays two key roles during OFT morphogenesis: population and proliferation of the endocardial cushions, and regulation of OFT myocardial proliferation. In response to signaling from the conal OFT myocardium, the endocardium undergoes EMT to give rise to a population of mesenchymal cells that seed the initially acellular endocardial cushions, which then remodel into the arterial valves [32].

Signaling between CNC and SHF cells is required for OFT development [33,34], and removal of SHF progenitors results in OFT defects [35]. These observations show the importance of multiple extra-cardiac and cardiac cell lineages needed for OFT development. Migration of extra-cardiac lineages into the heart and OFT requires precise temporal and spatial regulation and signaling [36].

3. Development of the OFT

The OFT extends from ventricular myocardium to the margin of the pericardial cavity and is made up of the infundibulum (conus) nearer the right ventricle, and the proximal aorta and pulmonary artery (truncus) nearer the branchial arches [37,38]. The lumen of the OFT is continuous with that of the aortic sac of the pharyngeal arch arteries.

The OFT is derived from CNC and FHF cells that give rise to endocardium and myocardium, as well as cells derived from the SHF, and from EMT of endothelial cells (Figure 3) [30,36,38]. Additionally, luminal endothelial cells of the OFT vessels undergo EMT to contribute to the endocardial cushions that, together with the migrating CNC cells, form the OFT septum [36]. The distal OFT originates from CNC-derived mesenchyme cells [39,40], whereas the proximal OFT originates from endocardial-derived mesenchyme [41]. During early embryogenesis, CNC cells migrate ventrally as mesenchymal cells to populate the distal OFT, where they merge with SHF and endocardial cells to form the aorto-pulmonary septum [39]. This septum divides the initially single embryonic OFT (also called truncus arteriosus) into aortic and pulmonary arteries, establishing separate systemic and pulmonary circulations.

Much of the development of the OFTs is confused by naming conventions of structures present during embryogenesis and by different interpretations of anatomical, histologic and lineage-tracing models in different species [42]. It also seems likely that some of the observations in quail-chick models are not applicable to primate embryogenesis and that mouse models offer better insight. Nonetheless, there are some well-established principles to cell origin and specification in the OFT.

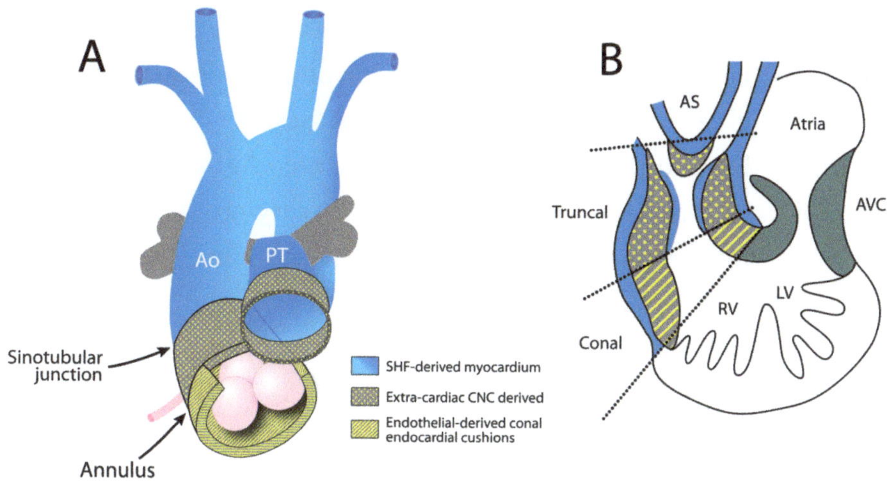

Figure 3. Genesis and cellular contributions to the outflow tract. Schematic shows the locations of outflow tract (OFT) colonization by the extra-cardiac cardiac neural crest (blue), vascular smooth muscle derived from the second heart field (dotted yellow) and the location of myocardium from derived from the second heart field (striped yellow). The aortic annulus or hinge region is formed where myocardial cells meet the vascular smooth muscle cells of the media of the aorta and pulmonary trunk and endothelial derived mesenchyme is the source of the fibroblastic annular tissue. The media of the aorta and pulmonary trunk is derived from secondary heart field proximally (dotted yellow) and the cardiac neural crest distally (blue). The interface between these populations is at the sinotubular junction. Abbreviations: Ao, aorta; AS, aortic sac; AVC, aorto-ventricular cushions; LV left ventricle; PT, pulmonary trunk; RV, right ventricle. Modified from [36] and [27]

3.1. Development of the Aorto-Pulmonary Trunk

Cells from the branchial mesenchyme, the paired 3rd/4th and 6th pharyngeal arteries, project into the pericardial cavity as an aortic sac. The 3rd and 4th pharyngeal arteries eventually form the aortic arch, while the initially paired 6th pharyngeal arteries fuse to form the pulmonary artery and ductus arteriosus. When the OFT is first formed, it has exclusively muscular walls that extend to the borders of the pericardial cavity, where the tract becomes continuous with the aortic sac. This sac is initially separated from the truncus but elongates to fuse with the distal truncus. Within the lumen, the endocardial jelly concentrates into pairs of facing cushions that continuously extend the length of the OFT, spiraling around one another as they run from the distal end of the right ventricle to the aortic sac. The cushions are proteoglycan-rich structures that eventually become populated by three mesenchymal cell populations: CNC-, SHF- and EMT-derived cells. The core of the protrusion is derived from the SHF, but it is covered by material derived from the neural crest [43].

Septation of the OFT requires formation of the truncal and conal cushions situated in the distal and proximal OFT, respectively. CNC cells form the mesenchyme of the truncal (right-superior and left-inferior) cushions that subsequently fuse to form the aortopulmonary septum, dividing the distal OFT into the aorta and pulmonary trunk [7]. Separation of the aortic and pulmonary trunk (aorto-pulmonary septation) occurs when the distal portions of the truncus swellings gradually fuse together in a cranial to caudal direction, to septation. By day 23–25 of human embryogenesis, the heart tube is formed and anterograde circulation begins, with development of the arterial pole over the next 5 days [20]. Septation of the aorto-pulmonary trunk results in the formation of the definitive intrapericardial pulmonary and aortic outflow channels, each of which possesses three segments, namely, the intrapericardial arterial trunks distal to the sinotubular junction, the arterial roots with their valves, and the subvalvar ventricular OFT. Separation of the aorta and pulmonary artery is completed by expansion of the aorto-pulmonary septum into the mesenchymal tissue of the proximal truncus swelling, separating the arterial valves (Figure 4). Mouse and chick studies have shown that abnormal EMT resulting in either deficient or excessive OFT cushion formation can give rise to structural OFT defects [36].

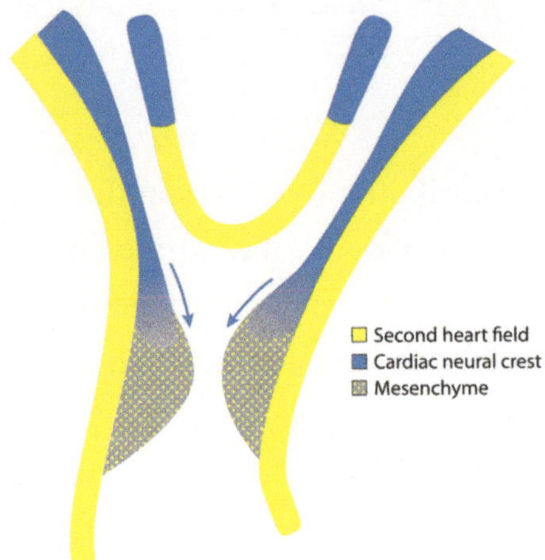

Figure 4. Remodeling of the endocardial cushions. Cardiac neural crest cells (blue) provide paracrine signals to second heart field cells (yellow) to orchestrate apoptosis (depicted as dark gray cells) and changes in extracellular matrix production during semilunar valve remodeling. Modified from [25].

3.2. Development of the Aortic and Pulmonary Valves

The boundary at the dog-leg bend in the OFT identifies the border of the primordial OFT destined to become the sinotubular junction [44]. The valves and their supporting sinuses develop from the proximal part of the tract. Aortic and pulmonary valve development begins at approximately days 31–35 in humans, from the endocardial cushions in the OFT and atrioventricular canal of the primitive heart tube [45]. In early stages of arterial valve development, endothelial cells overlying the primitive endocardial cushions invade the cushion matrix, resulting in relatively bulky and cellularized endocardial cushions [46].

The semilunar valves arise from the conotruncal and intercalated cushions of the OFT, with the conotruncal cushions give rise to the right and left leaflets of each of the valves. In the aorta, these are the right and left coronary leaflets, while in the pulmonary valve, these are the right and left cusps (Figure 5). From the opposite quadrants of the OFT, the right-posterior and the left-anterior intercalated cushions develop respectively into the posterior aortic (non-coronary cusp) and the anterior pulmonic (anterior cusp) leaflets. These semilunar valve leaflets also derive their mesenchyme primarily from the endocardium [47]. The muscular wall of the proximal OFT does not have a cellular contribution to the valve leaflets or their supporting arterial sinuses, but does contribute to their growth in paracrine fashion. The rudimentary arterial valve leaflets and sinuses are formed by creating "cavities" in the fused distal parts of the proximal endocardial cushions, along with similar cavities in the new cushions through apoptosis and alterations in the extracellular matrix (Figure 5) [48]. Cavitation of the cushions results in a central lumen of each cushion that separates the three valve leaflets, with the peripheral portion arterializing to form the wall of the supporting valve sinuses. Valvulogenesis continues with elongation and thinning of the endocardial cushions by remodeling and compartmentalizing into the collagen-rich fibrosa, proteoglycan-rich spongiosa, and elastin-rich atrialis/ventricularis layers [46]. The extracellular matrix composition and organization of the valve leaflets are critical for normal valve function, and dysregulation of extracellular matrix remodeling or structural components can lead to valve malformations [49].

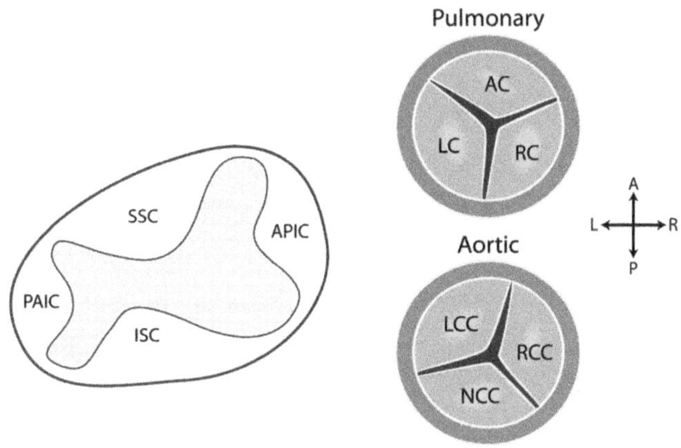

Figure 5. Development of the leaflets of the aortic and pulmonary valves. The semilunar valves arise from the conotruncal and intercalated cushions of the outflow tract. The conotruncal (superior and inferior septal) cushions give rise to the right and left leaflets of each of the semilunar valves. In the aorta, these are the right and left coronary leaflets, while in the pulmonary valve, these are the right and left cusps. The right-posterior and the left-anterior intercalated cushions develop respectively into the posterior aortic (non-coronary cusp of the aortic valve) and the anterior pulmonic (anterior cusp of the pulmonic valve) leaflets. Abbreviations: AL, anterior leaflet; APIC, anterior pulmonary intercalated cushion; CA, coronary artery; ISC, inferior septal cushion; LL, left leaflet; LCL, left coronary leaflet; NCL, non-coronary leaflet; PAIC, posterior aortic intercalated cushion; RCL, right coronary leaflet, RL, right leaflet

4. Transcriptional Regulation of Valvulogenesis

The gene regulatory network of valve progenitor cells in the endocardial cushions includes the complex spatial and temporal interplay of transcription factors involved in EMT and mesenchymal progenitor populations [50]. Endocardial cushion formation is initiated by signals from the OFT myocardium that cause adjacent endocardial cells to undergo EMT. Many transcription factors and signaling pathways have been implicated in EMT and cushion morphogenesis, including members of the TGF-β superfamily, Notch, BMP and Gata families, Nfatc1, Wnt/β-catenin, Twist-1, Sox9 and others (Figure 6). The complexity of cardiac structure and functioning cells types developed from an apparently few embryonic cell types is surprising. Similarly, the marked localization of single-gene defects to specific cardiac structures appears at odds with the presence of many of these proteins in numerous cell types of the heart and other organs [5].

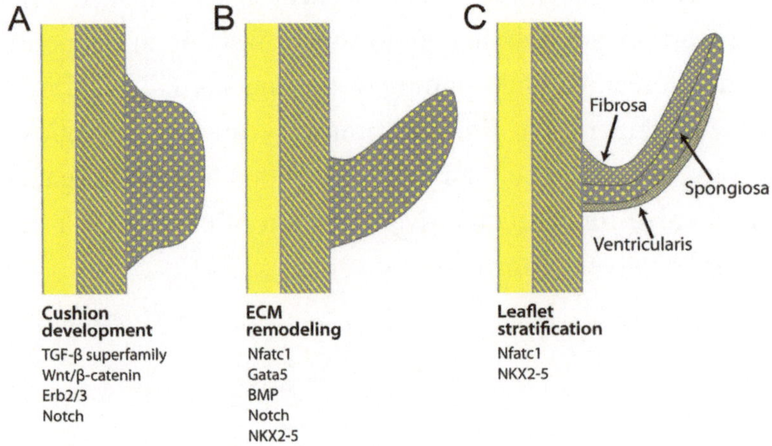

Figure 6. Transcription factors active in aortic valve development. (**A**) Endocardial cushions (purple) form in the cardiac outflow tract. Valve progenitor cells are generated by an endothelial-to-mesenchymal transition (EMT); (**B**) Endocardial cushions elongate to form valve primordia of individual valve leaflets. Extracellular matrix (ECM) remodeling and morphogenesis of the valve leaflets is dependent on Nfatc1 and Gata5; (**C**) ECM of the primordial semilunar valve thins, elongates and stratifies into fibrosa, spongiosa, and ventricularis layers. Modified from [45].

Ascertaining the timing and relative expression of these transcription factors is difficult and has been complicated by misinterpretation of results from older studies using less robust techniques and non-human models. Nevertheless, an expanding list of transcription factors appear to have important roles, or at least are well described. These factors overlap with genes that have been implicated in BAV, but to a limited extent.

4.1. Notch

Signaling factors, particularly from the Notch and TGF-β families, facilitate EMT and mesenchymal invasion of the OFT cushions [51]. The Notch pathway is involved in the majority of cardiac embryogenesis, notably including valve development [52]. *Notchl, 2* and *4* receptors and their ligands (Jag1/2 and Dll4) are expressed in the OFT and cushions throughout valvulogenesis [51,53–55]. When activated, the Notch intracellular domain (*NICD*) translocates to the nucleus where it creates a complex of *NICD*, *Rbpj*, and the inhibitor *MAML* leading to activation of *Notch* target genes. In the embryonic valve, *HES*, *HEY*, *Acta2*, *Snai2*, *Smad3*, and *Runx3* are direct Notch target genes [56]. Notch activation also inhibits TGF-β-induced *Smadl* and *Smad2* signaling, subsequently decreasing expression of their target genes [57]. Underscoring the importance of *NOTCH*, its inactivation or mutation leads to multiple forms of CHD, such as BAV [15], Alagille syndrome [58,59] and hypocellular endocardial cushions [57,60].

Several mouse models have been generated for *Notchl/2/4* and their downstream effectors to examine the functions of Notch signaling during valve development. In mice, *Notchl/2/4*, *Rbpj* and *Maml* knockouts are embryonic lethal, with affected embryos having OFT and other cardiac and non-cardiac abnormalities [51,57,61], whereas *Notch3* knockouts do not have an abnormal phenotype [62]. Demonstrating the complexity of pathways in aortic disease, haploinsufficiency of *Notch1* on a mouse *NOS3*$^{-/-}$ background causes marked aortic phenotypes, whereas each mutation alone has very limited phenotypic changes [63–65]. Interestingly, single-gene knockouts of the cardiac ligands of *Notch*—*Jag1*, *Jag2* and *Dll4*—also do not show valve abnormalities, perhaps indicating redundant signaling. Importantly, Notch has been implicated in mouse and human calcific aortic valve disease (CAVD), a common form of heart valve disease [66–68].

4.2. BMPs and TGF-β

BMPs 2–7 and TGF-βs are part of the TGF-β superfamily expressed in the embryonic heart. BMPs bind to cardiac BMP Type I receptors—ALK2 (activin-like kinase) and ALK3—and Type II receptors—BMPRII, ActRII or ActRIIB—that activate an intracellular canonical signaling pathway mediated by Smad4 [69,70]. Similarly, three TGF-β ligands (TGF-β 1/2/3) bind to cardiac Type I (ALK5) and Type II (TGFBRII) receptors to activate canonical TGF-β signaling [69] mediated by Smad2 and Smad3. This transcriptional pathway in conjunction with Smad inhibitory proteins regulates transcription of TGF-β superfamily-responsive genes [71]. BMP, Notch and TGF-β promote EMT, mesenchymal cell invasion into the cardiac cushions and remodeling of the valves [69,72]. Specific to formation of the arterial valves, TGF-β signaling plays an essential role in the initial promotion and cessation of EMT, and in cushion mesenchyme proliferation and in differentiation during heart valve development.

BMP, TGF-β and Notch are not only activators of these processes, but also transcriptional repressors via the *Snail* family of proteins that are required for the initial steps in EMT and cushion development [73]. As *BMP, TGF*-β and *Notch* all target *Snail* expression, Snail is likely a critical point of convergence for their signaling in valve development. In the adult heart, abnormal BMP signaling has been found in CAVD [74,75], implicating it in the pathogenesis of this condition. Numerous cardiac tissue–specific knock-down experiments have established the importance of the BMP pathway in the development of the endocardial cushions and valve development [76–78]. In contrast, cardiac tissue–specific knock-down of TGF-β1 yields little structural defect. Knock-down of TGF-β2 does produce structural OFT, septal and aortic arch defects [79,80], along with hypercellular cardiac cushions and valves [81]. Important to the initiation and progression of CAVD, TGF-β signaling is involved in the activation of valvular interstitial cells and their transformation to myofibroblasts in the adult valve [82].

4.3. Gata

The *Gata* family of zinc-finger transcription factors binds the "GATA" nucleotide motif and plays an essential role in cardiac development [83]. With relevance to the aortic valve, *Gata4* and *Gata5* are expressed in endocardial cells, endocardial cushions and OFT, and *Gata6* is expressed in CNC cells [84]. Abnormalities in mice with *GATA* mutations indicate that interaction between *Gata4* and *Gata5* is necessary for the endocardial cushions to develop, as *GATA4*$^{+/-}$ *GATA5*$^{+/-}$ double heterozygotes have enlarged semilunar valves compared with single *GATA4*$^{+/-}$ and *GATA5*$^{+/-}$

heterozygotes [84]. *Gata4* mutant mice and humans show septal defects, including both atrial and ventricular septal defects [8,85–88].

4.4. Nuclear Factor in Activated T-Cell, Cytoplasmic 1

In the embryonic heart, *Nfatc1* is expressed before EMT of the OFTs and is seen in endocardial cells, but not in transformed mesenchymal cells of the endocardial cushions [41]. It is also expressed after rudimentary valve formation, enabling elongation of the valve leaflets through degradation of the extracellular matrix of the endocardial cushions by enzymes such as cathepsin K [89]. *Nfatc1*-deficient (*nfatc1*$^{-/-}$) mice have normal endocardial cushion formation but fail to begin normal remodeling of the endocardial cushion for arterial valve development, and this deficiency is embryonic lethal [90].

In addition to its role in valve development, *Nfatc1* also controls NFκB ligand (*RANKL*), a member of the tumor necrosis factor ligand family that is a key factor for osteoclastogenesis and that signals through its receptor *RANK* to promote differentiation of bone-resorbing osteoclasts [91]. The transcription factor *Nfatc1* transduces signals from *RANKL* for differentiation of osteoclast-mediated bone resorption [91] by controlling expression of β3-integrin [92]. Thus, common defects involving *Nfatc1* may be at play in BAV, CAVD and ascending aortic aneurysm.

4.5. Nkx2-5

The homeodomain factor *NKX2-5* is the most commonly mutated single gene in human CHD, accounting for 1%–4% of specific malformations, including cardiac conduction and OFT abnormalities as well as atrial and ventricular septal defects. However, lack of mutational genotype-phenotype correlation points to an early role for this factor in development of the FHF and SHF, and possible phenotypic modification by downstream genes [93]. Although *Nkx2-5* is widely expressed in the developing heart, its most significant role appears to be in SHF development, specifically, directing SHF specification and morphogenesis of SHF-derived cardiac structures [94,95]. *Nkx2*-5 represses *Bmp2/Smad1* signaling and regulates SHF proliferation and OFT morphology [94], and appears to require *Mef2c* for its action [96]. However, for a gene associated with so much human CHD, we know little about its mechanisms of action in cardiac development, especially considering its importance in late natal and post-natal cardiac development [97].

4.6. Nitric Oxide

The first non-human BAV was observed in *NOS3* deficient mice, where the normal expression of *NOS3* expressed in aortic valve endothelium of adult mice was not observed [63]. Structural cardiovascular abnormalities of the aorta were not observed in *NOS3*$^{-/-}$ mice except when combined with haploinsufficiency of *NOTCH1* [65]. The role of *NOS3* in adult development of aortic aneurysm, coarctation or aortic valve stenosis is not clear as aortic wall NOS expression is lower in bicuspid aortic aneurysm [98] and in the aortic root [99] but not associated with aortic stenosis or aneurysm in *NOS3*$^{-/-}$ mice [100].

5. Etiology of BAV Disease

The mature aortic valve has cusps composed of three overlapping layers of highly organized extracellular matrix, embedded with valve interstitial cells and covered by a layer of valve endothelial cells [101]. The three layers are the fibrosa, spongiosa and ventricularis (Figure 6). The fibrosa, which is located on the arterial aspect of arterial valves, is composed predominantly of fibrillar collagens (Types I and III) that are circumferentially oriented and provide tensile stiffness [46–49]. The ventricularis layer, located on the ventricular side of the arterial valves, is composed primarily of radially oriented elastic fibers that facilitate tissue motion [50,51]. The middle layer, the spongiosa, is composed primarily of proteoglycans with interspersed collagen fibers. Proteoglycans, which are also present in the other layers, serve as an interface between the orthogonally arranged fibrosa and ventricularis layers to provide tissue compressibility and integrity.

Like other forms of congenital heart disease (CHD), although chromosomal (DiGeorge and Turner syndrome) and Mendelian (*NOTCH1*) causes of BAV have been identified, these account for a small percentage of BAV cases [102]. The genetic mechanisms underlying the majority of "sporadic" cases of BAV are not known. Even for these seemingly sporadic cases, epidemiological studies have demonstrated a roughly 10% increased risk of BAV in siblings and offspring, and a similar figure for the occurrence of aortic aneurysm in relatives with, or without, BAV, indicating the potential role of shared genes or even environmental causes [103,104].

The genetic architecture of sporadic BAV likely includes: (i) accumulation of rare and uncommon variants in cardiac developmental genes leading to a mutational load favoring BAV formation; (ii) epigenetic modification of cardiac developmental genes; (iii) common variants in genes that may not be obviously linked to cardiac development but have impact on their function; and perhaps; (iv) environmental causes. Complicating this scenario, many CHD-causing gene variants are likely selected against by a decrease in reproductive fitness. The resulting allelic heterogeneity reduces the power of GWAS for CHD. This may or may not be an issue for BAV, as its effect on reproductive fitness is thought to be limited. Nevertheless, these issues collectively make the discovery of the etiology of BAV difficult (Table 1).

Table 1. Factors that may confound discovery of BAV-associated genes.

Low frequency of individual variants causing BAV
High number of variants causing BAV
Variants of many structural types
Variants of many functional roles
Mixed inheritance patterns of disease
High fetal loss of CHD

BAV is commonly associated with aneurysm of the aortic sinuses, the ascending aorta, and aortic coarctation. Pathological examination of the BAV-associated aortic aneurysm often shows non-inflammatory degeneration of smooth muscle cells often described as cystic medial necrosis [105–107]. The co-occurrence of BAV with aortic aneurysm and coarctation of the aorta may imply a common genetic mechanism for these diseases. Dysregulation of the canonical TGF-β signaling axis in humans offers one such example. As described above, TGF-β signaling is a key pathway promoting EMT in valvulogenesis and cellular migration, activities critical to normal valvular development. Mutations in the canonical TGF-β signaling pathway may therefore be hypothesized to cause an enhanced rate of BAV. The human condition Loeys-Dietz syndrome (LDS) is caused by mutations in the genes encoding the TGF-β receptors 1 and 2 (*TGFBR1* and *TGFBR2*), the TGF-β ligands 2 and 3 (*TGFB2* and *TGFB3*), as well as in the downstream transducer of TGF-β signaling, SMAD3. BAV is frequently encountered in patients with LDS, as well as a nearly complete penetrance of thoracic aortic aneurysm [108,109]. While overt TGF-β dysregulation may be an uncommon mechanism for typical BAV-associated thoracic aortic aneurysm, minor variation in other pathways that overlap functionality between valvulogenesis and arterial development may be common in patients with BAV-associated thoracic aortic aneurysm. While one commonly encounters arguments that aortic aneurysms are solely the result of abnormal flow patterns around the valve, these arguments cannot properly account for observed individual variation and the lack of correlation between hemodynamic derangement and aneurysm size seen in BAV patients. Therefore it seems likely that genetic variation in addition to hemodynamic factors plays a major role in aneurysm susceptibility in typical BAV disease.

As previously mentioned, BAV is the most common of congenital valvular defects and is characterized by a valve having only two commissures (Figure 7). It is commonly associated with aneurysm of the aortic sinuses and the ascending aorta, and aortic coarctation. Pathological examination of the BAV-associated aortic aneurysm often shows non-inflammatory degeneration of neural crest-derived smooth muscle cells often described as cystic medial necrosis [105–107]. Nevertheless, experimental evidence supporting a common underlying developmental mechanism to explain the association of aortic valve and associated aortopathy is lacking.

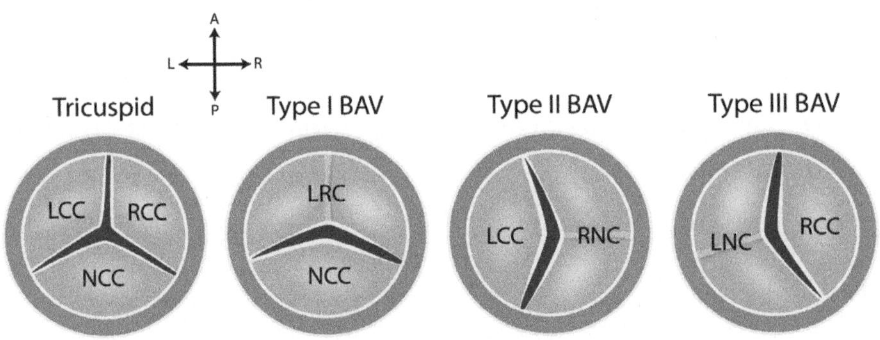

Figure 7. Anatomy of the bicuspid valve and potential pathways for its development. The bicuspid valve is classified as Type I: fusion of the right coronary cusp (RCC) and left coronary cusp (LCC) to create a fused left-right cusp (LRC). A Type I BAV results from persistent fusion of the left and right leaflets normally be formed by the superior and inferior septal cushions. Type II: fusion of the RCC and non-coronary cusp (NCC) to create a fused right-non-coronary cusp (RNC). Type III: fusion between the LCC and NCC to create a fused left-non-coronary cusp (LNC). Both Type II and Type III BAVs result from fusion of the posterior aortic interacted disc with either the inferior (Type II) or superior (Type III) septal cushion. These differences in anatomy imply differences in etiologic mechanisms [110].

Human BAV has been associated with chromosomal variation in DiGeorge syndrome ($22q11.2^{del}$) and Turner syndrome (Xp^{del}). The genetic basis of structural valve abnormalities in DiGeorge syndrome has been attributed to hemizygosity of *TBX1* and impaired downstream signaling by *Fgf8* [111,112], but the association is imperfect. The cause of BAV, often with coarctation, in 30% of women with Turner syndrome is unknown, although good evidence has implicated a haploinsufficient region lying distal to Xp11.4 [113–115]. The very high incidence of BAV in Turner women compared with XY men favors existence of autosomal modifier genes for this valvular disease and perhaps a homologous Y chromosomal gene [4]. BAV has also been associated with the primary ciliopathies, such as Joubert syndrome [116], and with ventricular non-compaction [117,118]. Using linkage, loci within the 5q15-21, 13q33-qter and 18q22.1 chromosomal regions have been identified [4,119], but the responsible genes have not.

Smaller abnormalities such as copy number variation, indels and single-nucleotide polymorphisms almost certainly have some responsibility for BAV in the general population, especially in sporadic cases not associated with extensive non-valvular phenotypes. Variants in *NKX2-5* (5q34) [120,121], *NOTCH1* (9q34.3) [15,16,122,123], *FBN1* (*15q21.1*) [124], *MATR3* (*5q31.2*) [125] and *GATA5* (20q13.33) [126–128] have been observed in individuals with BAV. However, some of these associations may result from co-existing disease, such as association of FBN1 with ascending aortic disease [129]. Unfortunately, none of these findings provide epiphanous insight into the causes of BAV.

Study of the cause(s) of BAV is a good example of the limitations of disease mapping using genetic variation to explore human complex disease (Table 1). There may be significant cost and time advantages to discerning the cause of BAV and its co-existing diseases using vertebrate models of the condition. Despite limitations in animal models of human disease, targeted "knock-in" candidate gene mutations in mice [130] and zebrafish [131] may provide useful insight by modeling human BAV better than gene knockout mouse models do [130]. These individual SNPs or small insertion/deletion mutations are far more frequently observed in human disease than whole-exome or whole-gene deletions. In addition, these smaller variants more accurately replicate human disease and thus have greater potential applicability. The value of large or whole-gene deletion is principally confined to identifying pathways of disease rather than the exact molecular biology of disease. Although these techniques are a necessary albeit limited step, they cannot explain biological functions of the candidate genes identified. Culturing of embryonic and aortic valve interstitial cells will be needed to validate these targets and identify their relationships to subsequent CAVD and aortic disease [3,130].

6. Summary

In this review, we have described the series of events from cellular and transcriptional embryogenesis of the heart, to development of the aortic valve. The frequent occurrence of BAV and its anatomically discrete but common co-existing diseases (ascending aortic disease, aortic stenosis and coarctation of the aorta) leads us to suspect a shared cellular origin. However, the extensive cell-cell signaling and interactions of cardiac embryogenesis preclude simplistic explanations of this disease.

Acknowledgments

This work was supported by a National Institutes of Health grants 1R01HL114823 (SCB), 1P30GM103342 (RAN), 8P20GM103444-07 (RAN), R01HL127692 (RAN, DM), American Heart Association 15GRNT25080052 (RAN).

Abbreviations

ALK = activin-like kinase; BAV = bicuspid aortic valve; BMP = bone morphogenic pathway; CAVD = calcific aortic valve disease; CHD = congenital heart disease; CNC = cardiac neural crest; EMT = epithelial to mesenchymal transition; FGF = fibroblast growth factor; FHF = first heart field; GWAS = genomewide association study; LPM = lateral plate mesoderm; Nfatc1 = nuclear factor in activated T-cell, cytoplasmic 1; NICD = Notch intracellular domain; OFT = outflow tract; SHF = second heart field; SNP = single nucleotide polymorphism; TGF-β = transforming growth factor-β; Wnt = wingless-related MMTV integration sites.

Conflicts of Interest

The authors declare no conflict of interest.

References

1. Michelena, H.I.; Prakash, S.K.; della Corte, A.; Bissell, M.M.; Anavekar, N.; Mathieu, P.; Bosse, Y.; Limongelli, G.; Bossone, E.; Benson, D.W.; *et al.* Bicuspid aortic valve: Identifying knowledge gaps and rising to the challenge from the international bicuspid aortic valve consortium (bavcon). *Circulation* **2014**, *129*, 2691–2704.
2. Della Corte, A.; Body, S.C.; Booher, A.M.; Schaefers, H.J.; Milewski, R.K.; Michelena, H.I.; Evangelista, A.; Pibarot, P.; Mathieu, P.; Limongelli, G.; *et al.* Surgical treatment of bicuspid aortic valve disease: Knowledge gaps and research perspectives. *J. Thorac. Cardiovasc. Surg.* **2014**, *147*, 1749–1757.
3. Yutzey, K.E.; Demer, L.L.; Body, S.C.; Huggins, G.S.; Towler, D.A.; Giachelli, C.M.; Hofmann-Bowman, M.A.; Mortlock, D.P.; Rogers, M.B.; Sadeghi, M.M.; *et al.* Calcific aortic valve disease: A consensus summary from the alliance of investigators on calcific aortic valve disease. *Arterioscler. Thromb. Vasc. Biol.* **2014**, *34*, 2387–2393.
4. Prakash, S.K.; Bosse, Y.; Muehlschlegel, J.D.; Michelena, H.I.; Limongelli, G.; della Corte, A.; Pluchinotta, F.R.; Russo, M.G.; Evangelista, A.; Benson, D.W.; *et al.* A roadmap to investigate the genetic basis of bicuspid aortic valve and its complications: Insights from the international bavcon (bicuspid aortic valve consortium). *J. Am. Coll. Cardiol.* **2014**, *64*, 832–839.
5. Srivastava, D.; Olson, E.N. A genetic blueprint for cardiac development. *Nature* **2000**, *407*, 221–226.
6. Maitra, M.; Koenig, S.N.; Srivastava, D.; Garg, V. Identification of gata6 sequence variants in patients with congenital heart defects. *Pediatr. Res.* **2010**, *68*, 281–285.
7. Srivastava, D. Making or breaking the heart: From lineage determination to morphogenesis. *Cell* **2006**, *126*, 1037–1048.

8. Hirayama-Yamada, K.; Kamisago, M.; Akimoto, K.; Aotsuka, H.; Nakamura, Y.; Tomita, H.; Furutani, M.; Imamura, S.; Takao, A.; Nakazawa, M.; *et al.* Phenotypes with Gata4 or NKX2.5 mutations in familial atrial septal defect. *Am. J. Med. Genet. A* **2005**, *135*, 47–52.
9. Li, C.; Li, X.; Pang, S.; Chen, W.; Qin, X.; Huang, W.; Zeng, C.; Yan, B. Novel and functional DNA sequence variants within the gata6 gene promoter in ventricular septal defects. *Int. J. Mol. Sci.* **2014**, *15*, 12677–12687.
10. Pang, S.; Liu, Y.; Zhao, Z.; Huang, W.; Chen, D.; Yan, B. Novel and functional sequence variants within the tbx2 gene promoter in ventricular septal defects. *Biochimie* **2013**, *95*, 1807–1809.
11. Yang, Y.Q.; Wang, J.; Liu, X.Y.; Chen, X.Z.; Zhang, W.; Wang, X.Z. Mutation spectrum of gata4 associated with congenital atrial septal defects. *Arch. Med. Sci.* **2013**, *9*, 976–983.
12. Aguayo-Gomez, A.; Arteaga-Vazquez, J.; Svyryd, Y.; Calderon-Colmenero, J.; Zamora-Gonzalez, C.; Vargas-Alarcon, G.; Mutchinick, O.M. Identification of copy number variations in isolated tetralogy of fallot. *Pediatr. Cardiol.* **2015**, in press.
13. Greenway, S.C.; Pereira, A.C.; Lin, J.C.; DePalma, S.R.; Israel, S.J.; Mesquita, S.M.; Ergul, E.; Conta, J.H.; Korn, J.M.; McCarroll, S.A.; *et al. De novo* copy number variants identify new genes and loci in isolated sporadic tetralogy of fallot. *Nat. Genet.* **2009**, *41*, 931–935.
14. Nguyen, H.H.; Jay, P.Y. A single misstep in cardiac development explains the co-occurrence of tetralogy of fallot and complete atrioventricular septal defect in down syndrome. *J. Pediatr.* **2014**, *165*, 194–196.
15. Garg, V.; Muth, A.N.; Ransom, J.F.; Schluterman, M.K.; Barnes, R.; King, I.N.; Grossfeld, P.D.; Srivastava, D. Mutations in notch1 cause aortic valve disease. *Nature* **2005**, *437*, 270–274.
16. McKellar, S.H.; Tester, D.J.; Yagubyan, M.; Majumdar, R.; Ackerman, M.J.; Sundt, T.M., 3rd. Novel notch1 mutations in patients with bicuspid aortic valve disease and thoracic aortic aneurysms. *J. Thorac. Cardiovasc. Surg.* **2007**, *134*, 290–296.
17. Olson, E.N. Gene regulatory networks in the evolution and development of the heart. *Science* **2006**, *313*, 1922–1927.
18. Wessels, A.; van den Hoff, M.J.; Adamo, R.F.; Phelps, A.L.; Lockhart, M.M.; Sauls, K.; Briggs, L.E.; Norris, R.A.; van Wijk, B.; Perez-Pomares, J.M.; *et al.* Epicardially derived fibroblasts preferentially contribute to the parietal leaflets of the atrioventricular valves in the murine heart. *Dev. Biol.* **2012**, *366*, 111–124.
19. Gittenberger-de Groot, A.C.; Bartelings, M.M.; Poelmann, R.E.; Haak, M.C.; Jongbloed, M.R. Embryology of the heart and its impact on understanding fetal and neonatal heart disease. *Semin. Fetal Neonatal Med.* **2013**, *18*, 237–244.
20. Buckingham, M.; Meilhac, S.; Zaffran, S. Building the mammalian heart from two sources of myocardial cells. *Nat. Rev. Genet.* **2005**, *6*, 826–835.
21. Kelly, R.G. The second heart field. *Curr. Top. Dev. Biol.* **2012**, *100*, 33–65.
22. Kelly, R.G.; Buckingham, M.E.; Moorman, A.F. Heart fields and cardiac morphogenesis. *Cold Spring Harb. Perspect. Med.* **2014**, *4*, doi:10.1101/cshperspect.a015750.
23. Cai, C.L.; Liang, X.; Shi, Y.; Chu, P.H.; Pfaff, S.L.; Chen, J.; Evans, S. ISL1 identifies a cardiac progenitor population that proliferates prior to differentiation and contributes a majority of cells to the heart. *Dev. Cell* **2003**, *5*, 877–889.

24. Lindsey, S.E.; Butcher, J.T.; Yalcin, H.C. Mechanical regulation of cardiac development. *Front. Physiol.* **2014**, *5*, 318, doi:10.3389/fphys.2014.00318.
25. Jain, R.; Engleka, K.A.; Rentschler, S.L.; Manderfield, L.J.; Li, L.; Yuan, L.; Epstein, J.A. Cardiac neural crest orchestrates remodeling and functional maturation of mouse semilunar valves. *J. Clin. Investig.* **2011**, *121*, 422–430.
26. Kirby, M.L.; Hutson, M.R. Factors controlling cardiac neural crest cell migration. *Cell Adh. Migr.* **2010**, *4*, 609–621.
27. Waldo, K.L.; Hutson, M.R.; Ward, C.C.; Zdanowicz, M.; Stadt, H.A.; Kumiski, D.; Abu-Issa, R.; Kirby, M.L. Secondary heart field contributes myocardium and smooth muscle to the arterial pole of the developing heart. *Dev. Biol.* **2005**, *281*, 78–90.
28. Bajolle, F.; Zaffran, S.; Kelly, R.G.; Hadchouel, J.; Bonnet, D.; Brown, N.A.; Buckingham, M.E. Rotation of the myocardial wall of the outflow tract is implicated in the normal positioning of the great arteries. *Circ. Res.* **2006**, *98*, 421–428.
29. Brade, T.; Pane, L.S.; Moretti, A.; Chien, K.R.; Laugwitz, K.L. Embryonic heart progenitors and cardiogenesis. *Cold Spring Harb. Perspect. Med.* **2013**, *3*, a013847.
30. Harris, I.S.; Black, B.L. Development of the endocardium. *Pediatr. Cardiol.* **2010**, *31*, 391–399.
31. Bu, L.; Jiang, X.; Martin-Puig, S.; Caron, L.; Zhu, S.; Shao, Y.; Roberts, D.J.; Huang, P.L.; Domian, I.J.; Chien, K.R. Human isl1 heart progenitors generate diverse multipotent cardiovascular cell lineages. *Nature* **2009**, *460*, 113–117.
32. Jain, R.; Rentschler, S.; Epstein, J.A. Notch and cardiac outflow tract development. *Ann. N. Y. Acad. Sci.* **2010**, *1188*, 184–190.
33. Kelly, R.G. The second heart field. In *Current Topics in Developmental Biology*; Benoit, G.B., Ed.; Academic Press: Waltham, MA, USA, 2012; Volume 100, pp 33–65.
34. Barnett, P.; van den Boogaard, M.; Christoffels, V. Localized and temporal gene regulation in heart development. *Curr. Top. Dev. Biol.* **2012**, *100*, 171–201.
35. Ward, C.; Stadt, H.; Hutson, M.; Kirby, M.L. Ablation of the secondary heart field leads to tetralogy of fallot and pulmonary atresia. *Dev. Biol.* **2005**, *284*, 72–83.
36. Neeb, Z.; Lajiness, J.D.; Bolanis, E.; Conway, S.J. Cardiac outflow tract anomalies. *Wiley Interdiscip. Dev. Biol.* **2013**, *2*, 499–530.
37. Restivo, A.; Piacentini, G.; Placidi, S.; Saffirio, C.; Marino, B. Cardiac outflow tract: A review of some embryogenetic aspects of the conotruncal region of the heart. *Anat. Rec. A Discov. Mol. Cell. Evol. Biol.* **2006**, *288*, 936–943.
38. Abu-Issa, R. Heart fields: Spatial polarity and temporal dynamics. *Anat. Rec.* **2014**, *297*, 175–182.
39. Kirby, M.L.; Gale, T.F.; Stewart, D.E. Neural crest cells contribute to normal aorticopulmonary septation. *Science* **1983**, *220*, 1059–1061.
40. Jiang, X.; Rowitch, D.H.; Soriano, P.; McMahon, A.P.; Sucov, H.M. Fate of the mammalian cardiac neural crest. *Development* **2000**, *127*, 1607–1616.
41. Wu, B.; Wang, Y.; Lui, W.; Langworthy, M.; Tompkins, K.L.; Hatzopoulos, A.K.; Baldwin, H.S.; Zhou, B. Nfatc1 coordinates valve endocardial cell lineage development required for heart valve formation. *Circ. Res.* **2011**, *109*, 183–192.

42. Okamoto, N.; Akimoto, N.; Hidaka, N.; Shoji, S.; Sumida, H. Formal genesis of the outflow tracts of the heart revisited: Previous works in the light of recent observations. *Congenit. Anom.* **2010**, *50*, 141–158.
43. Lin, C.J.; Lin, C.Y.; Chen, C.H.; Zhou, B.; Chang, C.P. Partitioning the heart: Mechanisms of cardiac septation and valve development. *Development* **2012**, *139*, 3277–3299.
44. Anderson, R.H.; Webb, S.; Brown, N.A.; Lamers, W.; Moorman, A. Development of the heart: (3) Formation of the ventricular outflow tracts, arterial valves, and intrapericardial arterial trunks. *Heart* **2003**, *89*, 1110–1118.
45. Wirrig, E.E.; Yutzey, K.E. Conserved transcriptional regulatory mechanisms in aortic valve development and disease. *Arterioscler. Thromb. Vasc. Biol.* **2014**, *34*, 737–741.
46. Hinton, R.B., Jr.; Lincoln, J.; Deutsch, G.H.; Osinska, H.; Manning, P.B.; Benson, D.W.; Yutzey, K.E. Extracellular matrix remodeling and organization in developing and diseased aortic valves. *Circ. Res.* **2006**, *98*, 1431–1438.
47. de Lange, F.J.; Moorman, A.F.; Anderson, R.H.; Manner, J.; Soufan, A.T.; de Gier-de Vries, C.; Schneider, M.D.; Webb, S.; van den Hoff, M.J.; Christoffels, V.M. Lineage and morphogenetic analysis of the cardiac valves. *Circ. Res.* **2004**, *95*, 645–654.
48. Butcher, J.T.; Markwald, R.R. Valvulogenesis: The moving target. *Philos. Trans. R Soc. Lond B Biol. Sci.* **2007**, *362*, 1489–1503.
49. Schoen, F.J. Evolving concepts of cardiac valve dynamics: The continuum of development, functional structure, pathobiology, and tissue engineering. *Circulation* **2008**, *118*, 1864–1880.
50. Combs, M.D.; Yutzey, K.E. Heart valve development: Regulatory networks in development and disease. *Circ. Res.* **2009**, *105*, 408–421.
51. Timmerman, L.A.; Grego-Bessa, J.; Raya, A.; Bertran, E.; Perez-Pomares, J.M.; Diez, J.; Aranda, S.; Palomo, S.; McCormick, F.; Izpisua-Belmonte, J.C.; *et al.* Notch promotes epithelial-mesenchymal transition during cardiac development and oncogenic transformation. *Genes Dev.* **2004**, *18*, 99–115.
52. Williams, R.; Lendahl, U.; Lardelli, M. Complementary and combinatorial patterns of notch gene family expression during early mouse development. *Mech. Dev.* **1995**, *53*, 357–368.
53. Loomes, K.M.; Taichman, D.B.; Glover, C.L.; Williams, P.T.; Markowitz, J.E.; Piccoli, D.A.; Baldwin, H.S.; Oakey, R.J. Characterization of notch receptor expression in the developing mammalian heart and liver. *Am. J. Med. Genet.* **2002**, *112*, 181–189.
54. Varadkar, P.; Kraman, M.; Despres, D.; Ma, G.; Lozier, J.; McCright, B. Notch2 is required for the proliferation of cardiac neural crest-derived smooth muscle cells. *Dev. Dyn.* **2008**, *237*, 1144–1152.
55. Benedito, R.; Duarte, A. Expression of dll4 during mouse embryogenesis suggests multiple developmental roles. *Gene Expr. Patterns* **2005**, *5*, 750–755.
56. Andersson, E.R.; Sandberg, R.; Lendahl, U. Notch signaling: Simplicity in design, versatility in function. *Development* **2011**, *138*, 3593–3612.
57. Fu, Y.; Chang, A.; Chang, L.; Niessen, K.; Eapen, S.; Setiadi, A.; Karsan, A. Differential regulation of transforming growth factor β signaling pathways by notch in human endothelial cells. *J. Biol. Chem.* **2009**, *284*, 19452–19462.

58. Loomes, K.M.; Underkoffler, L.A.; Morabito, J.; Gottlieb, S.; Piccoli, D.A.; Spinner, N.B.; Baldwin, H.S.; Oakey, R.J. The expression of Jagged1 in the developing mammalian heart correlates with cardiovascular disease in alagille syndrome. *Hum. Mol. Genet.* **1999**, *8*, 2443–2449.
59. Kamath, B.M.; Bauer, R.C.; Loomes, K.M.; Chao, G.; Gerfen, J.; Hutchinson, A.; Hardikar, W.; Hirschfield, G.; Jara, P.; Krantz, I.D.; *et al.* Notch2 mutations in alagille syndrome. *J. Med. Genet.* **2012**, *49*, 138–144.
60. Jia, Q.; McDill, B.W.; Li, S.Z.; Deng, C.; Chang, C.P.; Chen, F. Smad signaling in the neural crest regulates cardiac outflow tract remodeling through cell autonomous and non-cell autonomous effects. *Dev. Biol.* **2007**, *311*, 172–184.
61. High, F.A.; Lu, M.M.; Pear, W.S.; Loomes, K.M.; Kaestner, K.H.; Epstein, J.A. Endothelial expression of the notch ligand jagged1 is required for vascular smooth muscle development. *Proc. Natl. Acad. Sci. USA* **2008**, *105*, 1955–1959.
62. Krebs, L.T.; Xue, Y.; Norton, C.R.; Sundberg, J.P.; Beatus, P.; Lendahl, U.; Joutel, A.; Gridley, T. Characterization of notch3-deficient mice: Normal embryonic development and absence of genetic interactions with a notch1 mutation. *Genesis* **2003**, *37*, 139–143.
63. Lee, T.C.; Zhao, Y.D.; Courtman, D.W.; Stewart, D.J. Abnormal aortic valve development in mice lacking endothelial nitric oxide synthase. *Circulation* **2000**, *101*, 2345–2348.
64. Bosse, K.; Hans, C.P.; Zhao, N.; Koenig, S.N.; Huang, N.; Guggilam, A.; LaHaye, S.; Tao, G.; Lucchesi, P.A.; Lincoln, J.; *et al.* Endothelial nitric oxide signaling regulates notch1 in aortic valve disease. *J. Mol. Cell. Cardiol.* **2013**, *60*, 27–35.
65. Koenig, S.N.; Bosse, K.M.; Nadorlik, H.A.; Lilly, B.; Garg, V. Evidence of aortopathy in mice with haploinsufficiency of *Notch1* in *Nos3*-null background. *J. Cardiovasc. Dev. Dis.* **2015**, *2*, 17–30.
66. Acharya, A.; Hans, C.P.; Koenig, S.N.; Nichols, H.A.; Galindo, C.L.; Garner, H.R.; Merrill, W.H.; Hinton, R.B.; Garg, V. Inhibitory role of notch1 in calcific aortic valve disease. *PLoS ONE* **2011**, *6*, e27743.
67. Nigam, V.; Srivastava, D. Notch1 represses osteogenic pathways in aortic valve cells. *J. Mol. Cell. Cardiol.* **2009**, *47*, 828–834.
68. Nus, M.; MacGrogan, D.; Martinez-Poveda, B.; Benito, Y.; Casanova, J.C.; Fernandez-Aviles, F.; Bermejo, J.; de la Pompa, J.L. Diet-induced aortic valve disease in mice haploinsufficient for the notch pathway effector rbpjk/csl. *Arterioscler. Thromb. Vasc. Biol.* **2011**, *31*, 1580–1588.
69. Garside, V.C.; Chang, A.C.; Karsan, A.; Hoodless, P.A. Co-ordinating notch, bmp, and tgf-β signaling during heart valve development. *Cell. Mol. Life Sci.* **2013**, *70*, 2899–2917.
70. Thomas, P.S.; Sridurongrit, S.; Ruiz-Lozano, P.; Kaartinen, V. Deficient signaling via ALK2 (acvr1) leads to bicuspid aortic valve development. *PLoS ONE* **2012**, *7*, e35539.
71. Conway, S.J.; Doetschman, T.; Azhar, M. The inter-relationship of periostin, tgf β, and bmp in heart valve development and valvular heart diseases. *Sci.World J.* **2011**, *11*, 1509–1524.
72. Jiao, K.; Kulessa, H.; Tompkins, K.; Zhou, Y.; Batts, L.; Baldwin, H.S.; Hogan, B.L. An essential role of bmp4 in the atrioventricular septation of the mouse heart. *Genes Dev.* **2003**, *17*, 2362–2367.
73. Niessen, K.; Fu, Y.; Chang, L.; Hoodless, P.A.; McFadden, D.; Karsan, A. Slug is a direct notch target required for initiation of cardiac cushion cellularization. *J. Cell Biol.* **2008**, *182*, 315–325.

74. Steiner, I.; Kasparova, P.; Kohout, A.; Dominik, J. Bone formation in cardiac valves: A histopathological study of 128 cases. *Virchows Arch.* **2007**, *450*, 653–657.
75. Ankeny, R.F.; Thourani, V.H.; Weiss, D.; Vega, J.D.; Taylor, W.R.; Nerem, R.M.; Jo, H. Preferential activation of smad1/5/8 on the fibrosa endothelium in calcified human aortic valves—Association with low bmp antagonists and smad6. *PLoS ONE* **2011**, *6*, e20969.
76. Gaussin, V.; van de Putte, T.; Mishina, Y.; Hanks, M.C.; Zwijsen, A.; Huylebroeck, D.; Behringer, R.R.; Schneider, M.D. Endocardial cushion and myocardial defects after cardiac myocyte-specific conditional deletion of the bone morphogenetic protein receptor alk3. *Proc. Natl. Acad. Sci. USA* **2002**, *99*, 2878–2883.
77. Kruithof, B.P.; Duim, S.N.; Moerkamp, A.T.; Goumans, M.J. Tgfβ and bmp signaling in cardiac cushion formation: Lessons from mice and chicken. *Differentiation* **2012**, *84*, 89–102.
78. Delot, E.C.; Bahamonde, M.E.; Zhao, M.; Lyons, K.M. Bmp signaling is required for septation of the outflow tract of the mammalian heart. *Development* **2003**, *130*, 209–220.
79. Bartram, U.; Molin, D.G.; Wisse, L.J.; Mohamad, A.; Sanford, L.P.; Doetschman, T.; Speer, C.P.; Poelmann, R.E.; Gittenberger-de Groot, A.C. Double-outlet right ventricle and overriding tricuspid valve reflect disturbances of looping, myocardialization, endocardial cushion differentiation, and apoptosis in tgf-β(2)-knockout mice. *Circulation* **2001**, *103*, 2745–2752.
80. Sanford, L.P.; Ormsby, I.; Gittenberger-de Groot, A.C.; Sariola, H.; Friedman, R.; Boivin, G.P.; Cardell, E.L.; Doetschman, T. Tgfβ2 knockout mice have multiple developmental defects that are non-overlapping with other tgfβ knockout phenotypes. *Development* **1997**, *124*, 2659–2670.
81. Azhar, M.; Runyan, R.B.; Gard, C.; Sanford, L.P.; Miller, M.L.; Andringa, A.; Pawlowski, S.; Rajan, S.; Doetschman, T. Ligand-specific function of transforming growth factor β in epithelial-mesenchymal transition in heart development. *Dev. Dyn.* **2009**, *238*, 431–442.
82. Walker, G.A.; Masters, K.S.; Shah, D.N.; Anseth, K.S.; Leinwand, L.A. Valvular myofibroblast activation by transforming growth factor-β: Implications for pathological extracellular matrix remodeling in heart valve disease. *Circ. Res.* **2004**, *95*, 253–260.
83. Rivera-Feliciano, J.; Lee, K.H.; Kong, S.W.; Rajagopal, S.; Ma, Q.; Springer, Z.; Izumo, S.; Tabin, C.J.; Pu, W.T. Development of heart valves requires gata4 expression in endothelial-derived cells. *Development* **2006**, *133*, 3607–3618.
84. Laforest, B.; Nemer, M. Gata5 interacts with gata4 and gata6 in outflow tract development. *Dev. Biol.* **2011**, *358*, 368–378.
85. Garg, V.; Kathiriya, I.S.; Barnes, R.; Schluterman, M.K.; King, I.N.; Butler, C.A.; Rothrock, C.R.; Eapen, R.S.; Hirayama-Yamada, K.; Joo, K.; *et al.* Gata4 mutations cause human congenital heart defects and reveal an interaction with tbx5. *Nature* **2003**, *424*, 443–447.
86. Sarkozy, A.; Conti, E.; Neri, C.; D'Agostino, R.; Digilio, M.C.; Esposito, G.; Toscano, A.; Marino, B.; Pizzuti, A.; Dallapiccola, B. Spectrum of atrial septal defects associated with mutations of nkx2.5 and gata4 transcription factors. *J. Med. Genet.* **2005**, *42*, e16.
87. Rajagopal, S.K.; Ma, Q.; Obler, D.; Shen, J.; Manichaikul, A.; Tomita-Mitchell, A.; Boardman, K.; Briggs, C.; Garg, V.; Srivastava, D.; *et al.* Spectrum of heart disease associated with murine and human gata4 mutation. *J. Mol. Cell. Cardiol.* **2007**, *43*, 677–685.

88. Misra, C.; Sachan, N.; McNally, C.R.; Koenig, S.N.; Nichols, H.A.; Guggilam, A.; Lucchesi, P.A.; Pu, W.T.; Srivastava, D.; Garg, V. Congenital heart disease-causing Gata4 mutation displays functional deficits *in vivo*. *PLoS Genet.* **2012**, *8*, e1002690.
89. De la Pompa, J.L.; Timmerman, L.A.; Takimoto, H.; Yoshida, H.; Elia, A.J.; Samper, E.; Potter, J.; Wakeham, A.; Marengere, L.; Langille, B.L.; *et al.* Role of the nf-atc transcription factor in morphogenesis of cardiac valves and septum. *Nature* **1998**, *392*, 182–186.
90. Lin, C.Y.; Lin, C.J.; Chen, C.H.; Chen, R.M.; Zhou, B.; Chang, C.P. The secondary heart field is a new site of calcineurin/nfatc1 signaling for semilunar valve development. *J. Mol. Cell. Cardiol.* **2012**, *52*, 1096–1102.
91. Alexopoulos, A.; Bravou, V.; Peroukides, S.; Kaklamanis, L.; Varakis, J.; Alexopoulos, D.; Papadaki, H. Bone regulatory factors nfatc1 and osterix in human calcific aortic valves. *Int. J. Cardiol.* **2010**, *139*, 142–149.
92. Crotti, T.N.; Flannery, M.; Walsh, N.C.; Fleming, J.D.; Goldring, S.R.; McHugh, K.P. Nfatc1 regulation of the human β3 integrin promoter in osteoclast differentiation. *Gene* **2006**, *372*, 92–102.
93. Reamon-Buettner, S.M.; Borlak, J. Nkx2-5: An update on this hypermutable homeodomain protein and its role in human congenital heart disease (chd). *Hum. Mutat.* **2010**, *31*, 1185–1194.
94. Prall, O.W.; Menon, M.K.; Solloway, M.J.; Watanabe, Y.; Zaffran, S.; Bajolle, F.; Biben, C.; McBride, J.J.; Robertson, B.R.; Chaulet, H.; *et al.* An nkx2-5/bmp2/smad1 negative feedback loop controls heart progenitor specification and proliferation. *Cell* **2007**, *128*, 947–959.
95. Yang, Y.P.; Li, H.R.; Cao, X.M.; Wang, Q.X.; Qiao, C.J.; Ya, J. Second heart field and the development of the outflow tract in human embryonic heart. *Dev. Growth Differ.* **2013**, *55*, 359–367.
96. Vincentz, J.W.; Barnes, R.M.; Firulli, B.A.; Conway, S.J.; Firulli, A.B. Cooperative interaction of NKX2.5 and mef2c transcription factors during heart development. *Dev. Dyn.* **2008**, *237*, 3809–3819.
97. George, V.; Colombo, S.; Targoff, K.L. An early requirement for NKX2.5 ensures the first and second heart field ventricular identity and cardiac function into adulthood. *Dev. Biol.* **2015**, *400*, 10–22.
98. Aicher, D.; Urbich, C.; Zeiher, A.; Dimmeler, S.; Schafers, H.J. Endothelial nitric oxide synthase in bicuspid aortic valve disease. *Ann. Thorac. Surg.* **2007**, *83*, 1290–1294.
99. Mohamed, S.A.; Radtke, A.; Saraei, R.; Bullerdiek, J.; Sorani, H.; Nimzyk, R.; Karluss, A.; Sievers, H.H.; Belge, G. Locally different endothelial nitric oxide synthase protein levels in ascending aortic aneurysms of bicuspid and tricuspid aortic valve. *Cardiol. Res. Pract.* **2012**, *2012*, 165957, doi:10.1155/2012/165957.
100. El Accaoui, R.N.; Gould, S.T.; Hajj, G.P.; Chu, Y.; Davis, M.K.; Kraft, D.C.; Lund, D.D.; Brooks, R.M.; Doshi, H.; Zimmerman, K.A.; *et al.* Aortic valve sclerosis in mice deficient in endothelial nitric oxide synthase. *Am. J. Physiol. Heart Circ. Physiol.* **2014**, *306*, H1302–H1313.
101. Hinton, R.B.; Yutzey, K.E. Heart valve structure and function in development and disease. *Annu. Rev. Physiol.* **2011**, *73*, 29–46.
102. Pierpont, M.E.; Basson, C.T.; Benson, D.W., Jr.; Gelb, B.D.; Giglia, T.M.; Goldmuntz, E.; McGee, G.; Sable, C.A.; Srivastava, D.; Webb, C.L.; *et al.* Genetic basis for congenital heart defects: Current knowledge. *Circulation* **2007**, *115*, 3015–3038.

103. Huntington, K.; Hunter, A.G.; Chan, K.L. A prospective study to assess the frequency of familial clustering of congenital bicuspid aortic valve. *J. Am. Coll. Cardiol.* **1997**, *30*, 1809–1812.
104. Glick, B.N.; Roberts, W.C. Congenitally bicuspid aortic valve in multiple family members. *Am. J. Cardiol.* **1994**, *73*, 400–404.
105. Bonderman, D.; Gharehbaghi-Schnell, E.; Wollenek, G.; Maurer, G.; Baumgartner, H.; Lang, I.M. Mechanisms underlying aortic dilatation in congenital aortic valve malformation. *Circulation* **1999**, *99*, 2138–2143.
106. De Sa, M.; Moshkovitz, Y.; Butany, J.; David, T.E. Histologic abnormalities of the ascending aorta and pulmonary trunk in patients with bicuspid aortic valve disease: Clinical relevance to the ross procedure. *J. Thorac. Cardiovasc. Surg.* **1999**, *118*, 588–594.
107. Tadros, T.M.; Klein, M.D.; Shapira, O.M. Ascending aortic dilatation associated with bicuspid aortic valve: Pathophysiology, molecular biology, and clinical implications. *Circulation* **2009**, *119*, 880–890.
108. Loeys, B.L.; Chen, J.; Neptune, E.R.; Judge, D.P.; Podowski, M.; Holm, T.; Meyers, J.; Leitch, C.C.; Katsanis, N.; Sharifi, N.; *et al.* A syndrome of altered cardiovascular, craniofacial, neurocognitive and skeletal development caused by mutations in tgfbr1 or tgfbr2. *Nat. Genet.* **2005**, *37*, 275–281.
109. Loeys, B.L.; Schwarze, U.; Holm, T.; Callewaert, B.L.; Thomas, G.H.; Pannu, H.; de Backer, J.F.; Oswald, G.L.; Symoens, S.; Manouvrier, S.; *et al.* Aneurysm syndromes caused by mutations in the tgf-β receptor. *N. Engl. J. Med.* **2006**, *355*, 788–798.
110. Fernandez, B.; Duran, A.C.; Fernandez-Gallego, T.; Fernandez, M.C.; Such, M.; Arque, J.M.; Sans-Coma, V. Bicuspid aortic valves with different spatial orientations of the leaflets are distinct etiological entities. *J. Am. Coll. Cardiol.* **2009**, *54*, 2312–2318.
111. Keyte, A.; Hutson, M.R. The neural crest in cardiac congenital anomalies. *Differentiation* **2012**, *84*, 25–40.
112. Merscher, S.; Funke, B.; Epstein, J.A.; Heyer, J.; Puech, A.; Lu, M.M.; Xavier, R.J.; Demay, M.B.; Russell, R.G.; Factor, S.; *et al.* Tbx1 is responsible for cardiovascular defects in velo-cardio-facial/digeorge syndrome. *Cell* **2001**, *104*, 619–629.
113. Sachdev, V.; Matura, L.A.; Sidenko, S.; Ho, V.B.; Arai, A.E.; Rosing, D.R.; Bondy, C.A. Aortic valve disease in turner syndrome. *J. Am. Coll. Cardiol.* **2008**, *51*, 1904–1909.
114. Bondy, C.; Bakalov, V.K.; Cheng, C.; Olivieri, L.; Rosing, D.R.; Arai, A.E. Bicuspid aortic valve and aortic coarctation are linked to deletion of the x chromosome short arm in turner syndrome. *J. Med. Genet.* **2013**, *50*, 662–665.
115. Miller, M.J.; Geffner, M.E.; Lippe, B.M.; Itami, R.M.; Kaplan, S.A.; DiSessa, T.G.; Isabel-Jones, J.B.; Friedman, W.F. Echocardiography reveals a high incidence of bicuspid aortic valve in turner syndrome. *J. Pediatr.* **1983**, *102*, 47–50.
116. Karp, N.; Grosse-Wortmann, L.; Bowdin, S. Severe aortic stenosis, bicuspid aortic valve and atrial septal defect in a child with joubert syndrome and related disorders (jsrd)—A case report and review of congenital heart defects reported in the human ciliopathies. *Eur. J. Med. Genet.* **2012**, *55*, 605–610.

117. Imbalzano, E.; Ceravolo, R.; di Stefano, R.; Vatrano, M.; Saitta, A. Rare combination of left ventricular noncompaction, bicuspid aortic valve and myocardial bridging. Rare case or common genetic mutations? *Int. J. Cardiol.* **2014**, *171*, e90–e92.
118. Kalayci, A.; Guler, Y.; Karabay, C.Y.; Guler, A.; Aung, S.M.; Kirma, C. Noncompaction cardiomyopathy. Is it more than noncompaction? *Herz* **2013**, *38*, 216–218.
119. Martin, L.J.; Ramachandran, V.; Cripe, L.H.; Hinton, R.B.; Andelfinger, G.; Tabangin, M.; Shooner, K.; Keddache, M.; Benson, D.W. Evidence in favor of linkage to human chromosomal regions 18q, 5q and 13q for bicuspid aortic valve and associated cardiovascular malformations. *Hum. Genet.* **2007**, *121*, 275–284.
120. Beffagna, G.; Cecchetto, A.; dal Bianco, L.; Lorenzon, A.; Angelini, A.; Padalino, M.; Vida, V.; Bhattacharya, S.; Stellin, G.; Rampazzo, A.; *et al.* R25c mutation in the nkx2.5 gene in italian patients affected with non-syndromic and syndromic congenital heart disease. *J. Cardiovasc. Med.* **2013**, *14*, 582–586.
121. Qu, X.K.; Qiu, X.B.; Yuan, F.; Wang, J.; Zhao, C.M.; Liu, X.Y.; Zhang, X.L.; Li, R.G.; Xu, Y.J.; Hou, X.M.; *et al.* A novel NKX2.5 loss-of-function mutation associated with congenital bicuspid aortic valve. *Am. J. Cardiol.* **2014**, *114*, 1891–1895.
122. Freylikhman, O.; Tatarinova, T.; Smolina, N.; Zhuk, S.; Klyushina, A.; Kiselev, A.; Moiseeva, O.; Sjoberg, G.; Malashicheva, A.; Kostareva, A. Variants in the notch1 gene in patients with aortic coarctation. *Congenit. Heart Dis.* **2014**, *9*, 391–396.
123. Foffa, I.; Ait Ali, L.; Panesi, P.; Mariani, M.; Festa, P.; Botto, N.; Vecoli, C.; Andreassi, M.G. Sequencing of NOTCH1, GATA5, TGFBR1 and TGFBR2 genes in familial cases of bicuspid aortic valve. *BMC Med. Genet.* **2013**, *14*, 44, doi:10.1186/1471-2350-14-44.
124. Pepe, G.; Nistri, S.; Giusti, B.; Sticchi, E.; Attanasio, M.; Porciani, C.; Abbate, R.; Bonow, R.O.; Yacoub, M.; Gensini, G.F. Identification of fibrillin 1 gene mutations in patients with bicuspid aortic valve (bav) without marfan syndrome. *BMC Med. Genet.* **2014**, *15*, 23, doi:10.1186/1471-2350-15-23.
125. Quintero-Rivera, F.; Xi, Q.J.; Keppler-Noreuil, K.M.; Lee, J.H.; Higgins, A.W.; Anchan, R.M.; Roberts, A.E.; Seong, I.S.; Fan, X.; Lage, K.; *et al.* Matr3 disruption in human and mouse associated with bicuspid aortic valve, aortic coarctation and patent ductus arteriosus. *Hum. Mol. Genet.* **2015**, *24*, 2375–2389.
126. Padang, R.; Bagnall, R.D.; Richmond, D.R.; Bannon, P.G.; Semsarian, C. Rare non-synonymous variations in the transcriptional activation domains of gata5 in bicuspid aortic valve disease. *J. Mol. Cell. Cardiol.* **2012**, *53*, 277–281.
127. Shi, L.M.; Tao, J.W.; Qiu, X.B.; Wang, J.; Yuan, F.; Xu, L.; Liu, H.; Li, R.G.; Xu, Y.J.; Wang, Q.; *et al.* Gata5 loss-of-function mutations associated with congenital bicuspid aortic valve. *Int. J. Mol. Med.* **2014**, *33*, 1219–1226.
128. Bonachea, E.M.; Chang, S.W.; Zender, G.; LaHaye, S.; Fitzgerald-Butt, S.; McBride, K.L.; Garg, V. Rare gata5 sequence variants identified in individuals with bicuspid aortic valve. *Pediatr. Res.* **2014**, *76*, 211–216.

129. LeMaire, S.A.; McDonald, M.L.; Guo, D.C.; Russell, L.; Miller, C.C., 3rd; Johnson, R.J.; Bekheirnia, M.R.; Franco, L.M.; Nguyen, M.; Pyeritz, R.E.; *et al.* Genome-wide association study identifies a susceptibility locus for thoracic aortic aneurysms and aortic dissections spanning fbn1 at 15q21.1. *Nat. Genet.* **2011**, *43*, 996–1000.
130. Aida, T.; Imahashi, R.; Tanaka, K. Translating human genetics into mouse: The impact of ultra-rapid *in vivo* genome editing. *Dev. Growth Differ.* **2014**, *56*, 34–45.
131. Hisano, Y.; Ota, S.; Kawahara, A. Genome editing using artificial site-specific nucleases in zebrafish. *Dev. Growth Differ.* **2014**, *56*, 26–33.

13

Dynamic Heterogeneity of the Heart Valve Interstitial Cell Population in Mitral Valve Health and Disease

Tori E. Horne [1,†], Matthew VandeKopple [1,†], Kimberly Sauls [2], Sara N. Koenig [1], Lindsey J. Anstine [1], Vidu Garg [1,3], Russell A. Norris [2] and Joy Lincoln [1,3,*]

[1] Center for Cardiovascular and Pulmonary Research and The Heart Center at Nationwide Children's Hospital Research Institute, 575 Children's Drive, Research Building III, WB4239, Columbus, OH 43215, USA; E-Mails: horne.119@buckeyemail.osu.edu (T.E.H.); matthew.vandekopple@nationwidechildrens.org (M.V.); Sara.Koenig@nationwidechildrens.org (S.N.K.); lindsey.miller@nationwidechildrens.org (L.J.A.); vidu.garg@nationwidechildrens.org (V.G.)

[2] Department of Regenerative Medicine and Cell Biology, Medical University of South Carolina, Charleston, SC 29425, USA; E-Mails: saulsk@musc.edu (K.S.); norrisra@musc.edu (R.A.N.)

[3] Department of Pediatrics, The Ohio State University, Columbus, OH 43215, USA

† These authors contributed equally to this work.

* Author to whom correspondence should be addressed;
E-Mail: joy.lincoln@nationwidechildrens.org

Academic Editor: Cheryl L. Maslen

Abstract: The heart valve interstitial cell (VIC) population is dynamic and thought to mediate lay down and maintenance of the tri-laminar extracellular matrix (ECM) structure within the developing and mature valve throughout life. Disturbances in the contribution and distribution of valve ECM components are detrimental to biomechanical function and associated with disease. This pathological process is associated with activation of resident VICs that in the absence of disease reside as quiescent cells. While these paradigms have been long standing, characterization of this abundant and ever-changing valve cell population is incomplete. Here we examine the expression pattern of Smooth muscle α-actin, Periostin, Twist1 and Vimentin in cultured VICs, heart valves from healthy embryonic, postnatal and adult mice, as well as mature valves from human patients and established mouse models of disease. We show that the VIC population is highly heterogeneous and phenotypes are dependent on age, species, location, and disease state. Furthermore, we identify phenotypic diversity across common models of mitral valve disease. These studies significantly contribute to characterizing the VIC population in health and disease and provide insights into the cellular dynamics that maintain valve structure in healthy adults and mediate pathologic remodeling in disease states.

Keywords: mitral valve; valve interstitial cell; activation; Vimentin; Periostin; Twist1; smooth muscle α-actin

1. Introduction

The mature heart valve leaflets must open and close over 100,000 times a day to maintain unidirectional blood flow through the heart. This is largely achieved by an intricate and highly organized connective tissue system within the valve structures that provide all the necessary biomechanical properties. The three stratified layers of extracellular matrix (ECM) within the valve leaflets (mitral, tricuspid) or cusps (aortic, pulmonic) are essential for stretch, compression and strength in response to changes in the hemodynamic load [1]. This ECM architecture is established during embryonic development and postnatal growth, and maintained by valve interstitial cells (VICs) that reside within the core of the valve leaflet in the adult. Overlying the ECM and VIC population is a layer of valve endothelial cells (VECs) that provide a physical barrier against the hemodynamic environment, and *in vitro* have been shown to molecularly communicate with underlying VICs to regulate their phenotype [2–4]. Maintaining this structure-function relationship of the valve leaflet is essential as changes in the contribution and distribution of ECM components lead to valve disease and associated biomechanical failure.

The VIC population is the most abundant cell type within the valve and predominantly originates from a subset of cells that undergo endothelial-to-mesenchymal transformation (EMT) in the atrioventricular canal and outflow tract regions. EMT results in formation of endocardial cushions that remodel and later give rise to the mature valve structures [5]. While endothelial-derived cells have been shown to be major source of valve precursor cells, there are several lines of evidence to suggest that additional sources also exist (reviewed [2]). *In vivo*, newly transformed mesenchyme cells express traditional markers including Twist1 and Snai1 and *in vitro*, these cells are immunoreactive to smooth muscle α-actin (SMA) (reviewed in [2]). Following EMT, the embryonic VICs (eVICs) continue to proliferate and mediate the remodeling process which involves breakdown of the primitive proteoglycans (e.g., hyaluronan) within the endocardial cushion and deposition of more specialized matrices (collagens, proteoglycans, elastin) that will give rise to the tri-laminar layers after birth. The specialized role of eVICs within the valve primordia suggests maturation beyond a typical endocardial cushion mesenchymal cell, however phenotypes of intermediate eVICs have not been explored. Soon after birth, the postnatal VICs are less proliferative and minimally active [6,7] and remain in this quiescent (qVIC) state in the absence of disease throughout life to maintain ECM homeostasis [1,6].

In contrast to healthy valves, there is a wealth of evidence to suggest that VICs are no longer quiescent in disease but activated (aVIC) similar to myofibroblasts. Studies in humans [6,8,9] large animals [7,10,11], and mice [12–15] have demonstrated that in disease states VICs upregulate the myofibroblast marker SMA, which is thought to recapitulate embryonic phenotypes. Notably, activation is not ubiquitous to all resident VICs suggesting heterogeneity amongst the population and there is a diverse profile of "activated" markers that are increased in subsets of VICs depending on disease, age, sex and species [16]. In myxomatous mitral valves from human patients, Rabkin *et al.* observed increased SMA in addition to Vimentin, Desmin and Embryonic Smooth muscle myosin heavy chain (SMemb) protein levels [6]. Similar increases in SMA and Desmin expression were also noted in myxomatous disease in a canine model [10]. However, differential changes in these markers were not observed at the mRNA level in a more recent non-biased screen of human myxomatous patients [17]. Histological analysis of human calcific aortic valve disease also report increased SMA in pediatric and adult patients [9], with an additional study by Latif *et al.*, describing aberrant Calponin, SM22, Caldesmon, and Smooth muscle myosin heavy chain expression, reflecting a more diverse VIC population containing myofibroblast- and smooth muscle-like lineages in this disease type [8]. In this later study, changes in smooth muscle and myofibroblast markers were regionalized within the tri-laminar layers of the ECM and changes in protein expression were not uniform to all aVICs, highlighting the complexity of differential VIC phenotypes in disease. While VIC activation is characteristic of several different forms of valve pathology, the stimulus and function of this process remain poorly understood.

The mechanisms that underlie VIC activation in disease are not fully understood, but there is increasing evidence from *in vitro* studies to suggest molecular, cellular and biomechanical influences. Culture of VICs on stiff substrates significantly increases SMA expression [18–22] more robustly after passage 1 [11] and Xu *et al.*, reported decreased SMA in confluent porcine VICs [23]. Similar to fibroblast activation, Tgfβ1 is the most potent inducer of SMA expression in cultured VICs [24–26], which is largely mediated by canonical Smad, and non-canonical MAPK signaling [27,28]. In addition, increased RhoA and Rho kinase activity is sufficient to promote myofibroblast-related phenotypic markers [29]. In contrast, FGF-2 [27], reduced β-catenin [30], and knockdown of the actin filament stabilizer, cofilin [11] have all been shown to prevent Tgfβ1- and substrate-induced VIC activation. Interestingly, substrate-induced VIC activation can be reversed by transferring cells to a soft substrate [18], or adding polyunsaturated fatty acids to the growth medium [31], highlighting the plasticity of cultured aVICs and potential reversibility of activation. At the cellular level, substrate-induced VIC activation is significantly attenuated when co-cultured with VECs both in the presence [32], or absence [33] of physical interactions. While the dogma has been that VIC activation marked by SMA expression is a key process in the onset of progression of heart valve pathology, the role of aVICs in disease has not directly been tested and therefore remains unknown.

It has been long presumed that aVICs function to promote ECM remodeling of the adult valve similar to the embryo, however, unlike development, ECM remodeling in disease is poorly controlled and often leads to biomechanical failure. SMA-positive aVICs have been shown to co-express matrix metalloproteinases (MMPs) that are thought to break down healthy ECM within the valve, and subsequently replace it with an alternative matrix dependent on the disease type [6]. For example, myxomatous mitral valves disease contains an abundance of proteoglycans and fragmented collagen fibers [34], which together contribute to prolapsed biomechanics. While in calcific aortic valve disease the matrix is mineralized [35] leading to leaflet stiffening and stenosis. In this latter disease state, VICs have been shown to express osteogenic markers, such as Runx2 and *in vitro* this "transdifferentiation" process precedes increased SMA [36,37]. Worthy of mention, SMA is not always increased in valve pathology and there are reports of unchanged or decreased expression [17,38,39], suggesting that VIC activation is not always present in disease, or SMA is not a ubiquitous marker of this "activated" phenotype. These collective studies highlight the complexity of VIC biology and while insights from *in vitro* studies are informative, little is known of the phenotypic characteristics of VICs *in situ* in health and disease.

In this study, we sought to build on several previous studies and determine the phenotypes of VICs in embryonic, postnatal, adult wild type and diseased heart valves by examining the expression patterns of Twist1, Vimentin, Periostin and SMA. In doing this, we highlight the complex heterogeneity of this abundant cell population in health and disease and emphasize the need to understand the role of VIC phenotypes in maintaining healthy valve structures and promoting disease pathogenesis. These studies provide important insights into the cellular mechanisms underlying disease that can be used in the development of alternative, non-surgical based therapies to prevent, attenuate, and potentially reverse pathological processes.

2. Experimental Section

2.1. Generation of Mice

C57BL/6NJ wild type mice were purchased from Jackson Labs (Bar Harbor, ME, USA) (stock number 005304) and embryos and hearts were collected at embryonic day (E) 12.5, 13.5, 17.5, postnatal days (PND) 2 and 5, 6 weeks and 12 months of age. Hearts from 12-month-old $Fbn1^{C1039/+}$ mice and $Fbn1^{+/+}$ (wild type littermate) mice were a kind gift from Vidu Garg and generated as previously described [40]. Tissue sections from 15 month *Tie2-cre*; $FilaminA^{flox/flox}$ ($Filamin\ A^{-/-}$) and $Tie2\text{-}cre^{-}$; $FilaminA^{flox/flox}$ ($Filamin\ A^{+/+}$) mice were generously shared by Russell Norris [41].

2.2. Human Tissue

Human tissue was obtained from surgical specimens as part of a Leducq transatlantic network in collaboration with Russell Norris. All samples were harvested by offsite partners and were fixed, embedded and sectioned in their various laboratories. Sections were sent to The Research Institute at Nationwide Children's Hospital for histological and immunohistological assessment. Consent and Institutional Review Board (IRB) approval for these studies is in place at partnering institutions. Control valve biopsies were obtained from patients who perished as a result of either subarachnoid hemorrhage or intracranial bleeds. No structural heart defects were noted in these patients. Myxomatous valves were surgical cases obtained from patients who fit diagnostic criteria of myxomatous degeneration and mitral valve prolapse. This was defined by >2 mm atrial leaflet displacement in a parasternal long-axis view as well as >5 mm valve thickness. Patient samples involved in the study were men greater than 50 years of age.

2.3. Histological Analysis

Human tissue, E12.5 and E13.5 whole embryos and hearts from E17.5, PND2, PND5, 6 weeks, 9 and 12 months old wild type, or diseased mice were fixed overnight in 4% paraformaldehyde at 4 °C and processed for paraffin embedding. Seven-micrometer-thick sections were cut, deparaffinized and subject to Pentachrome staining (American Master Tech Scientific, Inc.; Lodi, CA, USA) according to the manufacturer's instructions. In sister sections, immunofluorescence was performed as previously described [42] by blocking tissue in 1% bovine serum albumin, 0.1% cold water fish skin gelatin, 0.1% Tween 20 and 0.05% NaN_3/PBS for 1 h at room temperature. For double staining, anti-SMA (A2547, 1:200, Sigma-Aldrich, St. Louis, MO, USA) was incubated overnight at 4 °C with Periostin (Abcam ab14041, 1:100), Twist1 (Sigma T6451, 1:200) or Vimentin (ab45939, 1:200, Abcam, Cambridge, MA, USA). Non-specific binding was washed in 1× PBS and tissue sections were incubated in Donkey-anti mouse-568 (Molecular Probes-Life Technologies, Grand Island, NY, USA) for 1 h at room temperature to detect SMA expression, followed by Goat-anti rabbit-488 (Periostin, Twist1, Vimentin) under the same conditions. Tissue sections were then washed in 1× PBS and mounted with DAPI. For anti-Twist1, antigen retrieval was performed by boiling for 10 min in Unmasking Solution (Vector Labs, Youngstown, OH, USA) prior to blocking. Images were visualized using an Olympus BX51 and captured using CellSens software. Image brightness, contrast and removal of autofluorescent red blood cells were edited using Adobe Photoshop CS5.

2.4. Cell Culture

Two mitral valves (4 leaflets) were isolated from two 7-week old Sprague-Dawley rats (Taconic, Hudson, NY, USA) and briefly washed in 1× PBS. Leaflets were digested for 10 min in 5 mL type II collagenase solution (Worthington Biochemical, 600 U/mL in 10% FBS DMEM) to remove the endothelial cell layer. Leaflets were then placed in 10 mL collagenase overnight at 37 °C with gentle agitation. Homogenized cells were washed once with fresh VIC media (DMEM, 10% FBS, 1% pen/streptomycin) and all isolated cells were plated in a T-75 flask. Media was changed every 2–3 days, and cells were passaged when they reached ~80% confluence. Cells were used between passages 2–5.

One-hundred thousand rat mitral VICs (rMVICs) were plated on collagen-coated Matrigen Softwell (Matrigen, Brea, CA, USA) 6-well plates of varying stiffness (2 kPa, 12 kPa) or collagen-coated tissue culture plastic (TCP) and allowed to adhere for 24 h. Serum was then removed for 48 h, after which cells were briefly washed with 1× PBS and fixed in 4% paraformaldehyde. Fixed cell cultures were processed for immunostaining as described above.

3. Results

VICs have been shown to display differential molecular profiles *in vitro* and *in vivo* depending on age, sex and disease state [16,43]. The goal of this study was to examine VIC phenotypes based on expression of mesenchyme of Twist1, Vimentin, Periostin and SMA in healthy embryonic, postnatal and adult valves, as well as valves from established mouse models of valve disease. We show that mesenchyme cells within the endocardial cushion at E12.5 express very low levels of SMA (Figure 1A,A'), relative to the surrounding myocardium (arrow, Figure 1A), and Periostin is only detectable in the distal region of the superior cushion (arrowhead, Figure 1A,A'). Twist1 is observed in the endocardium within the ventricles (arrow, Figure 1B), and in the cushion protein expression is enriched in the endothelial cell layer although largely cytoplasmic (arrowhead, Figure 1B'). In contrast, Vimentin is highly expressed in the mesenchyme and endothelial cells within the cushion (arrowheads, Figure 1C,C'), as well as the endocardium (arrow, Figure 1C). At E13.5, SMA is observed within the core region of the parietal leaflets of the developing mitral and tricuspid valves (arrows, Figure 1D,E), and expression is distinct from Periostin localized towards the atrial and ventricular surfaces (Figure 1D). In the superior cushion, Periostin is more widespread throughout with a few cells co-localizing with SMA towards the center of the superior cushion (arrowhead, Figure 1D). At this time, Twist1 continues to be localized at the endothelium (arrowhead, Figure 1E), and Vimentin expression remains highly expressed throughout (Figure 1F).

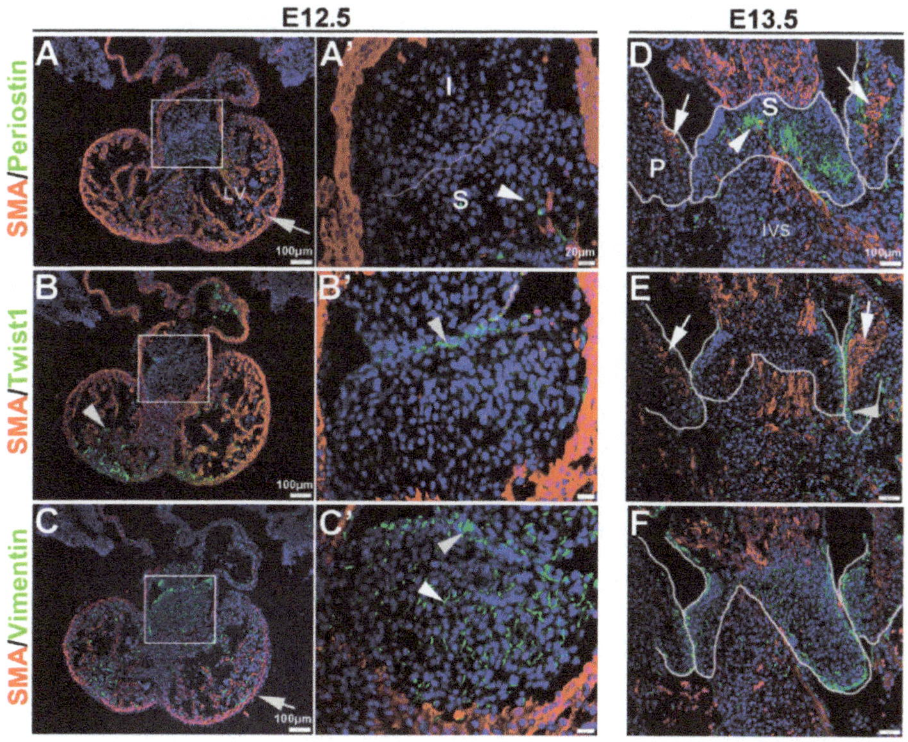

Figure 1. Characterization of VIC phenotypes during early heart valve development. Immunohistochemistry to show expression of smooth muscle α-actin (SMA) with Periostin (**A**,**A'**,**D**), Twist1 (**B**,**B'**,**E**) and Vimentin (**C**,**C'**,**F**) in cells within the inferior and superior endocardial cushions at E12.5 (**A–C'**) and atrioventricular valve primordia at E13.5 (**D–F**). Arrows indicate SMA expression (red) and arrowheads indicate Periostin (**A**,**A'**,**D**) Twist1 (**B**,**B'**,**E**) and Vimentin (**C**,**C'**,**F**) shown in green. The boxed areas in A-C are shown at higher magnification in (**A'–C'**). The white lines highlight the developing valve regions. I, inferior cushion; IVS, intraventricular septum; LV, left ventricle; P, parietal leaflets; S, superior cushion.

In the remodeling valve at E17.5, the eVICs have matured beyond a mesenchymal phenotype and are thought to be actively remodeling the ECM towards a tri-laminar structure. At this time, SMA is localized to the atrial (arrow, Figure 2A') and ventricular (Figure 2B') surface of the mural mitral valve leaflet, and noticeably SMA-positive cells are negative for Periostin seen throughout the leaflet core (arrowhead, Figure 2A'). Similar to E13.5, Twist1 remains enriched at the endothelium (arrowheads, Figure 2B') and Vimentin is highly expressed in the majority of VECs and VICs (Figure 2C').

These studies show that, *in vivo*, mesenchyme cells at E12.5 and eVICs of the remodeling valve widely express Vimentin, but are largely negative for SMA and Periostin until E13.5 when non-overlapping expression domains are observed. Twist1 however, is localized to the valve endothelium throughout valvulogenesis and low levels of expression are observed in the interstitial cell population.

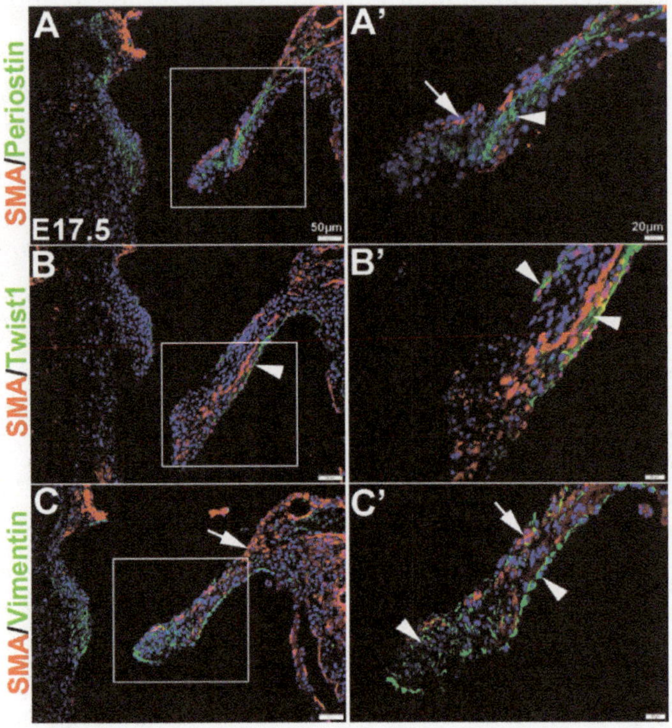

Figure 2. Characterization of VIC phenotypes in remodeling mitral heart valve structures. Immunohistochemistry to show expression of smooth muscle α-actin (SMA) with Periostin (**A**,**A'**), Twist1 (**B**,**B'**) and Vimentin (**C**,**C'**) in cells within the elongating mitral valve leaflet (mural). Arrows indicate SMA expression (red) and arrowheads indicate Periostin (**A**,**A'**) Twist1 (**B**,**B'**) and Vimentin (**C**,**C'**) shown in green. The boxed areas in A-C are shown at higher magnification in (**A'**–**C'**).

Once the tri-laminar structure has been established after birth, postnatal VICs become quiescent and remain this way throughout adulthood to maintain physiological valve structure and function [43]. Here we show that by PND2 and PND5, VICs continue to express SMA along the atrial surface of the mitral valve leaflets (arrows, Figure 3A–F). While Periostin is downregulated by PND5, as is Twist1 although low levels are still detected in the endothelium (arrowheads, Figures 3B',E). Vimentin remains highly detectable in most, but not all VICs and VECs at PND2 and many positive VICs co-express SMA (Figure 3C,C'). By PND5, Vimentin is notably downregulated (Figure 3F). At 6 weeks and 12 months of age, Periostin is undetected (Figure 4A,D) and SMA expression is rare (Figure 4A–F). Twist1 remains endothelial at both these later time points (Figure 4B,E), and Vimentin appears higher at 6 weeks compared to PND5, however by 12 months immunoreactivity is observed in few cells (Figure 4F). In conclusion, Vimentin commonly marks the VIC and VEC population at all stages prior to 12 months, while Twist1 is largely cytoplasmic and enriched at the endothelium. SMA and Perisotin are detectable from E13.5 and mark distinct and localized VIC populations until postnatal growth and remodeling are complete.

Similar to cardiac fibroblasts, VICs spontaneously express SMA when cultured on stiff substrates such as tissue culture plastic (TCP) and considered activated [11,18–22]. Furthermore, cell passage number and density can further affect SMA levels [11,23]. To characterize the phenotype of cultured VICs relative to observations made from *in vivo* studies (Figures 1–4), adult rat mitral VICs (rMVICs) were isolated and 100,000 cells were cultured at passage number 2–5 on 3D nanofiber (polycaprolactone) scaffolds coated with collagen (Nanofiber Solutions) with substrate rigidities of 2 and 12 kPa, in addition to collagen-coated tissue culture plastic (TCP). As shown in Figure 5, rVICs cultured on 2 kPa express low levels of SMA and Periostin (Figure 5A), while nuclear Twist1 is prominent (Figure 5D) and Vimentin is highly expressed (Figure 5G). Similar to *in vivo* studies (Figures 1–4), Vimentin continues to be expressed in VICs under all conditions and overlaps with SMA expression that increases and forms stress fibers on stiffer substrate surfaces (12 kPa, TCP) (Figure 5G–I). In contrast, Periostin remains at low levels around the nuclei on 12 kPa and TCP substrates (Figure 5B,C) and Twist1 expression is reduced with substrate stiffness (Figure 5E,F). These data suggest that on softer substrates, rMVICs are Twist1 and Vimentin positive and morphologically undifferentiated, while as stiffness increases, VICs increase SMA and form organized actin stress fibers.

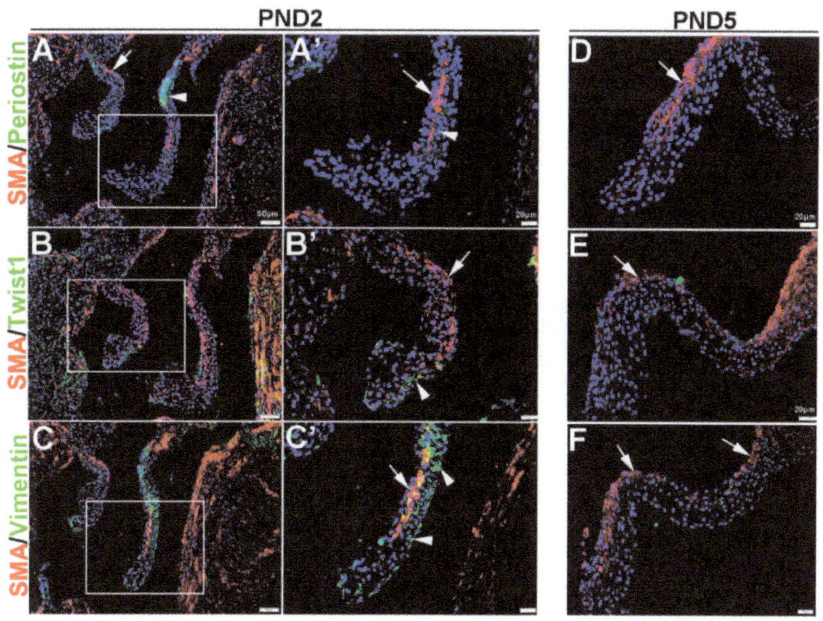

Figure 3. Characterization of VIC phenotypes in postnatal mitral valve leaflets. Immunohistochemistry to show expression of smooth muscle α-actin (SMA) with Periostin (**A**,**A'**,**D**), Twist1 (**B**,**B'**,**E**) and Vimentin (**C**,**C'**,**F**) in cells within the maturing mitral valve leaflet at postnatal day (PND) 2 (**A**–**C'**) and PND5 (**D**–**F**). Arrows indicate SMA expression (red) and arrowheads indicate Periostin (**A**,**A'**) Twist1 (**B**,**B'**) and Vimentin (**C**,**C'**) shown in green. The boxed areas in A–C are shown at higher magnification in (**A'**–**C'**).

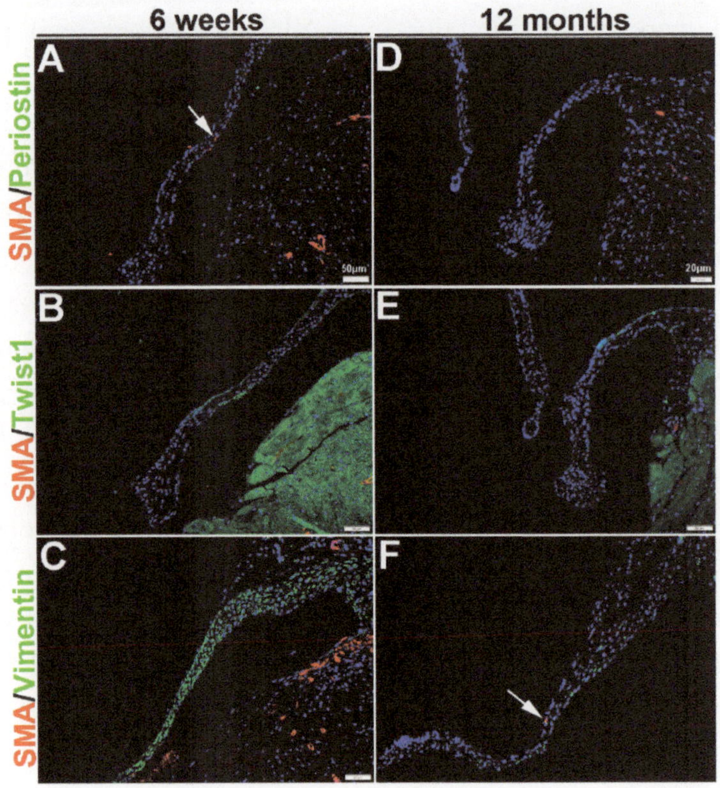

Figure 4. Characterization of VIC phenotypes in adult and aging mitral valves. Immunohistochemistry to show expression of smooth muscle α-actin (SMA) with Periostin (**A**,**D**), Twist1 (**B**,**E**) and Vimentin (**C**,**F**) in cells within the mature mitral valve leaflets. Arrows indicate SMA expression (red).

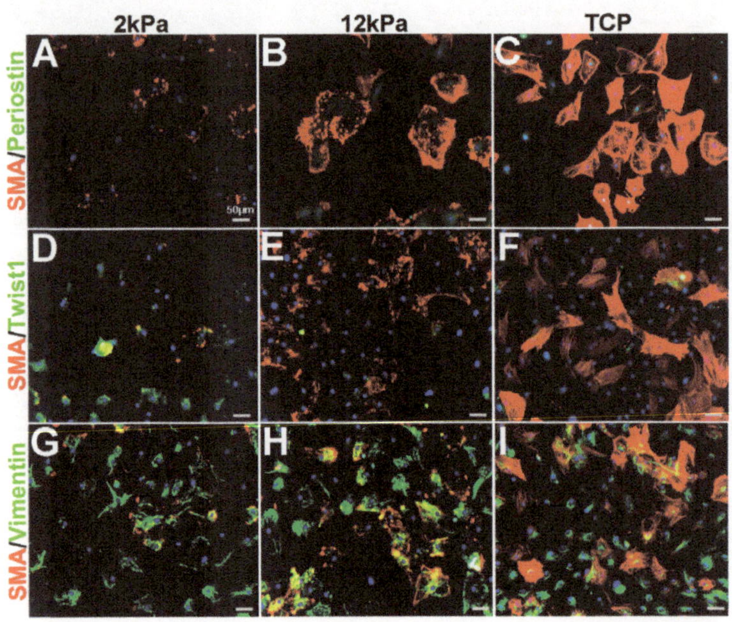

Figure 5. Expression profiles of rat mitral VICs cultured on increasing substrate stiffness. Immunohistochemistry to show expression of smooth muscle α-actin (SMA) with Periostin (**A–C**), Twist1 (**D–F**)) and Vimentin (**G–I**) in isolated rat mitral VICs cultured on 3D nanofiber (polycaprolactone) scaffolds coated with collagen (Nanofiber Solutions) with substrate rigidities of 2 kPa (**A**,**D**,**G**), 12 kPa (**B**,**E**,**H**) and tissue culture plastic (TCP) (**C**,**F**,**I**).

In heart valve disease, changes in VIC phenotypes have been described [6,43]. Here, we examine VIC phenotypes in established mouse models of mitral valve disease using SMA, Periostin, Twist1 and Vimentin expression. *Filamin* $A^{-/-}$ mice develop myxomatous mitral valve disease by 2 months of age, characterized by significant leaflet thickening and pathologic ECM remodeling (Figure 6A,B) [41].

At 15 months of age, these myxomatous changes are associated with increased proteoglycans (Figure 6B). In addition, SMA is detected in subsets of VICs but not all (arrows, Figure 6D), and increased Twist1 appears to be ectopically expressed in SMA-positive VICs (arrowheads, Figure 6F). Periostin was not significantly detected in wild type or diseased mice (Figure 6C,D) and Vimentin expression appears similar (Figure 6G,H).

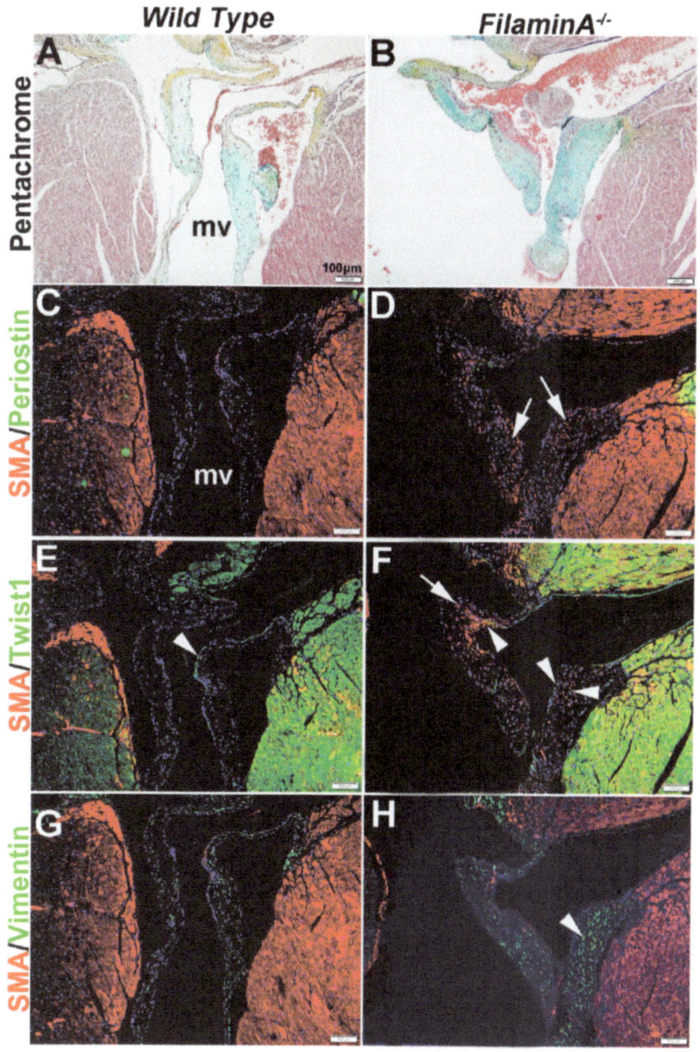

Figure 6. Characterization of VIC phenotypes in myxomatous mitral valves from 15 month old *Filamin* $A^{-/-}$ mice. Pentachrome staining to show extracellular matrix composition and organization in 15 month wild type (*Filamin* $A^{+/+}$) (**A**) and *Filamin* $A^{-/-}$ (**B**) mice. (**C–H**) Immunohistochemistry to detect expression of smooth muscle α-actin (SMA) with Periostin (**C**,**D**), Twist1 (**E**,**F**) and Vimentin (**G**,**H**) in cells within the mitral valve leaflet of wild type (**C**,**E**,**G**) and *Filamin* $A^{-/-}$ (**D**,**F**,**H**) mice. Arrows indicate SMA expression (red) and arrowheads indicate Twist1 (**E**,**F**) and Vimentin (**G**,**H**) shown in green. mv: mitral valve

Mice carrying a cysteine substitution mutation in *Fibrillin-1* (*Fbn1*) serve as a model for Marfan Syndrome. Homozygous *Fbn1*$^{C1039/C1039}$ mice die soon after birth from aortic dissection, but heterozygotes are viable and exhibit mitral valve thickening and functional prolapse by 9 months of age [40]. In Figure 7, we show that in diseased mitral valves from *Fbn1*$^{C1039/+}$ mice SMA (arrow, Figure 7D) and Periostin (arrowhead, Figure 7D) are increased in different VIC subsets. In addition, Twist1 reactivity is also increased at the endothelium (arrowhead, Figure 7F). Vimentin remains highly expressed in the majority of VICs in *Fbn1*$^{C1039/+}$ mice (arrowhead, Figure 7H), overlapping with SMA expression in several places. These observations made from Figures 6 and 7 highlight the diversity of VIC phenotypes in mouse models of mitral valve disease.

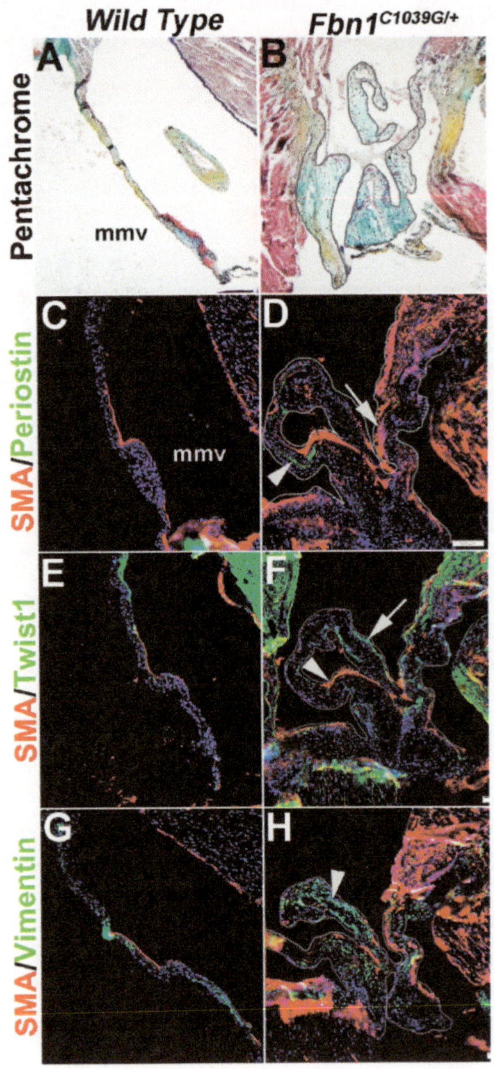

Figure 7. Characterization of VIC phenotypes in diseased mitral valves from 12 month old *Fbn1*$^{C1039/+}$ mice. Pentachrome staining to show extracellular matrix composition and organization in 12 month wild type (*Fbn1*$^{+/+}$ mice) (**A**) and *Fbn1*$^{C1039/+}$ (**B**) mice. (**C–H**) Immunohistochemistry to detect expression of smooth muscle α-actin (SMA) with Periostin (**C**,**D**), Twist1 (**E**,**F**) and Vimentin (**G**,**H**) in cells within the mitral valve leaflet of wild type (**C**,**E**,**G**) and *Fbn1*$^{C1039/+}$ (**D**,**F**,**H**) mice. Arrows indicate SMA expression (red) and arrowheads indicate Periostin (**C**,**D**), Twist1 (**E**,**F**) and Vimentin (**G**,**H**) shown in green. mmv, mural mitral valve.

To extend these studies into humans, expression patterns were examined in control and myxomatous mitral valve biopsies from human patients (male, aged >50 years old). By Pentachrome staining, myxomatous valves are histologically thickened with excess abundance of proteoglycans (Figure 8H) as compared to control subjects that died from subarachnoid hemorrhage or intracranial bleeds (Figure 8A). Due to the large size, human mitral valves were divided into top, middle and base regions (See Figure 8A,H) and myxomatous valves were further subdivided into atrial and ventricular zones (Figure 8H). Control mitral valves express high levels of SMA along the atrial surface (arrowheads Figure 8C,D,F,G) with Periostin enriched on the ventricular side, particularly at the base (Figure 8D). Little staining of any marker, other than Vimentin is observed in the tip region (Figure 8E). In myxomatous valves, SMA expression on the atrial surface is diminished, although expression is noted in VICs within the middle and base regions (Figure 8J,K,M,N). Periostin is significantly increased at the atrial (Figure 8K) and ventricular (Figure 8N) surfaces in disease, and Vimentin reactivity remains throughout the valve leaflet (Figure 8O,R). These observations suggest that SMA and Periostin are differentially expressed in human myxomatous mitral valves which may reflect phenotypic changes in the VIC population.

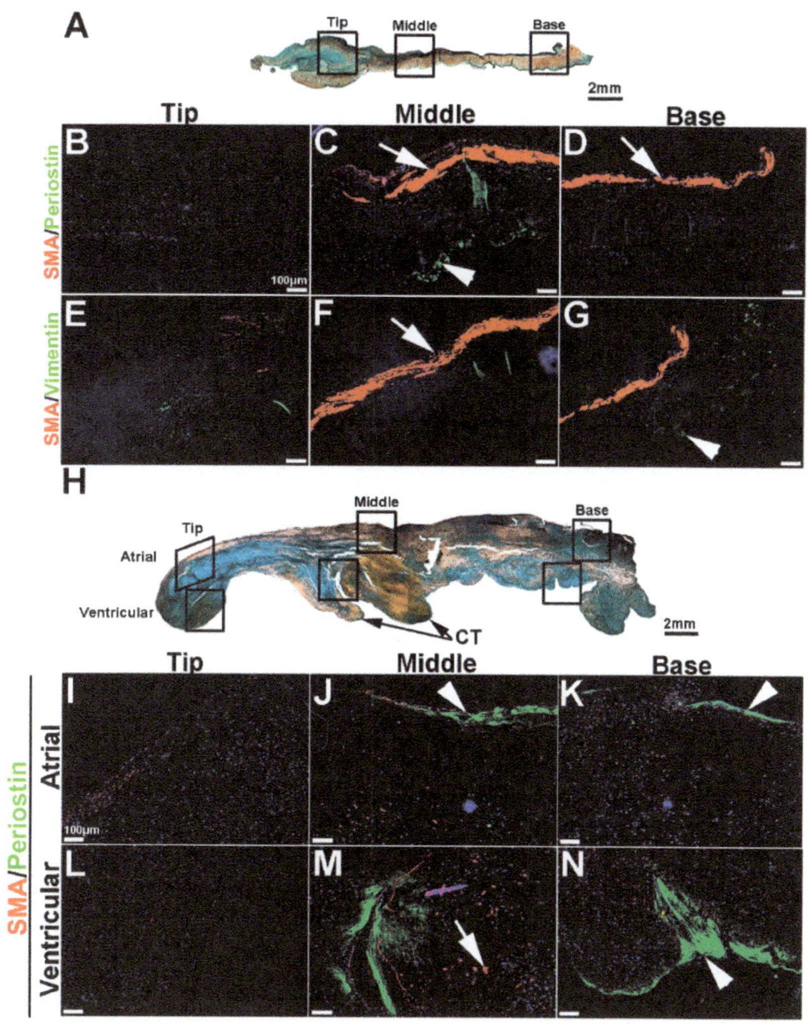

Figure 8. *Cont.*

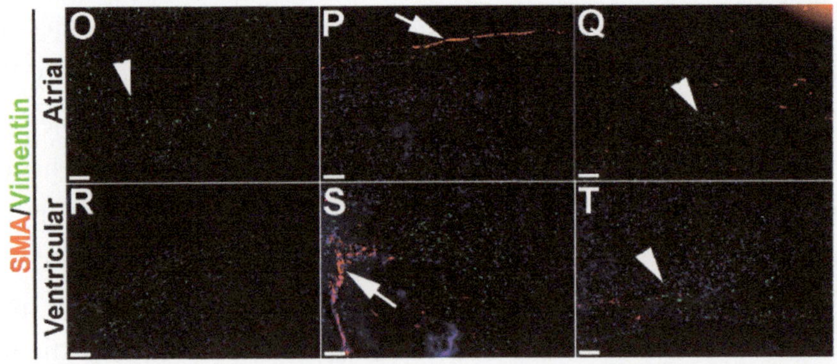

Figure 8. VIC phenotypes in diseased human myxomatous mitral valve biopsies. (**A,H**) Pentachrome staining to show extracellular matrix composition and organization in control (**A**) and myxomatous (**H**) mitral valves from human patients. (**B–G,I–T**) Immunohistochemistry to detect expression of smooth muscle α-actin (SMA) with Periostin (**B–D,I–N**) and Vimentin (**E–G,O–T**) in cells within the mitral valve leaflet of control (**B–G**) and myxomatous (**I–T**) patients. Arrows indicate SMA expression (red) and arrowheads indicate Periostin (green) expression. Boxed areas in A and H highlight the regions of immunostaining of cells within the tip, middle and base regions of both control and diseased valves. CT, chordae tendineae.

4. Discussion

The phenotypic characterization of VICs is incomplete and therefore the goal of this study was to use molecular markers to "road map" the VIC population in embryonic, postnatal and adult heart valves from wild type and diseased mice. In 2007, a review by Liu *et al.*, described five phenotypes of the VIC population: embryonic progenitor endothelial/mesenchyme cells, quiescent, activated, progenitor and osteoblastic. Here, we extend these studies and demonstrate the complex, age-, species- and disease-dependent heterogeneity of VICs within the valve structures. It is apparent that eVICs are dynamic: in the endocardial cushion the newly transformed cells are considered mesenchymal in phenotypes based on their molecular profiles and morphology (reviewed in [44]). However, it should be noted that even at this stage, studies have demonstrated heterogeneity as well as differentiation beyond mesenchyme phenotype in subsets of cushion cells [45]. Interestingly, SMA is expressed in newly transformed mesenchyme cells from endocardial cushion assays *in vitro* [46–51], yet, *in vivo*, we detected only low levels of SMA expression at E12.5 (Figure 1). It can be speculated that this discrepancy could be due to the *in vitro* environment that favors SMA induction, including growth factor enriched media (containing Tgfβ) and/or artificial biomechanical stiffness. Beyond the cushion stage, the nomenclature of interstitial cells has not been well defined. Here we show that SMA is expressed in subsets of cells within the elongating superior cushion and parietal leaflets at E13.5 (Figure 1D–F) and along the atrial surface of the valve from E17.5 (Figures 2 and 3) to PND5 in mice. These SMA-positive cells may represent a myofibroblast-like phenotype that promotes physiological remodeling of the valve primordia during development and tri-laminar formation after birth [1,5]. In contrast, the Perisotin-positive cells at late embryonic and postnatal stages are distinct from the myofibroblasts and may represent fibroblast- or protofibroblast-like phenotypes. There are also many cells that do not express SMA or Periostin, but are Vimentin positive, suggesting an alternative phenotype. However, the ubiquitous expression pattern of Vimentin until late postnatal stages suggest that this is a generic and less informative marker of the ever-changing VIC population. Although, Vimentin along with Twist1 have previously been noted as markers of mesenchyme cells, yet we observe additional expression in the endothelium and therefore these should proteins be considered as endothelial and interstially expressed. The nomenclature of interstitial cells within the developing valve beyond the endocardial cushion stage has not been assigned, but the dynamic heterogeneity of these cells suggests maturation beyond mesenchyme cells types and therefore eVIC deems appropriate. As described [43], adult VICs in the mouse are quiescent (qVICs) with rare SMA expression observed and undetectable Periostin (Figure 4A,F). However in adult human valves, we observed high levels of SMA expression along the atrial surface and Periostin enriched at the ventricular surface (Figure 8), suggesting species dependency. These expression profiles of postnatal VICs *in vivo* are different to cultured rMVICs (Figure 5) but somewhat similar to mesenchyme cushion cells at E12.5 (Figure 1). However, adult qVICs have lower proliferation and migratory indices and are functionally diverse from cushion mesenchyme cells and therefore further work is required to phenotypically characterize adult qVICs at molecular and functional levels.

Valve disease is commonly associated with VIC activation of otherwise quiescent cells. The gold standard marker of these cells has been SMA, however increased expression is not always observed in disease [17,38,39]. Therefore, it is considered that pathological ECM remodeling by VICs may not require SMA expression, or as our data suggests there are additional markers of disease-causing VICs *in vivo*; many of which remain unknown. Here, we show that VICs from human patients and two mouse models of mitral valve disease express diverse molecular profiles, yet commonly exhibit myxomatous phenotypes associated with excess proteoglycan accumulation. In 15 month old *Filamin* $A^{-/-}$ mice (Figure 5D) SMA is highly expressed in VICs throughout the valve leaflets, while increased SMA in affected mitral valves from *Fbn1*$^{C1039/+}$ mice is localized to atrial regions (Figure 6D and Figure 7D).

In addition, Periostin is not significantly expressed in *Filamin* $A^{-/-}$ mice (Figure 6D), but highly detected in *Fbn1*$^{C1039/+}$ mitral valves (Figure 7D), similar to human disease (Figure 8). Twist1 was not highly detectable in healthy, adult or cultured VICs, yet it is observed in a small subset of VICs in *Filamin* $A^{-/-}$ mice (Figure 6F) and in VECs and sub-endothelial VICs in the *Fbn1*$^{C1039/+}$ model (Figure 7F), characteristic of more mesenchyme-type phenotypes. These discrepancies between disease models could be due to the differential pathological stimuli underlying mitral valve disease in these mice. For example, substitute mutations in *Fbn1* and increased Tgfβ signaling are thought to promote changes in mitral valve structure in *Fbn1*$^{C1039/+}$ mice [40], while rescue of altered cross-talk between the cytoskeleton protein *Filamin A,* with decreased serotonylation of Filamin A underlies mitral valve abnormalities in deficient mice [41]. The take home message from these studies suggests that despite similar mitral valve phenotypes, the VIC molecular profiles are diverse. In contrast to this conclusion, increased SMA is common to both calcific and myxomatous disease types, yet in these states the biomechanical phenotypes of the valve are very different; stenotic *versus* prolapsed [6,8]. The reason for this is not clear, but in calcific aortic valve disease deposition of the mineralized ECM is driven by VICs expressing osteoblast markers that precede increased SMA expression *in vitro* [36,37]. A comparative post-SMA-positive VIC in myxomatous disease has not been described but warrants further investigation.

While this current descriptive study and others previous are highly informative they do not delineate the differences between cause and effect of VIC phenotypes on disease processes. Studies by Rabkin *et al.* support a causative role for SMA-positive VICs in driving pathological changes in the valve ECM [6]. However, it remains unclear what induces SMA in disease and we are left to speculate that localized changes in the hemodynamic environment as a result of structural defects, or biomechanics following pathologic ECM remodeling might play a role [37]. Furthermore it is considered that SMA may not only mark resident aVICs but also represent newly transformed mesenchymal cells recently shown to be present in disease as a result of adult EMT [33,50,52]. However, data shown here (Figure 1) suggests that SMA is not highly expressed in EMT-derived cells within the endocardial cushion and this would therefore suggest that pathological-EMT may not recapitulate developmental events, although further work is required to determine this.

5. Conclusions

In conclusion, these studies have highlighted the heterogeneity of VIC phenotypes in developing and maturing mitral valve structures in healthy mice over time. Furthermore, we have identified that increased SMA expression is not commonly observed in mouse models of mitral valve disease and other cell lineages (mesenchyme-, fibroblast-like) may also contribute to valve disease pathology. However, it is recognized that aortic valve disease was not included in these studies and due to the differential hemodynamic environment and structure VIC behavior may be different in the outflow valve sets. For advancements in the treatment of valve disease to occur, it is imperative that we delineate the function of the diverse VIC populations in disease types and identify the pathological stimuli promoting phenotypic changes in VICs. Furthermore, understanding the plasticity of adult VICs in disease will determine if promoting quiescence would be an effective approach in the development of non-surgical therapeutics. In addition, as age, sex and disease state have all been shown to influence VIC phenotypes, the need for personalized medicine will be essential when considering diagnostic and prognostic treatment programs.

Acknowledgments

We thank Blair Austin for technical assistance. This work was sponsored by The National Institute of Health (R01HL127033 (J.L.), C06 RR018823 (R.A.N.), COBRE 1P30 GM103342 (R.A.N.), 8P20 GM103444-07 (R.A.N.), R01HL127692 (R.A.N.)), National Center for Advancing Translational Sciences (TL1TR001069 (S.N.K.)), and The American Heart Association (14GRNT19630003 (J.L.), 15GRNT25080052 (R.A.N.)).

Author Contributions

Data collection was generated by T.E.H., M.V.K., L.J.A. and J.L., S.N.K, and K.S. were involved with collection of murine valve tissue from disease mouse models with supervision from V.G. and R.A.N. Data was analyzed and the manuscript prepared by J.L.

Conflicts of Interest

The authors declare no conflict of interest.

References

1. Hinton, R.B., Jr.; Lincoln, J.; Deutsch, G.H.; Osinska, H.; Manning, P.B.; Benson, D.W.; Yutzey, K.E. Extracellular matrix remodeling and organization in developing and diseased aortic valves. *Circ. Res*. **2006**, *98*,1431–1438.
2. Tao, G.; Kotick, J.D.; Lincoln, J. Heart valve development, maintenance, and disease: The role of endothelial cells. *Curr. Top. Dev. Biol*. **2012**, *100*, 203–232.
3. Butcher, J.T.; Nerem, R.M. Valvular endothelial cells regulate the phenotype of interstitial cells in co-culture: Effects of steady shear stress. *Tissue Eng*. **2006**, *12*, 905–915.
4. Bosse, K.; Hans, C.P.; Zhao, N.; Koenig, S.N.; Huang, N.; Guggilam, A.; LaHaye, S.; Tao, G.; Lucchesi, P.A.; Lincoln, J.; *et al*. Endothelial nitric oxide signaling regulates Notch1 in aortic valve disease. *J. Mol. Cell. Cardiol*. **2013**, *60*, 27–35.
5. Lincoln, J.; Alfieri, C.M.; Yutzey, K.E. Development of heart valve leaflets and supporting apparatus in chicken and mouse embryos. *Dev. Dyn*. **2004**, *230*, 239–250.
6. Rabkin, E.; Aikawa, M.; Stone, J.R.; Fukumoto, Y.; Libby, P.; Schoen, F.J. Activated interstitial myofibroblasts express catabolic enzymes and mediate matrix remodeling in myxomatous heart valves. *Circulation*. **2001**, *104*, 2525–2532.
7. Olsson, M.; Rosenqvist, M.; Nilsson, J. Expression of HLA-DR antigen and smooth muscle cell differentiation markers by valvular fibroblasts in degenerative aortic stenosis. *J. Am. Coll. Cardiol*. **1994**, *24*, 1664–1671.
8. Latif, N.; Sarathchandra, P.; Chester, A.H.; Yacoub, M.H. Expression of smooth muscle cell markers and co-activators in calcified aortic valves. *Eur. Heart J*. **2015**, *36*, 1335–1345.
9. Wirrig, E.E.; Hinton, R.B.; Yutzey, K.E. Differential expression of cartilage and bone-related proteins in pediatric and adult diseased aortic valves. *J. Mol. Cell. Cardiol*. **2011**, *50*, 561–569.
10. Disatian, S.; Ehrhart, E.J., III; Zimmerman, S.; Orton, E.C. Interstitial cells from dogs with naturally occurring myxomatous mitral valve disease undergo phenotype transformation. *J. Heart Valve Dis*. **2008**, *17*, 402–411.
11. Pho, M.; Lee, W.; Watt, D.R.; Laschinger, C.; Simmons, C.A.; McCulloch, C.A. Cofilin is a marker of myofibroblast differentiation in cells from porcine aortic cardiac valves. *Am. J. Physiol. Heart Circ. Physiol*. **2008**, *294*, H1767–H1778.
12. Munjal, C.; Opoka, A.M.; Osinska, H.; James, J.F.; Bressan, G.M.; Hinton, R.B. TGF-beta mediates early angiogenesis and latent fibrosis in an Emilin1-deficient mouse model of aortic valve disease. *Dis. Model. Mech*. **2014**, *7*, 987–996.
13. Hinton, R.B.; Adelman-Brown, J.; Witt, S.; Krishnamurthy, V.K.; Osinska, H.; Sakthivel, B.; James, J.F.; Li, D.Y.; Narmoneva, D.A.; Mecham, R.P.; *et al*. Elastin haploinsufficiency results in progressive aortic valve malformation and latent valve disease in a mouse model. *Circ. Res*. **2010**, *107*, 549–557.

14. Matsumoto, Y.; Adams, V.; Jacob, S.; Mangner, N.; Schuler, G.; Linke, A. Regular exercise training prevents aortic valve disease in low-density lipoprotein-receptor-deficient mice. *Circulation* **2010**, *121*, 759–767.
15. Tanaka, K.; Sata, M.; Fukuda, D.; Suematsu, Y.; Motomura, N.; Takamoto, S.; Hirata, Y.; Nagai, R. Age-associated aortic stenosis in apolipoprotein E-deficient mice. *J. Am. Coll. Cardiol.* **2005**, *46*, 134–141.
16. McCoy, C.M.; Nicholas, D.Q.; Masters, K.S. Sex-related differences in gene expression by porcine aortic valvular interstitial cells. *PLoS ONE* **2012**, *7*, e39980.
17. Thalji, N.M.; Hagler, M.A.; Zhang, H.; Casaclang-Verzosa, G.; Nair, A.A.; Suri, R.M.; Miller, J.D. Nonbiased Molecular Screening Identifies Novel Molecular Regulators of Fibrogenic and Proliferative Signaling in Myxomatous Mitral Valve Disease. *Circ. Cardiovasc. Genet.* **2015**, *8*, 516–528.
18. Quinlan, A.M.; Billiar, K.L. Investigating the role of substrate stiffness in the persistence of valvular interstitial cell activation. *J. Biomed. Mater. Res. A*. **2012**, *100*, 2474–2482.
19. Chen, J.H.; Simmons, C.A. Cell-matrix interactions in the pathobiology of calcific aortic valve disease: Critical roles for matricellular, matricrine, and matrix mechanics cues. *Circ. Res.* **2011**, *108*, 1510–1524.
20. Gould, S.T.; Anseth, K.S. Role of cell-matrix interactions on VIC phenotype and tissue deposition in 3D PEG hydrogels. *J. Tissue Eng. Regen. Med.* **2013**, doi:10.1002/term.1836.
21. Cushing, M.C.; Liao, J.T.; Jaeggli, M.P.; Anseth, K.S. Material-based regulation of the myofibroblast phenotype. *Biomaterials* **2007**, *28*, 3378–3387.
22. Duan, B.; Hockaday, L.A.; Kapetanovic, E.; Kang, K.H.; Butcher, J.T. Stiffness and adhesivity control aortic valve interstitial cell behavior within hyaluronic acid based hydrogels. *Acta Biomater.* **2013**, *9*, 7640–7650.
23. Xu, S.; Liu, A.C.; Kim, H.; Gotlieb, A.I. Cell density regulates *in vitro* activation of heart valve interstitial cells. *Cardiovasc. Pathol.* **2012**, *21*, 65–73.
24. Liu, A.C.; Gotlieb, A.I. Transforming growth factor-beta regulates *in vitro* heart valve repair by activated valve interstitial cells. *Am. J. Pathol.* **2008**, *173*, 1275–1285.
25. Cushing, M.C.; Liao, J.T.; Anseth, K.S. Activation of valvular interstitial cells is mediated by transforming growth factor-beta1 interactions with matrix molecules. *Matrix Biol.* **2005**, *24*, 428–437.
26. Walker, G.A.; Masters, K.S.; Shah, D.N.; Anseth, K.S.; Leinwand, L.A. Valvular myofibroblast activation by transforming growth factor-β: Implications for pathological extracellular matrix remodeling in heart valve disease. *Circ. Res.* **2004**, *95*, 253–260.
27. Cushing, M.C.; Mariner, P.D.; Liao, J.T.; Sims, E.A.; Anseth, K.S. Fibroblast growth factor represses Smad-mediated myofibroblast activation in aortic valvular interstitial cells. *FASEB J.* **2008**, *22*, 1769–1777.
28. Hutcheson, J.D.; Ryzhova, L.M.; Setola, V.; Merryman, W.D. 5-HT(2B) antagonism arrests non-canonical TGF-beta1-induced valvular myofibroblast differentiation. *J. Mol. Cell. Cardiol.* **2012**, *53*, 707–714.
29. Gu, X.; Masters, K.S. Role of the Rho pathway in regulating valvular interstitial cell phenotype and nodule formation. *Am. J. Physiol. Heart Circ. Physiol.* **2011**, *300*, H448–H458.

30. Chen, J.H.; Chen, W.L.; Sider, K.L.; Yip, C.Y.; Simmons, C.A. Beta-catenin mediates mechanically regulated, transforming growth factor-β1-induced myofibroblast differentiation of aortic valve interstitial cells. *Arterioscler. Thromb. Vasc. Biol.* **2011**, *31*, 590–597.
31. Witt, W.; Buttner, P.; Jannasch, A.; Matschke, K.; Waldow, T. Reversal of myofibroblastic activation by polyunsaturated fatty acids in valvular interstitial cells from aortic valves. Role of RhoA/G-actin/MRTF signalling. *J. Mol. Cell. Cardiol.* **2014**, *74*, 127–138.
32. Gould, S.T.; Matherly, E.E.; Smith, J.N.; Heistad, D.D.; Anseth, K.S. The role of valvular endothelial cell paracrine signaling and matrix elasticity on valvular interstitial cell activation. *Biomaterials* **2014**, *35*, 3596–3606.
33. Shapero, K.; Wylie-Sears, J.; Levine, R.A.; Mayer, J.E., Jr.; Bischoff, J. Reciprocal interactions between mitral valve endothelial and interstitial cells reduce endothelial-to-mesenchymal transition and myofibroblastic activation. *J. Mol.Cell. Cardiol.* **2015**, *80*, 175–185.
34. Gupta, V.; Barzilla, J.E.; Mendez, J.S.; Stephens, E.H.; Lee, E.L.; Collard, C.D.; Laucirica, R.; Weigel, P.H.; Grande-Allen, K.J. Abundance and location of proteoglycans and hyaluronan within normal and myxomatous mitral valves. *Cardiovasc. Pathol.* **2009**, *18*, 191–197.
35. Rajamannan, N.M.; Gersh, B.; Bonow, R.O. Calcific aortic stenosis: From bench to the bedside—Emerging clinical and cellular concepts. *Heart* **2003**, *89*, 801–805.
36. Poggio, P.; Sainger, R.; Branchetti, E.; Grau, J.B.; Lai, E.K.; Gorman, R.C.; Sacks, M.S.; Parolari, A.; Bavaria, J.E.; Ferrari, G. Noggin attenuates the osteogenic activation of human valve interstitial cells in aortic valve sclerosis. *Cardiovasc. Res.* **2013**, *98*, 402–410.
37. Chen, J.; Ryzhova, L.M.; Sewell-Loftin, M.K.; Brown, C.B.; Huppert, S.S.; Baldwin, H.S.; Merryman, W.D. Notch1 Mutation Leads to Valvular Calcification Through Enhanced Myofibroblast Mechanotransduction. *Arterioscler. Thromb. Vasc. Biol.* **2015**, *35*, 1597–1605.
38. Dupuis, L.E.; Osinska, H.; Weinstein, M.B.; Hinton, R.B.; Kern, C.B. Insufficient versican cleavage and Smad2 phosphorylation results in bicuspid aortic and pulmonary valves. *J. Mol. Cell. Cardiol.* **2013**, *60*, 50–59.
39. Monzack, E.L.; Masters, K.S. Can valvular interstitial cells become true osteoblasts? A side-by-side comparison. *J. Heart Valve Dis.* **2011**, *20*, 449–463.
40. Ng, C.M.; Cheng, A.; Myers, L.A.; Martinez-Murillo, F.; Jie, C.; Bedja, D.; Gabrielson, K.L.; Hausladen, J.M.; Mecham, R.P.; Judge, D.P.; *et al.* TGF-beta-dependent pathogenesis of mitral valve prolapse in a mouse model of Marfan syndrome. *J. Clin. Investig.* **2004**, *114*, 1586–1592.
41. Sauls, K.; de Vlaming, A.; Harris, B.S.; Williams, K.; Wessels, A.; Levine, R.A.; Slaugenhaupt, S.A.; Goodwin, R.L.; Pavone, L.M.; Merot, J.; *et al.* Developmental basis for filamin-A-associated myxomatous mitral valve disease. *Cardiovasc. Res.* **2012**, *96*, 109–119.
42. Levay, A.K.; Peacock, J.D.; Lu, Y.; Koch, M.; Hinton, R.B., Jr.; Kadler, K.E.; Lincoln, J. Scleraxis is required for cell lineage differentiation and extracellular matrix remodeling during murine heart valve formation *in vivo*. *Circ. Res.* **2008**, *103*, 948–956.
43. Liu, A.C.; Joag, V.R.; Gotlieb, A.I. The emerging role of valve interstitial cell phenotypes in regulating heart valve pathobiology. *Am. J. Pathol.* **2007**, *171*, 1407–1418.
44. Person, A.D.; Klewer, S.E.; Runyan, R.B. Cell biology of cardiac cushion development. *Int. Rev. Cytol.* **2005**, *243*, 287–335.

45. Lincoln, J.; Alfieri, C.M.; Yutzey, K.E. BMP and FGF regulatory pathways control cell lineage diversification of heart valve precursor cells. *Dev. Biol.* **2006**, *292*, 292–302.
46. Liebner, S.; Cattelino, A.; Gallini, R.; Rudini, N.; Iurlaro, M.; Piccolo, S.; Dejana, E. β-Catenin is required for endothelial-mesenchymal transformation during heart cushion development in the mouse. *J. Cell Biol.* **2004**, *166*, 359–367.
47. Sakabe, M.; Ikeda, K.; Nakatani, K.; Kawada, N.; Imanaka-Yoshida, K.; Yoshida, T.; Yamagishi, T.; Nakajima, Y. Rho kinases regulate endothelial invasion and migration during valvuloseptal endocardial cushion tissue formation. *Dev. Dyn.* **2006**, *235*, 94–104.
48. Okagawa, H.; Markwald, R.R.; Sugi, Y. Functional BMP receptor in endocardial cells is required in atrioventricular cushion mesenchymal cell formation in chick. *Dev. Biol.* **2007**, *306*, 179–192.
49. Sugi, Y.; Yamamura, H.; Okagawa, H.; Markwald, R.R. Bone morphogenetic protein-2 can mediate myocardial regulation of atrioventricular cushion mesenchymal cell formation in mice. *Dev. Biol.* **2004**, *269*, 505–518.
50. Paranya, G.; Vineberg, S.; Dvorin, E.; Kaushal, S.; Roth, S.J.; Rabkin, E.; Schoen, F.J.; Bischoff, J. Aortic valve endothelial cells undergo transforming growth factor-beta-mediated and non-transforming growth factor-beta-mediated transdifferentiation *in vitro*. *Am. J. Pathol.* **2001**, *159*, 1335–1343.
51. Nakajima, Y.; Mironov, V.; Yamagishi, T.; Nakamura, H.; Markwald, R.R. Expression of smooth muscle alpha-actin in mesenchymal cells during formation of avian endocardial cushion tissue: A role for transforming growth factor beta3. *Dev. Dyn.* **1997**, *209*, 296–309.
52. Bischoff, J.; Aikawa, E. Progenitor cells confer plasticity to cardiac valve endothelium. *J. Cardiovasc. Transl. Res.* **2011**, *4*, 710–719.

14

Increased Infiltration of Extra-Cardiac Cells in Myxomatous Valve Disease

Kimberly Sauls [1], Katelynn Toomer [1], Katherine Williams [1], Amanda J. Johnson [1], Roger R. Markwald [1], Zoltan Hajdu [2] and Russell A. Norris [1,*]

[1] Department of Regenerative Medicine and Cell Biology, Children's Research Institute, Medical University of South Carolina, 171 Ashley Ave, Charleston, SC 29425, USA; E-Mails: saulsk@musc.edu (K.S.); toomerk@musc.edu (K.T.); willilin@musc.edu (K.W.); johnaj@musc.edu (A.J.J.); markwald@musc.edu (R.R.M.)

[2] Department of Bioengineering, Clemson University, 200 C Patewood Drive, Greenville, SC 29615, USA; E-Mail: zhajdu@clemson.edu

* Author to whom correspondence should be addressed; E-Mail: norrisra@musc.edu

Academic Editor: Cheryl L. Maslen

Abstract: Mutations in the actin-binding gene *Filamin-A* have been linked to non-syndromic myxomatous valvular dystrophy and associated mitral valve prolapse. Previous studies by our group traced the adult valve defects back to developmental errors in valve interstitial cell-mediated extracellular matrix remodeling during fetal valve gestation. Mice deficient in *Filamin-A* exhibit enlarged mitral leaflets at E17.5, and subsequent progression to a myxomatous phenotype is observed by two months. For this study, we sought to define mechanisms that contribute to myxomatous degeneration in the adult *Filamin-A*-deficient mouse. *In vivo* experiments demonstrate increased infiltration of hematopoietic-derived cells and macrophages in adolescent *Filamin-A* conditional knockout mice. Concurrent with this infiltration of hematopoietic cells, we show an increase in Erk activity, which localizes to regions of MMP2 expression. Additionally, increases in cell proliferation are observed at two months, when hematopoietic cell engraftment and signaling are pronounced. Similar changes are observed in human myxomatous mitral valve tissue, suggesting that infiltration of hematopoietic-derived cells and/or increased Erk signaling may contribute to myxomatous valvular dystrophy. Consequently, immune cell targeting and/or suppression of pErk activities may represent an effective therapeutic option for mitral valve prolapse patients.

Keywords: Filamin-A; myxomatous valve disease; hematopoietic cells; macrophage

1. Introduction

Mitral Valve Prolapse (MVP) is a common, degenerative cardiovascular disease that occurs in 2.4% of the population. MVP occurs when enlarged and weakened mitral leaflets billow back into the left atrium and fail to properly coapt during ventricular systole, which can lead to mitral regurgitation, congestive heart failure, and even sudden cardiac death. Histologically, the valves are characterized as myxomatous due to progressive fragmentation of collagen, expansion of the proteoglycan-rich spongiosa, and increased cell proliferation. These molecular and cellular changes result in enlarged mitral leaflets that are mechanically weakened over time and become ineffective at preventing the backflow of blood. There are no known nonsurgical cures for MVP, and, as such, it is currently the most common cause of mitral valve surgery. This is likely due to poor understanding of disease etiology and progression. However, previous studies have demonstrated that mutations in the *FLNA* (*Filamin-A*) gene are causal to a rare X-linked myxomatous valvular dystrophy in humans and may provide critical clues to disease inception and pathogenetic manifestation.

The Filamin family consists of three homologous proteins: A, B and C. Filamins A and B are widely expressed, while Filamin-C expression is predominantly restricted to cardiac and skeletal muscle. Filamin exists as a homo- or hetero-dimer where it functions in crosslinking actin filaments, mechano-sensing through cell surface-bound integrins, and by means of these interactions regulates cell adhesion and migration [1,2]. Filamin-A has been shown to directly interact with a variety of intracellular proteins and can function as a scaffold for second messengers in signal transduction. Specifically, Filamin-A has been shown to directly bind the TGFβ signaling mediators Smad and R-ras [3,4]. Complete genetic removal of Filamin-A in the mouse results in embryonic lethality by embryonic day 14 due to vascular hemorrhaging and severe cardiac malformations [5,6]. Our recent studies have shown that Filamin-A is highly expressed in the mitral valve during development and is significantly diminished after birth, suggesting an important role for Filamin-A during valve development [7]. We previously reported the developmental importance for Filamin-A in the valves by generating conditional knockout mice. In these studies, Filamin-A was genetically removed from endothelial-derived tissue of the atrioventricular valves, and resulted in enlarged mitral leaflets that progressed to myxomatous degeneration by two months of age. The developmental defects were attributed to alterations in valvular interstitial cell contractility and impaired ability to remodel the maturing valve matrix. These studies importantly defined a developmental etiology for myxomatous valves and have provided a clinically relevant model to study mechanisms of disease pathogenesis. Thus, in this report we build on these previous studies and interrogate postnatal mechanisms by which myxomatous degeneration occurs using the Filamin-A-deficient mouse as the model for the disease.

2. Experimental Section

2.1. Gene Targeted Mice

All mouse experiments were performed as previously described [8]. Briefly, female mice homozygous for a conditional "floxed" allele of *FLNA* (*Filamin-A$^{f/f}$*) were bred with male transgenic mice expressing Cre under control of the *Tie2* promoter (*Tie2$^{Cre(+)}$*), which will target valve endocardium and endocardial-derived mesenchyme, resulting in a (*Tie2$^{Cre(+)}$*; *Filamin-A$^{f/y}$*) conditional knockout (cKO) mouse [9].

2.2. Histology, Immunohistochemistry/Immunofluorescence

Standard histological and immunochemical methods were used as previously described [8]. All mouse immunofluorescence was performed on 5-micron sections of 2-month-old adolescent wildtype (WT) and cKO mice. Human immunofluorescence was performed on 5-micron sections of posterior leaflet from the mitral valve of normal (control) and diseased (myxomatous) tissue. Human tissues were obtained from surgical specimens as part of a Leducq transatlantic network. All samples were harvested by offsite partners and were fixed, embedded and sectioned in their various laboratories. Sections were sent to our group at the Medical University of South Carolina (MUSC) for histological assessment. Consent and Institutional Review Board (IRB) approval for these studies is in place at partnering institutions. For human tissue analyses, 3 control and 5 myxomatous valves were analyzed. Control valve biopsies were obtained from patients who perished as a result of either subarachnoid hemorrhage or intracranial bleeds. Myxomatous valves were surgical cases obtained from patients who fit diagnostic criteria of myxomatous degeneration and mitral valve prolapse. This was defined by >2 mm atrial leaflet displacement in a parasternal long-axis view as well as >5 mm valve thickness. All patient samples involved in the study were men greater than 50 years of age. For immunohistochemistry (IHC): Antigen retrieval was performed for 10 min using antigen unmasking solution (Vector Laboratories, Burlingame, CA, USA, Cat#H-3300) by pressure cooker (Cuisinart, Stamford, CT, USA). Antibodies and their dilutions used for immunological experiments include: Collagen I (MD Biosciences, St. Paul, MN, USA, Cat#203002, 1:200), HaBP (EMD Millipore, Billerica, MA, USA, Cat#385911, 1:200), pERK1/2 (Cell Signaling Technology, Danvers, MA, USA, Cat#4370, 1:50), MMP2 (Abcam, Cambridge, MA, USA, Cat#ab37150, 1:250), MF20 (DSHB, Iowa City, IA, USA, Concentrate, 1:50), Ki67 (Abcam, Cat#ab16667, 1:250), Filamin-A (Abcam, Cat#ab76289, 1:250), MMP3 (Abcam, Cat#ab38907, 1:250), Versican (gift from Stan Hoffman, Medical University of South Carolina, 1:250), MMP7 (Abcam, Cat#ab38996, 1:500), CD45 (Abcam, Cat#ab10558, 1:100, for mouse), and CD45 (EMD Millipore, Cat#05-1410, 1:100, for human). For fluorescent detection of the primary antibodies, Alexa fluor 568 and Alexa fluor 488 secondary antibodies were used (Life Technologies, Rockville, MD, USA). Hyaluronan-binding protein (HaBP) was visualized by streptavidin-fluorescein (Life Technologies, Cat#S-32354, 1:100). Nuclei were counterstained with Hoechst (Life Technologies, Cat#H3569, 1:10,000) for 10 min and slides were coverslipped with SlowFade mounting medium (Life Technologies, Cat#S36937). Images were acquired with a Leica fluorescent microscope (Leica Biosystems, Buffalo Grove, IL, USA); $n > 3$ for each experiment.

2.3. Western Blotting

Isolated mitral leaflets from 2-month old mice were placed in SDS-PAGE buffer and boiled at 95 °C for 7 min before being run on a 4%–20% gradient polyacrylamide gel by electrophoresis (Biorad, , Cat#456-1094). A single leaflet per lane was used for Western blot experiments. Gels were transferred to a nitrocellulose membrane (Biorad, Cat#170-4158) and blocked for 1 h in 5% block (Biorad, Cat#170-6404) dissolved in 1X tris-buffered saline with Tween20 (BDH Chemicals, Poole Dorset, UK). Primary antibodies were incubated at (1:1000) dilution overnight at 4 °C. Primary antibodies used were pERK1/2 (Cell signaling, Cat#4370), pJNK1/2 (Cell Signaling, Cat#9255S), Erk (Cell Signaling, Cat#4695), JNK (Cell Signaling, Cat#9258S), MMP2 (Abcam, Cat#ab51125), MMP13 (Abcam, Cat#ab51072), and Actin (EMD Millipore, Cat#mab1501). Appropriate HRP-conjugated secondary antibodies were used at (1:10,000) in 5% block and incubated for 1 h at room temperature. Protein was detected using a chemiluminescent substrate (Life Technologies, Cat#34095). The entire process of tissue extraction to detection occurs within 18 h. We have determined that the rapidity of these experiments is critical in obtaining reproducible Western blots from single murine leaflets due to the small size and relative amounts of protein present in the extracts. Exact numbers of replicates are denoted in figure legends.

2.4. Statistics

Statistical significance was determined using a student's *t*-test (two-tailed, type 2), with significance ($p < 0.05$). Statistical data are presented as standard deviations from the mean.

3. Results and Discussion

3.1. Adolescent Filamin-A cKO Mice Exhibit Myxomatous Changes by Two Months

As a model for myxomatous valvular dystrophy, the *Filamin-A$^{f/f}$* mouse was bred onto the *Tie2$^{Cre(+)}$* background to genetically remove Filamin-A from all endothelial and endothelial-derived cells [8]. Since the mitral valve is largely derived from endothelium, the *Tie2$^{Cre(+)}$*; *Filamin-A$^{f/y}$* cKO mouse, previously described by our group, provides a model to study mechanisms that lead to the progression of myxomatous degeneration [8]. Histological analysis demonstrates enlarged mitral leaflets in the cKO mouse compared to the thin and elongated leaflets of the WT by two months of age (Figure 1). Movat's, Masson's, and immunohistochemistry (IHC), for collagen I and HaBP, demonstrate characteristics of myxomatous leaflets in the cKO, with an increase in the proteoglycan-rich regions and disruption of normal matrix organization.

3.2. Filamin-A-Deficient Mice Exhibit Increased Erk Signaling Concurrent with Increased MMP Expression and Cell Proliferation

To determine pathogenic mechanisms that contribute to the enlarged and myxomatous mitral valve in the cKO mouse, we performed an *in vivo* analysis examining alterations in signaling. Filamin-A functions in the regulation of various growth signaling pathways, including TGFβ, through direct interactions with downstream signaling mediators [1]. We hypothesized that loss of Filamin-A would result in the disruption of Erk1/2 signaling and that this may be pathogenic in myxomatous degeneration. By Western blot quantification of phospho/total Erk1/2 and phospho/total JNK in 2-month-old isolated anterior leaflets, and by IHC, we demonstrate that cKO mice have increased pErk1/2 and pJNK in the mitral valve (Figure 2A–C). Concurrent with these signaling activities, we observe increases in expression of the matrix metalloproteinases MMP2 and MMP13 in both mitral leaflets of the cKO compared to WT littermates (Figure 2D). Additionally, pErk localizes to regions of high MMP2 expression, suggesting excessive pErk1/2 may be an upstream signal promoting MMP expression in the diseased valve (Figure 2E), consistent with previous reports [10]. In addition to MMP expression, nuclear translocation of phospho-Erk1/2 has been reported to promote cell proliferation thorough activation of cell cycle regulatory proteins [11]. Since we see increased Erk1/2 signaling in our cKO mouse, we examined proliferation by immunostaining for ki67, and quantified proliferating cells. As shown in Figure 2F,G, proliferation was significantly increased in the cKO compared to the WT in both anterior and posterior leaflets.

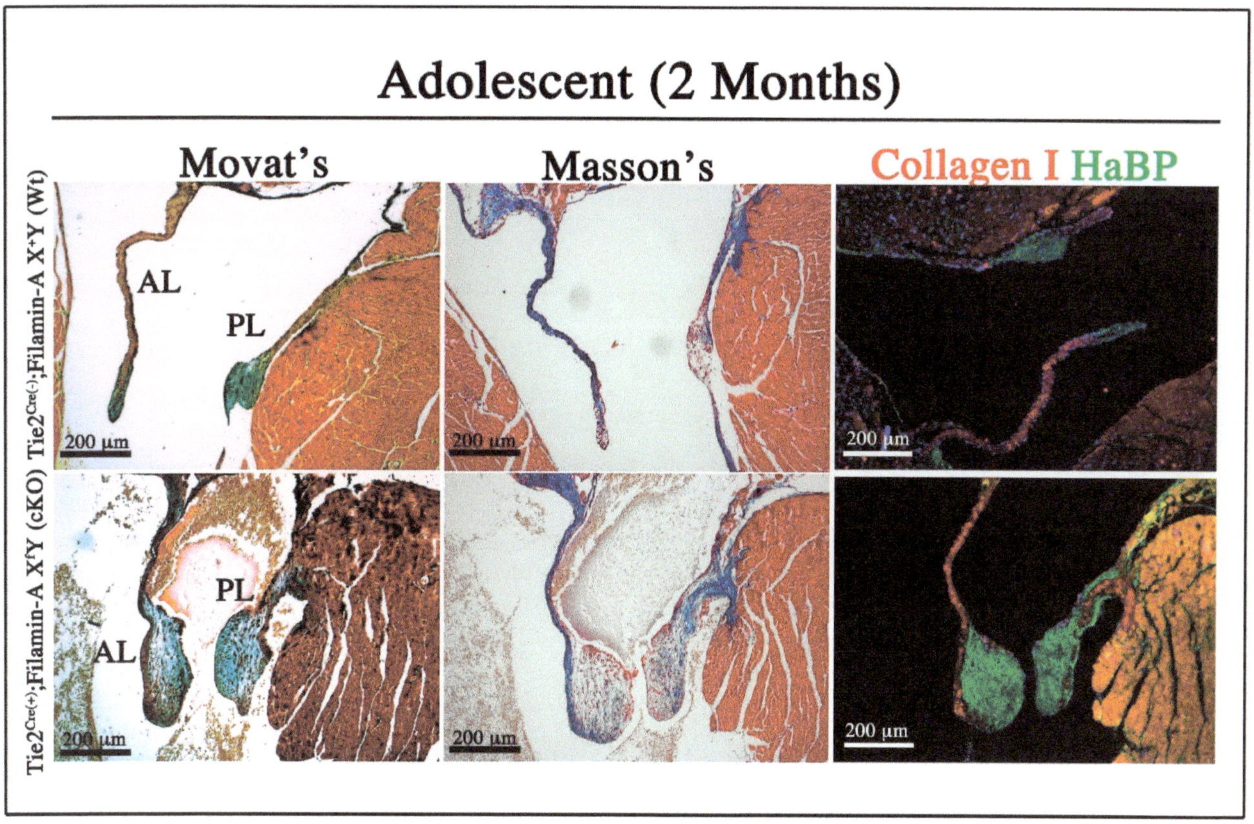

Figure 1. Filamin-A-deficient Mice Exhibit Myxomatous Mitral Leaflets. Adolescent 2-month-old mice were analyzed by Movat's Pentachrome, Masson's Trichrome, and Immunofluorescence for Collagen I (**red**) and Hyaluronan-binding protein (HaBP) (**green**). Movat's: Collagen (**yellow**), proteoglycans (**blue**), elastin/nuclei (**black**), muscle (red). Masson's: Collagen (blue), nuclei (black), muscle (red). Filamin-A-deficient mice exhibit increased proteoglycan content and disrupted matrix organization characteristic of myxomatous degeneration.

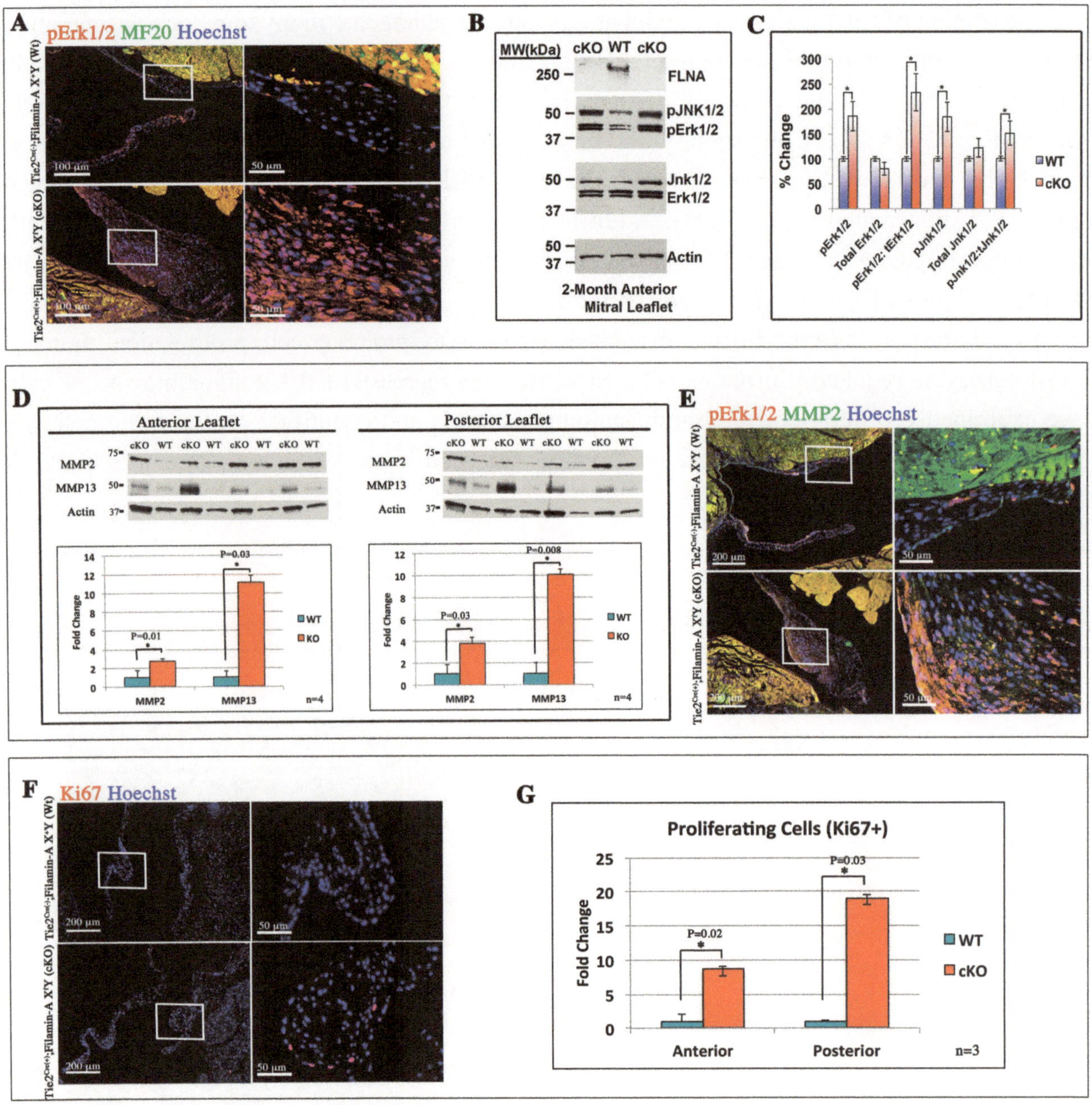

Figure 2. Erk1/2 Signaling, MMP expression, and Cell Proliferation are Increased in the Filamin-A cKO (**A**) IHC for phospho-Erk1/2 (**red**), MF20 (**green**), and nuclei (**blue**) demonstrate increased pErk accumulation in the 2-month-old cKO mitral valve; (**B**) Isolated anterior mitral leaflets from 2-month-old animals were analyzed individually by Western blot and demonstrate increased pErk1/2 and pJNK in relation to total protein, in the cKO compared to the WT; (**C**) Quantification of Western blot with * $p < 0.05$, $n > 4$; (**D**) Isolated anterior and posterior leaflets of cKO animals show increased expression of MMP2 and MMP13 compared to WT animals. All significant values are * $p < 0.05$, $n = 4$; (**E**) Immunofluorescence shows co-localization of pErk1/2 (**red**) with MMP2 expression (green); (**F**) Proliferating cells marked by Ki67 (**red**) and nuclei (**blue**) were quantified; (**G**) in both anterior and posterior leaflets. All significant values are * $p < 0.05$, $n = 3$.

3.3. Increased Infiltration of Hematopoietic-Derived Cells in Myxomatous Valves Contribute to Disease

To account for molecular changes (pErk, pJNK) and downstream consequences (MMP expression, proliferation) that contribute to disease in two-month-old cKO mice, the possibility that extra-cardiac cells may be promoting these pathogenic changes was examined. Hematopoietic cells have been shown to engraft into the murine adult mitral valve, and exhibit synthetic properties characteristic of fibroblasts as a part of normal valve homeostasis [12,13]. We hypothesized that in the Filamin-A model of myxomatous mitral valve disease, alterations in hematopoietic cell engraftment would be present in diseased valves and that these cells contribute to disease pathogenesis. Using CD45 as a marker for hematopoietic-derived cells, we observed an increase in the number of CD45-positive cells in the mitral leaflets of the cKOs compared to WT littermates (Figure 3A). CD45-positive cells engrafted primarily in the sub-endocardial region of the WT mouse, which is consistent with other reports in WT mice [12,13]. The cKO mice exhibited increased engraftment of hematopoietic-derived cells not only sub-endocardially, but also in the valvular interstitum [12]. To determine if these cells could be contributing to the myxomatous phenotype, we examined MMP expression as it related to the CD45-positive cells. Extracellular MMP2 localized to regions surrounding CD45-positive cells, suggesting these cells may be a significant source of MMPs (Figure 3B).

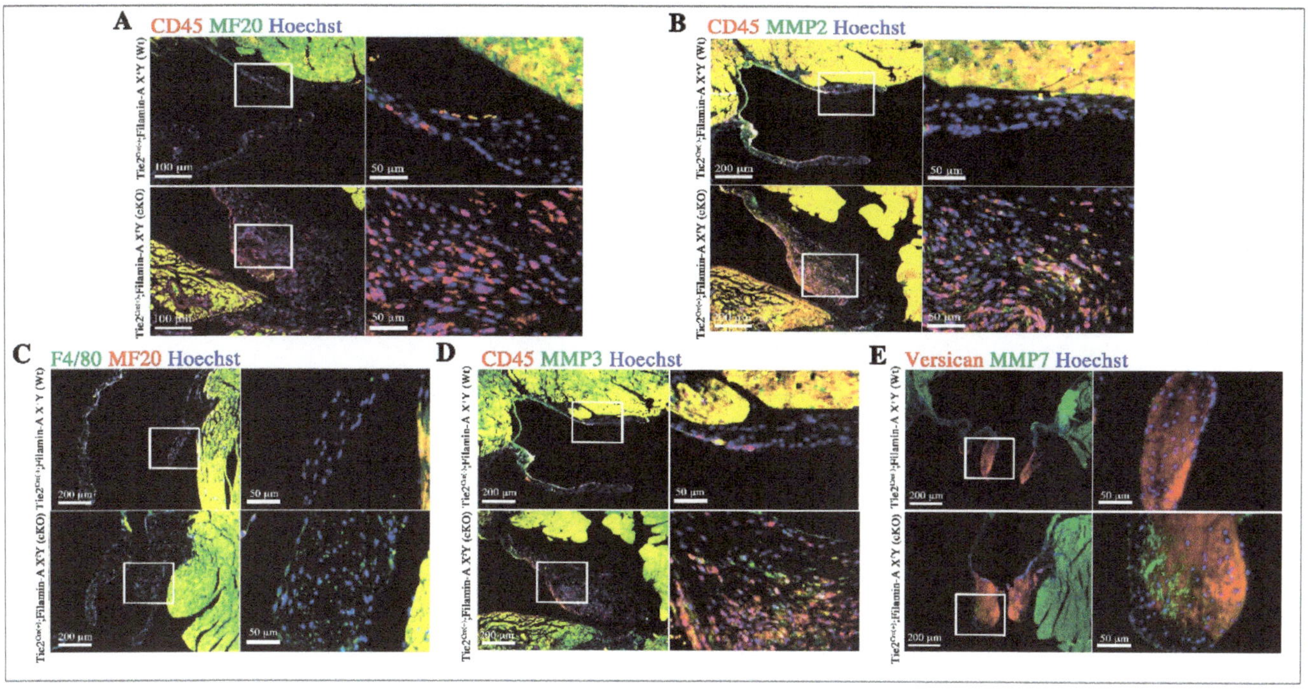

Figure 3. CD45-positve Cells Increased in the Filamin-A cKO mouse and may Contribute to Myxomatous Degeneration. (**A**) CD45-positive cells (**red**) are increased in the cKO compared to WT littermates; (**B**) CD45 cells (red) localize to MMP2 (**green**) expression in the posterior leaflet; (**C**) The macrophage marker F4/80 (green) is increased in the cKO posterior leaflet compared to the WT; (**D**) CD45-positive cells (red) express MMP3 and are localized to regions of secreted MMP3; (**E**) MMP7 (green) is increased in the CKO and co-localizes with versican expression (**red**).

Hematopoietic-derived cells that express CD45 are highly plastic and have been shown to develop into fully differentiated macrophages [14,15]. Since we see an increase in CD45-positive cells, we used the pan-macrophage marker F4/80 to determine if macrophage infiltration is also increased. Histologically, we observe an increase in expression of F4/80 in the cKO compared to the WT. This correlation between increased CD45 and F4/80 expressing cells suggests infiltrating CD45-positive cells may also be macrophages (Figure 3C).

To determine if there is an association between extra-cardiac cells and pathogenic mechanisms of disease, further characterization by IHC was performed. Macrophages are known to express MMPs at high levels, and have been specifically associated with MMP3 and MMP7 [16]. Our CKO mice show increased expression of both MMP3 (Figure 3D) and MMP7 (Figure 3E). Additionally, elevated levels of MMP3 were found in regions enriched with CD45-positive cells in cKO valves (Figure 3D). MMP7 distribution was primarily localized to the proteoglycan-enriched region of the leaflets, indicating a potential role in proteoglycan cleavage (Figure 3E). This data further suggests CD45-positive cells present in the mitral valve are involved in matrix remodeling and degradation.

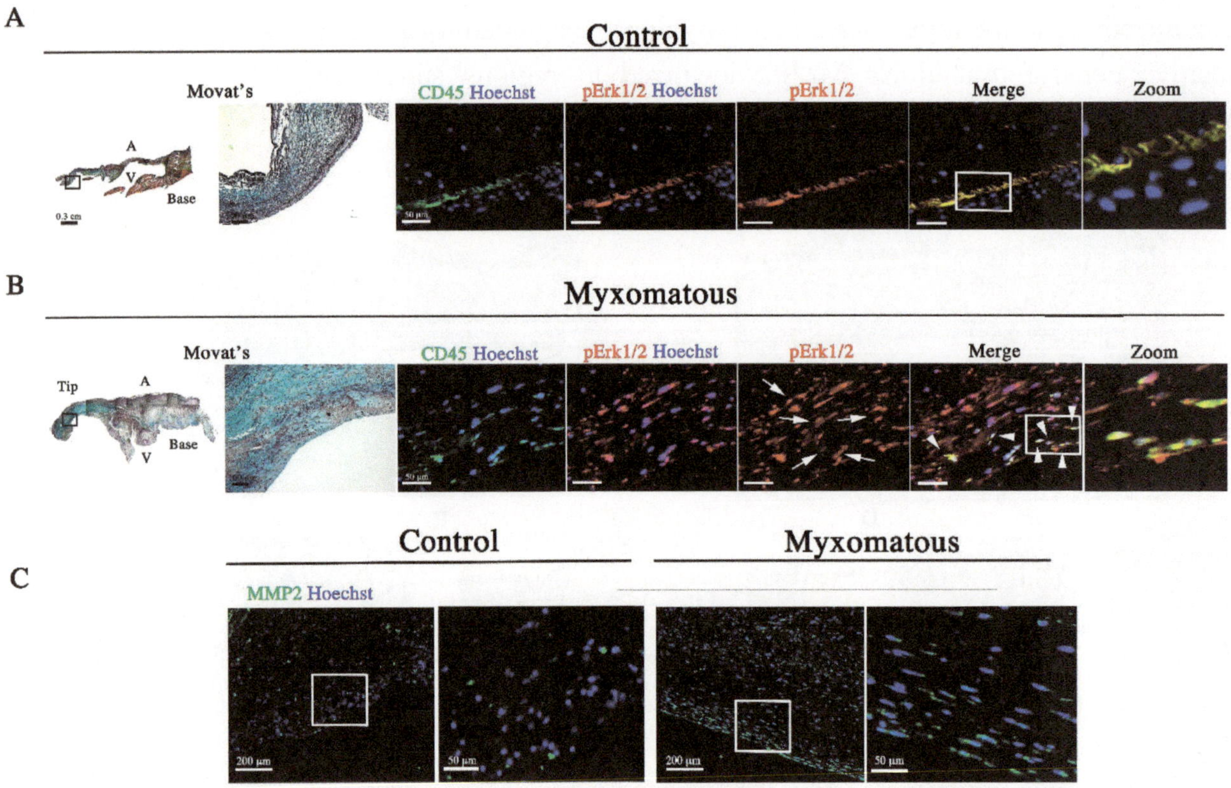

Figure 4. Myxomatous Human Mitral Leaflets Show Increased Infiltration of CD45-positive Cells. (**A**) IHC for CD45 (**green**) and pErk1/2 (**red**) and Movat's depicting elastin/nuclei (**black**), collagen (**yellow**), proteoglycans (**blue**), in the posterior leaflet from a normal human mitral valve; (**B**) Movat's and IHC in a myxomatous mitral leaflet form a human patient shows increased pErk1/2 (**red**) and CD45 cell (**green**) infiltration compared to control. CD45-positive cells also express pErk1/2 (**arrowheads**) and pErk1/2 is nuclear (**arrows**); (**C**) IHC for MMP2 (**green**) shows increased expression in the human myxomatous posterior leaflet. All images depict similar anatomical regions of the posterior leaflet.

To determine if the cellular and molecular changes observed in the cKO mouse are relevant to human disease, pErk, CD45, and MMP expression were examined in myxomatous and normal mitral valve tissue obtained from patients who underwent mitral valve surgery or autopsy respectively. In normal mitral tissue (control), pErk1/2 was present but restricted to the ventricularis layer and localized to the sub-endocardial region (Figure 4A). Myxomatous leaflets displayed increased pErk1/2 activity and in contrast to the control, pErk1/2 was active throughout all layers of the leaflet and was nuclear in localization compared to the primarily cytoplasmic expression in the control (Figure 4A,B). Additionally, CD45 positive cell infiltration was present in both the control and myxomatous leaflets, and these cells also express pErk1/2. Control leaflets exhibited restricted pErk1/2 activation in the region where CD45-positive cells reside. In contrast, myxomatous leaflets exhibit pErk1/2 activation not only in CD45-positive cells themselves, but also in proximal valve interstitial cells, suggesting the extra-cardiac cells may exhibit potential paracrine effects. MMP2 expression was also increased in the myxomatous valve compared to the control, and its localization was consistent with the pErk1/2 seen in the myxomatous valve (Figure 4C).

3.4. Discussion

Our results demonstrate that myxomatous changes occur by two months of age in the $Tie2^{Cre(+)}$; *Filamin-A-X^{f}Y* conditional knockout model of myxomatous mitral valve disease. Previous studies have established a link between increased growth factor signaling and syndromic forms of myxomatous mitral valve disease. For instance, patients with Marfan syndrome, a connective tissue disease that can result in myxomatous mitral valves and MVP, have indicated increased Erk1/2 signaling as a potential pathogenic mediator of the disease [17–21]. Marfan syndrome is caused by mutations in *FBN1* (*Fibrillin-1*), which result in excessive TGFβsignaling due to diminished binding of the latent form of the growth factor. This aberrant regulation of TGFβ results in alterations in pErk and pSmad2/3 activity accompanied by increased MMPs and cell proliferation [17]. As Filamin-A is known to interact with TGFβ signaling components, and mutations in FLNA cause a myxomatous valve disease that is similar to the mitral valve phenotype in Marfan syndrome, we hypothesized that Erk and Jnk signaling may also be elevated in the mitral leaflets of the Filamin-A deficient mouse. Indeed, our results presented here demonstrate increased Erk and Jnk activity in the mitral valve when Filamin-A is lost and that this signaling correlates with regions of MMP expression. Although TGFβ can initiate Erk signaling, we cannot directly tie increased Erk activity seen in our cKO mouse to TGFβ since many growth factors are known to be upstream of Erk signaling. These upstream signals include epidermal growth factor (EGF), fibroblast growth factor (FGF), and vascular endothelial growth factor (VEGF) [22]. It is yet to be determined whether these additional factors can activate the Erk/Jnk pathway in myxomatous valves. Regardless, upon activation Erk is translocated to the nucleus where it is known to promote expression of multiple genes, including MMPs [22]. The gelatinase MMP2, matrilysn MMP7 and the collagenase MMP13, were both significantly increased in the Filamin-A cKO valves. Increased expression of these enzymes are therefore likely candidates for contributing to myxomatous mitral valve degeneration and may contribute to the progressive deterioration of the structure and function of the valve over time. Additionally, previous studies have demonstrated that MMP-9 is also activated in cardiac and heart valve remodeling [23–25]. Together, these findings support a putative global stimulation of MMP expression and builds additional support for this class of enzymes in aberrant matrix destruction and remodeling in valve disease.

During normal valve homeostasis, hematopoietic-derived cells that exhibit synthetic processes characteristic of fibroblasts have been shown to engraft into the mitral valve [12]. In human myxomatous tissue, increased CD45-positive cells and blood-derived fibrocytes with matrix-altering abilities have also been observed [12,26,27]. Our data demonstrate an increase in hematopoietic cell engraftment in the context of human and murine myxomatous valve disease, and we show these cells may contribute |to myxomatous degeneration through matrix disruption (*i.e.*, MMP expression). In the mouse, regional localization patterns of hematopoietic cells differed between genotypes, where cells in the WT are localized sub-endocardially, while cells in the cKO integrate into the interstitial region of the leaflets. Correlated with infiltrating CD45-positive cells were significant increases in MMP2 expression in myxomatous leaflets, suggesting these cells may be a source. Additionally, increased MMP expression was observed throughout the leaflets and correlated regionally with CD45-positive cell infiltration, suggesting these cells may be a source of growth factors and promote myxomatous degeneration through paracrine mechanisms that alter the behavior of valvular interstitial cells.

To further characterize the hematopoietic cell population in the myxomatous mitral valve, we examined the possibility that these cells are monocytes/macrophages. In support of the idea that an immune response is initiated in myxomatous mitral valve disease, previous studies have identified serum increases in monocyte chemoattractant protein-1 (MCP-1) and additional increases in mast cells in dogs with myxomatous mitral leaflets [28,29]. In our cKO model, we observe an increase in macrophages in diseased mitral leaflets. This increase correlates with an increase in CD45-positive cells, suggesting these cells may also be macrophages. Expression of MMP3 by hematopoietic-derived cells further suggests these cells are TH-1 polarized M1 macrophages, which are classically associated with a pro-inflammatory phenotype and MMP expression [16]. To further support this, we show increased expression of MMP7, another macrophage-expressed metalloproteinase in M1 polarized macrophages. Expression of MMP7 preferentially corresponds to proteoglycan-rich regions of the mitral leaflets and is largely absent in the WT. Since MMP7 can cleave proteoglycans, this may be a mechanism by which proteoglycans are disrupted during disease. Both MMP-3 and MMP-7 degrade a number of ECM components including adhesive glycoproteins such as, laminin, fibronectin, tenascin, and some types of collagen [30]. Additionally, macrophages secrete factors that can have paracrine effects on the surrounding tissue. Previous studies have demonstrated this effect in dermal fibroblasts subjected to factors produced by M1 macrophages, where these cells show enhanced degradation properties in response to conditioned media [31]. Macrophages up-regulate MMPs in response to contact with different ECM components including collagen, laminin and fibronectin [32]. The mitral valve, which is composed of different matrix components, is an environment that would likely trigger up-regulation of MMPs in macrophages.

To determine if the molecular and cellular changes observed in the Filamin-A model of myxomatous valvular dystrophy are relevant to non-syndromic myxomatous disease in humans, we examined human resected mitral leaflets by IHC. Consistent with our murine studies, increases in pErk signaling were observed in human myxomatous posterior leaflets compared to normal tissue. Localization of pErk1/2 was confined to the ventricularis, sub-endocardial region of control leaflets and was primarily cytoplasmic, in contrast to the myxomatous leaflets, which displayed nuclear pErk1/2 activation throughout the entirety of the leaflet. Cellular populations of hematopoietic cells were increased in the human myxomatous leaflets and displayed co-expression of nuclear pErk1/2. MMP2 expression was also increased in myxomatous leaflets and observed in regions that encompass CD45 positive cells. Our results are consistent with previous reports that show increases in MMP2 activity in human mitral leaflets with myxomatous, floppy valves [33]. Taken together, our mouse and human data support the hypothesis that increased hematopoietic cell infiltration contributes to disease.

4. Conclusions

Loss of Filamin-A in the mitral leaflets of the mouse results in developmental defects in the structural architecture of the mitral valve. Post-natally, myxomatous degeneration occurs by two months of age and is accompanied by an increase in hematopoietic-derived cells, a sub-population of which are likely macrophages. These infiltrating extra-cardiac cells correlate with increased activation of Erk1/2 as well as putative downstream targets such as MMPs and genes that regulate and promote cell proliferation. Similar changes are observed in human myxomatous mitral valve tissue, whereby CD45-positive cells express nuclear pErk1/2. These murine and human studies suggest that infiltration of hematopoietic-derived cells and/or increased Erk1/2 signaling may be pathogenic to myxomatous valvular dystrophy. Consequently, immune cell targeting and/or suppression of pErk1/2 activities may represent an effective therapeutic option for mitral valve prolapse patients.

Acknowledgments

The work was performed in a facility constructed with support from the National Institutes of Health, Grant Number C06 RR018823 from the Extramural Research Facilities Program of the National Center for Research Resources. This work was supported by the Fondation Leducq (Paris, France) Mitral Transatlantic Network of Excellence grant 07CVD04. Other funding sources: National Heart Lung and Blood Institute: R01-HL33756 (RRM), COBRE 1P30 GM103342 (RRM, RAN), 8P20 GM103444-07 (RRM, ZH, RAN), R01-HL127692 (RAN), American Heart Association 15GRNT25080052 (RAN).

Author Contributions

K.S. and R.A.N. wrote the paper and were responsible for carrying out the experiments and data collection; K.T., K.W. and A.J. assisted in carrying out experiments and mouse husbandry; Z.H. and R.R.M. were involved in helpful discussions. R.A.N. led the project, assisted in experimental design and scientific advising.

Conflicts of Interest

The authors declare no conflict of interest.

References

1. Zhou, A.X.; Hartwig, J.H.; Akyurek, L.M. Filamins in cell signaling, transcription and organ development. *Trends Cell Biol.* **2010**, *20*, 113–123.

2. Kim, H.; Sengupta, A.; Glogauer, M.; McCulloch, C.A. Filamin A regulates cell spreading and survival via β1 integrins. *Exp. Cell Res.* **2008**, *314*, 834–846.
3. Sasaki, A.; Masuda, Y.; Ohta, Y.; Ikeda, K.; Watanabe, K. Filamin associates with Smads and regulates transforming growth factor-β signaling. *J. Biol. Chem.* **2001**, *276*, 17871–17877.
4. Griffiths, G.S.; Grundl, M.; Allen, J.S., III; Matter, M.L. R-Ras interacts with filamin a to maintain endothelial barrier function. *J. Cell. Physiol.* **2011**, *226*, 2287–2296.
5. Hart, A.W.; Morgan, J.E.; Schneider, J.; West, K.; McKie, L.; Bhattacharya, S.; Jackson, I.J.; Cross, S.H. Cardiac malformations and midline skeletal defects in mice lacking filamin A. *Hum. Mol. Genet.* **2006**, *15*, 2457–2467.
6. Feng, Y.; Chen, M.H.; Moskowitz, I.P.; Mendonza, A.M; Vidali, L.; Nakamura, F.; Kwiatkowski, D.J.; Walsh, C.A. Filamin A (FLNA) is required for cell-cell contact in vascular development and cardiac morphogenesis. *Proc. Natl. Acad. Sci. USA* **2006**, *103*, 19836–19841.
7. Norris, R.A.; Moreno-Rodriguez, R.; Wessels, A.; Merot, J.; Bruneval, P.; Chester, A.H.; Yacoub, M.H.; Hagège, A.; Slaugenhaupt, S.A.; Aikawa, E.; *et al.* Expression of the familial cardiac valvular dystrophy gene, filamin-A, during heart morphogenesis. *Dev. Dyn.* **2010**, *239*, 2118–2127.
8. Sauls, K.; de Vlaming, A.; Harris, B.S.; Williams, K.; Wessels, A.; Levine, R.A.; Slaugenhaupt, S.A.; Goodwin, R.L.; Pavone, L.M.; Merot. J.; *et al.* Developmental basis for filamin-A-associated myxomatous mitral valve disease. *Cardiovasc. Res.* **2012**, *96*, 109–119.
9. Kisanuki, Y.Y.; Hammer, R.E.; Miyazaki, J.; Williams, S.C.; Richardson, J.A.; Yanagisawa, M. Tie2-Cre transgenic mice: A new model for endothelial cell-lineage analysis *in vivo*. *Dev. Biol.* **2001**, *230*, 230–242.
10. Kuo, L.; Chang, H.C.; Leu, T.H.; Maa, M.C.; Hung, W.C. Src oncogene activates MMP-2 expression via the ERK/Sp1 pathway. *J. Cell. Physiol.* **2006**, *207*, 729–734.
11. Torii, S.; Nakayama, K.; Yamamoto, T.; Nishida, E. Regulatory mechanisms and function of ERK MAP kinases. *J. Biochem.* **2004**, *136*, 557–561.
12. Hajdu, Z.; Romeo, S.J.; Fleming, P.A.; Markwald, R.R.; Visconti, R.P.; Drake, C.J. Recruitment of bone marrow-derived valve interstitial cells is a normal homeostatic process. *J. Mol. Cell. Cardiol.* **2011**, *51*, 955–965.
13. Visconti, R.P.; Ebihara, Y.; LaRue, A.C.; Fleming, P.A.; McQuinn, T.C.; Masuya, M.; Minamiguchi, H.; Markwald, R.R.; Ogawa, M.; Drake, C.J. An *in vivo* analysis of hematopoietic stem cell potential: Hematopoietic origin of cardiac valve interstitial cells. *Circ. Res.* **2006**, *98*, 690–696.
14. Reddy, K.; Zhou, Z.; Schadler, K.; Jia, S.F.; Kleinerman, E.S. Bone marrow subsets differentiate into endothelial cells and pericytes contributing to Ewing's tumor vessels. *Mol. Cancer Res.* **2008**, *6*, 929–936.
15. Xu, J.; Kisseleva, T. Bone marrow-derived fibrocytes contribute to liver fibrosis. *Exp. Biol. Med.* **2015**, *240*, 691–700.
16. Martinez, F.O.; Gordon, S. The M1 and M2 paradigm of macrophage activation: Time for reassessment. *F1000Prime Rep.* **2014**, *6*, doi:10.12703/P6-13.
17. Ng, C.M.; Cheng, A.; Myers, L.A.; Martinez-Murillo, F.; Jie, C.; Bedja, D.; Gabrielson, K.L.; Hausladen, J.M.; Mecham, R.P.; Judge, D.P.; *et al.* TGF-β-dependent pathogenesis of mitral valve prolapse in a mouse model of Marfan syndrome. *J. Clin. Investig.* **2004**, *114*, 1586–1592.

18. Dugan, S.L.; Temme, R.T.; Olson, R.A.; Mikhailov, A.; Law, R.; Mahmood, H.; Noor, A.; Vincent, J.B. New recessive truncating mutation in LTBP3 in a family with oligodontia, short stature, and mitral valve prolapse. *Am. J. Med. Genet. A* **2015**, *167*, 1396–1399.
19. Doyle, A.J.; Doyle, J.J.; Bessling, S.L.; Maragh, S.; Lindsay, M.E.; Schepers, D.; Gillis, E.; Mortier, G.; Homfray, T.; Sauls, K.; *et al.* Mutations in the TGF-β repressor SKI cause Shprintzen-Goldberg syndrome with aortic aneurysm. *Nat. Genet.* **2012**, *44*, 1249–1254.
20. Malev, E.G.; Zemtsovskiĭ, E.V.; Omel'chenko, M.I.; Vasina, L.V. The role of transforming growth factor-β in the pathogenesis of mitral valve prolapse. *Kardiologiia* **2012**, *52*, 34–39.
21. Boileau, C.; Guo, D.C.; Hanna, N.; Regalado, E.S.; Detaint, D.; Gong, L.; Varret, M.; Prakash, S.K.; Li, A.H.; d'Indy, H.; Braverman, A.C.; *et al. TGFB2* mutations cause familial thoracic aortic aneurysms and dissections associated with mild systemic features of Marfan syndrome. *Nat. Genet.* **2012**, *44*, 916–921.
22. Roskoski, R., Jr. ERK1/2 MAP kinases: Structure, function, and regulation. *Pharmacol. Res.* **2012**, *66*, 105–143.
23. Cheng, X.W.; Shi, G.P.; Kuzuya, M.; Sasaki, T.; Okumura, K.; Murohara, T. Role for cysteine protease cathepsins in heart disease: Focus on biology and mechanisms with clinical implication. *Circulation* **2012**, *125*, 1551–1562.
24. Cheng, X.W.; Huang, Z.; Kuzuya, M.; Okumura, K.; Murohara, T. Cysteine protease cathepsins in atherosclerosis-based vascular disease and its complications. *Hypertension* **2011**, *58*, 978–986.
25. Jiang, H.; Cheng, X.W.; Shi, G.P.; Hu, L.; Inoue, A.; Yamamura, Y.; Wu, H.; Takeshita, K.; Li, X.; Huang, Z. *et al.* Cathepsin K-mediated Notch1 activation contributes to neovascularization in response to hypoxia. *Nat. Commun.* **2014**, *5*, 3838, doi:10.1038/ncomms4838.
26. Barth, P.J.; Koster, H.; Moosdorf, R. $CD34^+$ fibrocytes in normal mitral valves and myxomatous mitral valve degeneration. *Pathol. Res. Pract.* **2005**, *201*, 301–304.
27. Geirsson, A.; Singh, M.; Ali, R.; Abbas, H.; Li, W.; Sanchez, J.A.; Hashim, S.; Tellides, G. Modulation of transforming growth factor-β signaling and extracellular matrix production in myxomatous mitral valves by angiotensin II receptor blockers. *Circulation* **2012**, *126*, S189–S197.
28. Han, R.I.; Black, A.; Culshaw, G.J.; French, A.T.; Else, R.W.; Corcoran, B.M. Distribution of myofibroblasts, smooth muscle-like cells, macrophages, and mast cells in mitral valve leaflets of dogs with myxomatous mitral valve disease. *Am. J. Vet. Res.* **2008**, *69*, 763–769.
29. Zois, N.E.; Moesgaard, S.G.; Kjelgaard-Hansen, M.; Rasmussen, C.E.; Falk, T.; Fossing, C.; Häggström, J.; Pedersen, H.D.; Olsen, L.H. Circulating cytokine concentrations in dogs with different degrees of myxomatous mitral valve disease. *Vet. J.* **2012**, *192*, 106–111.
30. Stamenkovic, I. Extracellular matrix remodelling: The role of matrix metalloproteinases. *J. Pathol.* **2003**, *200*, 448–464.
31. Ploeger, D.T.; Hosper, N.A.; Schipper, M.; Koerts, J.A.; de Rond, S.; Bank, R.A. Cell plasticity in wound healing: Paracrine factors of M1/M2 polarized macrophages influence the phenotypical state of dermal fibroblasts. *Cell Commun. Signal.* **2013**, *11*, 29, doi:10.1186/1478-811X-11-29.
32. Khan, K.M.; Howe, L.R.; Falcone, D.J. Extracellular matrix-induced cyclooxygenase-2 regulates macrophage proteinase expression. *J. Biol. Chem.* **2004**, *279*, 22039–22046.

33. Togashi, M.; Tamura, K.; Nitta, T.; Ishizaki, M.; Sugisaki, Y.; Fukuda, Y. Role of matrix metalloproteinases and their tissue inhibitor of metalloproteinases in myxomatous change of cardiac floppy valves. *Pathol. Int.* **2007**, *57*, 251–259.

15

MVP-Associated Filamin A Mutations Affect FlnA-PTPN12 (PTP-PEST) Interactions

Damien Duval [1], Pauline Labbé [1], Léa Bureau [1], Thierry Le Tourneau [1], Russell A. Norris [2], Roger R. Markwald [2], Robert Levine [3], Jean-Jacques Schott [1], Jean Mérot [1,*]

[1] Institut du thorax, Inserm UMR 1087, CNRS UMR 6291, 8 Quai Moncousu, Nantes F-44007, France; E-Mails: damien.duval@etu.univ-nantes.fr (D.D.); pauline.labbe@etu.univ-nantes.fr (P.L.); bureau.lea@gmail.com (L.B.); thletourneau@yahoo.fr (T.L.T.); jjschott@univ-nantes.fr (J.-J.S.)

[2] Department of Cell Biology and Anatomy, Medical University of South Carolina, Charleston, SC 29425, USA; E-Mails: norrisra@musc.edu (R.A.N.); markwald@musc.edu (R.R.M.)

[3] Harvard Medical School, Massachusetts General Hospital, Boston, MA 02114-2696 USA; E-Mail: rlevine@partners.org

* Author to whom correspondence should be addressed; E-Mail: jean.merot@univ-nantes.fr

Academic Editor: Cheryl L. Maslen

Abstract: Although the genetic basis of mitral valve prolapse (MVP) has now been clearly established, the molecular and cellular mechanisms involved in the pathological processes associated to a specific mutation often remain to be determined. The *FLNA* gene (encoding Filamin A; FlnA) was the first gene associated to non-syndromic X-linked myxomatous valvular dystrophy, but the impacts of the mutations on its function remain un-elucidated. Here, using the first repeats (1–8) of FlnA as a bait in a yeast two-hybrid screen, we identified the tyrosine phosphatase PTPN12 (PTP-PEST) as a specific binding partner of this region of FlnA protein. In addition, using yeast two-hybrid trap assay pull down and co-immunoprecipitation experiments, we showed that the MVP-associated FlnA mutations (G288R, P637Q, H743P) abolished FlnA/PTPN12 interactions. PTPN12 is a key regulator of signaling pathways involved in cell-extracellular matrix (ECM) crosstalk, cellular responses to mechanical stress that involve integrins, focal adhesion transduction pathways, and actin cytoskeleton dynamics. Interestingly, we showed that the FlnA mutations impair the activation status of two PTPN12 substrates, the focal adhesion associated kinase Src, and the RhoA specific activating protein p190RhoGAP. Together, these data point to PTPN12/FlnA interaction and its weakening by FlnA mutations as a mechanism potentially involved in the physiopathology of FlnA-associated MVP.

Keywords: Filamin-A; PTPN12; mitral valve prolapse; p190RhoGAP; Src

1. Introduction

The mitral valve prolapse (MVP), the most common form of cardiac disease, involves approximately 2%–3% of the population and remains one of the major causes of valve surgery. In parallel to syndromic forms, the familial inheritance of non-syndromic MVP has now been clearly established [1]. Indeed, the syndromic forms of MVP have been linked to several genes such as *FBN1* (Fibrillin-1) in Marfan syndrome [2], *TGFBRs* (TGFβ receptors) in Loeys-Dietz syndrome [3], *COL-1* (Collagen-1) in Ehlers-Danlos syndrome [4], while the *FLNA* (Filamin A) gene was associated to non-syndromic X-linked myxomatous valvular dystrophy (XMVD) [5,6]. However, although recent studies have unraveled the molecular, cellular, and physiopathological processes in few syndromic MVPs, including Marfan syndrome, and lead to potential therapeutic treatments for better healthcare of these patients [7,8], the deleterious mechanisms at work in FlnA-associated MVP remain to be elucidated.

In the late 1990s we mapped X-linked myxomatous valvular dystrophy to chromosome Xq28 gene locus in a large French family and identified in 2007, in all affected members, a first mutation encoding p.Pro637Gln residue substitution (P637Q) in the *FLNA* gene [5,6]. In addition, three other FlnA mutations encoding two residue substitutions, p.Gly288Arg (G288R), p.Val711Asp (V711D), and a 1944-bp genomic deletion were subsequently identified in four other families around the world. Although FlnA mutations have been associated to important and various congenital developmental diseases, including periventricular heterotopy (PVH) [9], Melnick-Needles syndrome (MNS) [10], and otopalatodigital syndrome (OPD), it is important to note that the patients bearing MVP-associated FlnA mutations only suffer from valvular affections, suggesting similar but specific mechanisms are at work for these MVP-associated FlnA-mutations. As a matter of fact, common clinical traits were shared in the different families, including early onset of poly-valvular defects sometimes detectable in newborns, typical features of myxomatous disease with marked thickening of the mitral valve (thickness was superior to 4 mm), and alterations of the sub-valvular apparatus. Interestingly, we also detected similar defects in targeted FlnA knockout mice model which exhibited abnormal valvular development and hyperplasic mitral valves, strongly suggesting that the MVP FlnA mutations we identified are loss of function mutations [11,12].

Filamin A (FlnA) is the first actin filament cross-linking protein identified in non-muscle cells. It organizes actin filaments in orthogonal networks to stabilize the cellular actin cortex, and many previous studies defined central roles for FlnA in mechano-protection, cell adhesion, spreading, and migration [13-17]. The FlnA protein consists of a conserved N-terminal actin binding region followed by 24 immunoglobulin-like (Igl) repeated domains, among which the 24th is involved in non-covalent protein dimerization [15]. Over 90 FlnA interacting protein partners have now been identified attesting to the implication of FlnA in the regulation of many signaling cascades involving actin cytoskeleton regulation. Interestingly, only few of these binding partners were shown to interact with the first N-terminal Igl repeats region of FlnA (Igl-1–8) that are targeted by the MVP-associated FlnA mutations suggesting the pathological effects of the latter may arise from interactions with new, yet unknown, binding partners [18,19].

To identify binding partners specifically interacting with the FlnA region targeted by the MVP mutations we performed a yeast two-hybrid screen of a cDNA library using the FlnA Igl repeats 1–8 region as a bait (Figure 1A). This screen identified a key regulator of cellular cytoskeleton and cell-extracellular matrix interaction signaling pathway, the tyrosine phosphatase non-receptor type PTPN12/PTP-PEST, as a binding partner of FlnA-1–8 repeats [20-22]. Furthermore, using yeast two-hybrid, pulldown and co-immunoprecipitation assays, we showed that FlnA-G288R and P637Q mutations and a recently-identified mutation p.His743Pro (H743P) affect FlnA/PTPN12 interactions, supporting a potential role of altered FlnA/PTPN12 interactions in the physio-pathological mechanisms of FlnA-associated MVP.

2. Experimental Section

2.1. cDNAs, Mutagenesis, and Reagents

The cDNA encoding FlnA Igl repeats 1–8 fused to its Hinge 2 domain and its 24th Igl repeat (FlnA-1–8,24, see Figure 1A), was a kind gift of Dr F. Nakamura [15]. Human PTPN12 cDNA was obtained from Source Bioscience (Nottingham, UK) and C-terminally EGFP tagged FlnA from Dr D. Calderwood (Yale University, New Haven, CT, USA). pPC97, pPC86 vectors and the pPC97-CT7 (encoding the *GAL4* DNA binding domain fused to the C-terminal tail of mGluR7a glutamate receptor *GAL4*-BD-CT7), and pPC86-PICK1 (encoding *GAL4*-AD-PICK1 fusion) constructs used as positive controls in interaction assay were a kind gift of Dr H. Boudin (INSERM U913, Nantes, France) [23]. The construct encoding GST-RhoQ63L was a kind gift of Dr C. Guilluy (INSERM U1087, Nantes, France). All the mutations described below were made using PCR-based mutagenesis kits (Quickchange kit from Agilent Tech, Les Ulis, France). Polyclonal antibodies for GAPDH (1:10,000) and HRP-conjugated antibodies (1:10,000) were purchased from Santa Cruz. Monoclonal antibodies were purchased from Chemicon (anti-filamin A, 1:1000, Merck Millipore, Milsheom, France), Clontech (anti-EGFP, 1:1000, Saint-Germain-en-Laye, France), Roche (anti-HA, 1:1000), BD Bioscience (p190RhoGAP, 1:500, Le Pont de Claix, France), and Cell Signaling (Src and phospho-Src-Y416, 1:500 both, Merck Millipore).

2.2. Cell Culture and Transfection

The maintenance and the production of melanoma cells stably transfected with wild-type and mutant FlnAs were previously described in [24]. Hek293 cells were cultured in DMEM, supplemented with 10% fetal calf serum (FCS) and L-glutamine. The cells were transfected using Lipofectamine (Invitrogen, Illkirch, France) or Genecellin (BiocellChallenge, Toulon, France) according to the manufacturers' specifications.

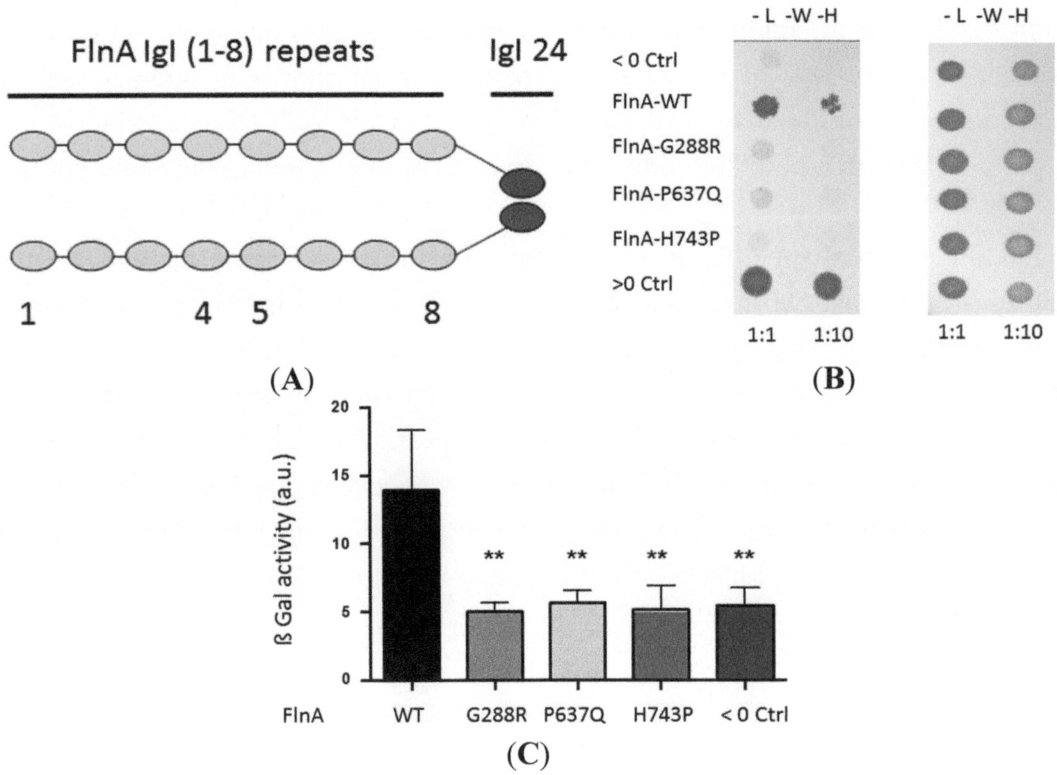

Figure 1. Effects of Filamin A mutations on FlnA/PTPN12 interaction. Yeast two-hybrid assay. (**A**) Schematic cartoon of the bait used in the two-hybrid library screening and interaction assay of FlnA mutations. The bait consists in the first eight IgI repeats fused to the second hinge and the 24th repeat of FlnA; (**B**) the left-hand image shows yeasts co-transfected with *GAL4*-AD-PTPN12 and, from top to bottom lane, *GAL4*-BD-CT7 (negative control; Neg Ctrl), *GAL4*-BD-FlnA-WT, G288R, P637Q or H743P or co-transfected with *GAL4*-AD-PICK1 and *GAL4*-BD-CT7 (positive control, Pos Ctrl) growing on histidine-free medium (interaction assay) or histidine-supplemented plates (growth assay, right-hand image). Two dilutions of 1:1 and 1:10 were spotted; (**C**) quantification of FlnA/PTPN12 interaction in β galactosidase assay. Results are presented in arbitrary units (au). ** indicates significant differences ($p < 0.01$, $n = 4$) *vs.* FlnA-WT.

2.3. Migration Assays: Wound Healing Assays

In wound healing assays, confluent cell monolayers were scratched with a pipette tip, washed with phosphate-buffered saline (PBS), and cell migration monitored using a Leica DMI6000B microscope (Nanterre, France) equipped for time-lapse video microscopy. Wound closure was monitored for 24–28 h on three fields per well and the data are presented as % of closure of FlnA-WT cells' monolayer wound closure at t = 24 h. Snapshots of migrating cells presenting trailing tails were extracted from these experiments.

2.4. Yeast Two-Hybrid Library Screening

Yeast two-hybrid screening was performed by Hybrigenics (Hybrigenics Services, Paris, France). The coding sequence of FlnA-1–8,24 was PCR-amplified and cloned into pB27 as a C-terminal fusion to LexA (*N*-LexA-FlnA-1–8,24-C). The construct was checked by sequencing the entire insert and used as a bait to screen a random-primed human placenta cDNA library constructed into pP6. pB27 and pP6 derive from the original pBTM116 and pGADGH plasmids, respectively. 79.4 million clones (eight-fold the complexity of the library) were screened using a mating approach with YHGX13 (Y187 ade2-101: loxP-kanMX-loxP, matα) and L40ΔGal4 (mata) yeast strains as previously described in [25]. 129 His + colonies were selected on a medium lacking tryptophan, leucine, and histidine. The prey fragments of the positive clones were amplified by PCR and sequenced at their 5′ and 3′ junctions. The resulting sequences were used to identify the corresponding interacting proteins in the GenBank database (NCBI, http://www.ncbi.nlm.nih.gov/) using a fully automated procedure. A confidence score (PBS, for Predicted Biological Score) was attributed to each interaction as previously described in [26]. The PBS relies on two different levels of analysis. Firstly, a local score takes into account the redundancy and independency of prey fragments, as well as the distribution of reading frames and stop codons in overlapping fragments. Secondly, a global score which takes into account the interactions found in all of the screens performed at Hybrigenics using the same library. This global score represents the probability of an interaction being nonspecific.

2.5. Yeast Two-Hybrid Interaction Assays

WT-FlnA-1–8,24 cDNA and those encoding G288R, H743P, and P637Q mutations (G288R, H743P, P637Q-FlnA-1–8,24, respectively) were PCR amplified and cloned in frame (5′-SalI, NotI-3′) with the DNA binding domain of *GAL4* in the pPC97 derived vector containing *LEU2* selection reporter (*GAL4*-BD-FlnA). The cDNA encoding the T587-N753 peptide region of PTPN12 identified in the library screen was PCR amplified and cloned in frame (5′-SalI, NotI-3′) with the activation domain of *GAL4* in the pPC86 vector containing *TRP1* selection reporter (*GAL4*-AD-PTPN12). The yeast reporter strain PJ69-4A was used and sequentially transfected with recombinant pPC97 and pPC86 plasmids using the lithium acetate method. Cells were patched onto selective (leucine; tryptophan and histidine-deprived $L^-W^-H^-$) plates that were incubated at 30 °C for 2–6 days. Standard colorimetric β-galactosidase assays performed on liquid cultures were used to verify and quantify the strength of the interaction between the different binding partners tested.

2.6. Co-Immunoprecipitation and Immunoblotting

Hek293 cells transfected with C-terminally EGFP-tagged FlnA-WT or FlnA-P637Q were lysed in NETF buffer containing: 100 mM NaCl, 2 mM EGTA, 50 mM Tris pH 7.5, 50 mM NaF, 1% NP-40, 1 mM PMSF, 1 mM Na_3VO_4, 1× protease inhibitor cocktail (Roche, Boulogne-Billancourt, France), and lysates clarified by centrifugation (15,000× *g* for 15 min at 4 °C). The cell lysates (500 µg) were incubated with 6 µg of anti-HA for 2 h at 4 °C and then with 30 µL of protein A conjugated beads (Dynabeads, Invitrogen, Illkirch, France) for 1 h at 4 °C. The immunoprecipitates were washed four times with NETF buffer, separated by SDS-PAGE, and transferred to a nitrocellulose membrane (Bio-Rad Transblot, Marnes-la-Coquette, France). Immunoblots were probed with appropriate antibodies and revealed using an enhanced chemiluminescence kit (GE Healthcare, Buc, France). Chemiluminescence signals were quantified using an Imager system (Roche Diagnostic, Boulogne-Billancourt, France) and the data normalized with respect to GAPDH.

2.7. Pulldown Experiments

The cDNA fragment encoding the peptide region of hum-PTPN12 (Pro600-Asp709) was PCR amplified and cloned in PGEX-6P1 vector to produce GST-PTPN12 fusion protein. The GST-PTPN12 and GST-PTPN12-ΔPro in which the proline-rich region (674-PPPLPERTP-682) of PTPN12 was deleted, were produced in BL21 *Escherichia coli* (*E. Coli*) and purified using glutathione agarose 4B beads (Macherey-Nagel, Hoerdt, France) as previously described in [24]. The GST-fusion proteins (30 μg) were incubated for 1 h at 4 °C with 500 μg of cleared cellular lysates prepared from melanoma cells stably transfected with FlnA-WT or FlnA-P637Q in NETF buffer containing: 100 mM NaCl, 2 mM EGTA, 50 mM Tris pH 7.5, 50 mM NaF, 1% NP-40, 1 mM PMSF, 1 mM Na_3VO_4, and 1× protease inhibitor cocktail (Roche). The beads were washed four times with cell lysis buffer and bound proteins separated by SDS-PAGE. Bound FlnAs were detected by immunoblotting using an anti-FlnA antibody. A similar protocol using GST-RhoA-Q63L and anti-p190RhoGAP antibody was performed to test p190RhoGAP activation status.

3. Results

3.1. A Yeast Two-Hybrid Library Screen Identified PTPN12 as A FlnA Binding Partner

Based on (1) the observation that all MVP-associated FlnA mutations target the same N-terminal region of the protein namely: the Igl-1 (G288R), Igl-4 (P637Q), Igl-5 (V711D and H743P), and Igl-6–7 (Δ761-943); (2) the fact that FlnA-associated MVP patients shared very similar clinical features; (3) the notion that the dimerization of FlnA polypeptides determines its association with specific binding partners [27]; and (4) the impossibility to use the full-length FlnA because of its size, we chose to use the first eight repeats of FlnA fused to its dimerization domain (24th Igl) as a bait to screen a human placental cDNA library in a LexA-based yeast two-hybrid assay (Figure 1A). 79.4 million clones (eight-fold the complexity of the library) were screened and HIS-positive clones isolated on leucine-, tryptophan-, and histidine-free selection medium. The sequencing of one of the positive clones identified the region (residue 587–753) of the tyrosine phosphatase PTPN12/PTP-PEST. Interestingly, this domain of PTPN12 encodes a proline-rich motif that was shown to participate to FlnA/PTPN12 interaction, suggesting the Igl repeat 1–8 region of FlnA constitute its yet unknown interaction domain with PTPN12 [28]. We then tested the impact of the FlnA-MVP mutations on FlnA/PTPN12 interactions.

3.2. MVP-Associated FlnA Mutations Impede its Interactions with PTPN12

3.2.1. Yeast Two-Hybrid Assay

To confirm the FlnA/PTPN12 interaction we observed using the LexA-based two-hybrid system, and to test the effects of the mutations on this interaction, we used another yeast two-hybrid assay based on the *GAL4* transcription factor. As illustrated on Figure 1, the yeasts co-expressing *GAL4*-AD-PTPN12 and *GAL4*-BD-FlnA-WT grew on the selective $L^-W^-H^-$ plates (Figure 1B, second lane) although less rapidly than those co-transfected with the two strongly-interacting partners used as a positive control, *GAL4*-AD-Pick1 and *GAL4*-BD-CT7 (Figure 1B, bottom lane). These data confirmed the direct PTN12/FlnA interaction and showed it could also be detected using this interaction trap assay. We then tested the effects of the MVP-FlnA mutations. Interestingly, neither FlnA-G288R, P637Q, H743P, nor CT7 (used as a negative control, top lane) enabled growth of PTPN12-expressing yeasts in the $L^-W^-H^-$ selection medium (Figure 1B). Importantly, all the yeasts grew equally well when the medium was supplemented with histidine, excluding potential toxicity biases due to exogenous protein overexpression (Figure 1B, right-hand image). The loss of interaction was quantified using β-galactosidase assay performed on liquid culture. As shown on Figure 1C, the FlnA mutations leveled down the galactosidase activity, which represents the PTPN12/FlnA-WT binding strength, to that measured with the negative control (CT7), suggesting a complete loss of interaction with PTPN12.

3.2.2. Pulldown and Co-Immunoprecipitation Assays

FlnA/PTPN12 interactions were then challenged in a pulldown assay using the interaction domain of PTPN12 fused to GST protein and melanoma cell lines stably expressing FlnA-WT and FlnA-P637Q [24]. In this assay (Figure 2), FlnA-WT was specifically retained on GST-PTPN12 (Figure 2, lane three) but not by GST or the mutant GST-PTPN12 construct in which the proline-rich domain (674-PPPLPERTP-682) of PTPN12 previously shown to participate to PTPN12-FlnA interactions (GST-PTPN12-ΔPro), was deleted (Figure 2 lanes one and five, respectively). Importantly, FlnA-P637Q did not interact with any of these GST constructs (Figure 2) even when larger amount of FlnA-P637Q was loaded on the beads (see input signals). Quantification revealed over 75% reduction of the FlnA-P637Q pulled down with respect to FlnA-WT (histogram on Figure 2).

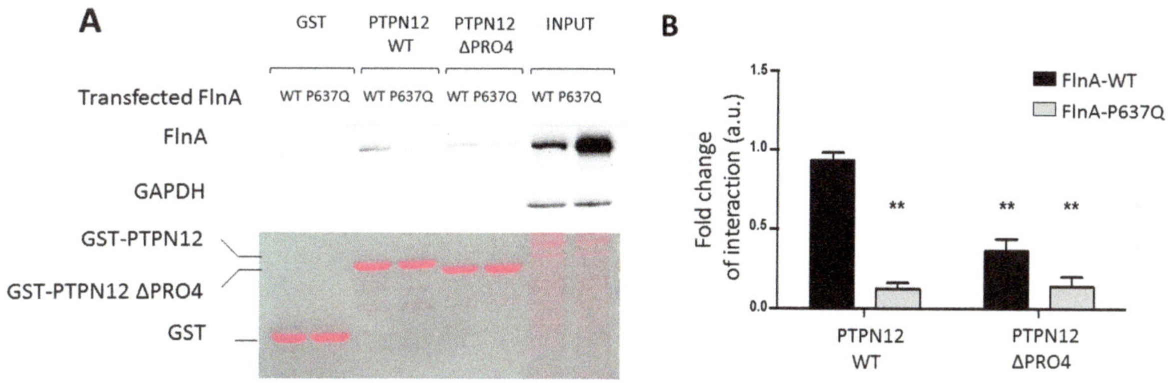

Figure 2. Effects of Filamin A mutations on FlnA/PTPN12 interaction. A) Pull-down assay. Equal amounts of GST, GST-PTPN12 or GST-PTPN12-ΔPro (lower image Red Ponceau coloration) were incubated with lysates of cells expressing FlnA-WT or FlnA-P637Q. Despite much larger expression of P637Q mutant in this experiment (input lanes), only FlnA-WT was readily detectable in GST-PTPN12 pulldown (lanes three and five). Deletion of the proline-rich domain of PTPN12 abolished PTPN12/FlnA interaction. Note the absence of detectable GAPDH contamination in the pulldown assays, which attests to low background and absence of unspecific binding in these experiments. B) Quantification from four similar experiments. ** indicates significant differences in the amount of retained FlnAs *vs.* FlnA-WT using GST-PTPN12 ($p < 0.01$, $n = 4$).

The interactions were then tested in a cellular context. Full-length HA-tagged PTPN12 was co-transfected with GFP-tagged-FlnA-WT, G288R or P637Q in Hek293 cells. As shown in Figure 3, both mutations significantly reduced by more than 60% ($p < 0.01$, $n = 4$) the FlnA co-immunoprecipitated with HA-PTPN12 using anti-HA antibody.

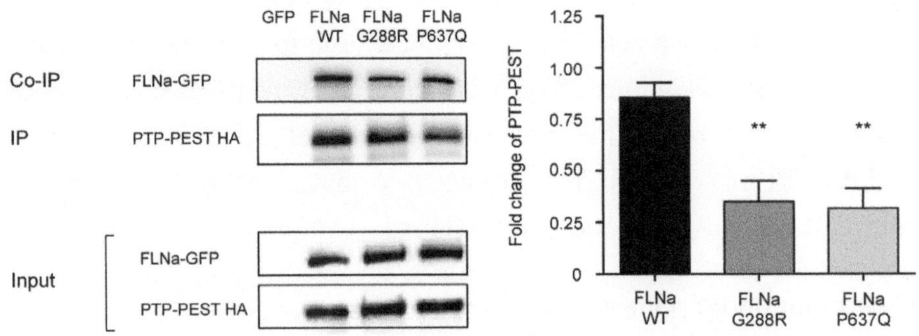

(A) (B)

Figure 3. Effects of Filamin A mutations on FlnA/PTPN12. (**A**) Co-immunoprecipitation assay. HA-tagged PTPN12 (HA-PTPN12) was co-transfected with GFP or GFP-tagged-FlnAs in Hek293 cells and immunoprecipitated using anti-HA antibody (IP). G288R and P637Q mutations significantly reduced the amount of FlnA co-IPed with PTPN12 (Co-IP) (lanes 3,4 upper blot). (**B**) Quantification of four similar experiments. ** indicates significant differences in the amount of co-immunoprecipitated FlnAs *vs.* FlnA-WT ($p < 0.01$, $n = 4$).

Together, these data are consistent with a model according to which FlnA repeats domain 1–8 constitute a structural element that interacts with the proline-rich region of PTPN12, and that the mutations G288R, P637Q, and potentially H743P, affect this molecular interface. We then analyzed the effects of FlnA mutations on the phosphorylation status of PTPN12 target substrates potentially affected in the physiopathological context of MVP.

3.3. PTPN12-FlnA Interactions Participate to p190RhoGAP and Src Regulation

In our previous studies we showed that the MVP-FlnA mutations tilt the RhoA/Rac1 GTPases balance toward increased RhoA activity and impede the cellular adhesion and migration capacities [24]. On the other hand, PTPN12 is known to regulate the tyrosine phosphorylation status and the activity of key actors of the RhoA GTPase pathway, extracellular matrix/cell interaction, cell adhesion, and migration signaling pathways, including the RhoA GTPase activating protein p190RhoGAP and the Src family kinase [20,29]. We, thus, investigated the impact of the FlnA mutations on these two actors. p190RhoGAP activity was tested in a set of pulldown experiments using the GST fused to activated RhoA as a bait (GST-RhoA-Q63L) to specifically isolate active RhoA-GAP regulators, including p190RhoGAP [30]. As shown in Figure 4A, and consistent with an increased cellular RhoA activity [24], a significantly lower amount of p190RhoGAP (40% decrease $p < 0.01$, $n = 4$) was isolated in FlnA-P637Q cells compared to FlnA-WT cells. On the other hand, the close inspection of cell morphologies during migration corroborated these results and suggested that FlnA-PTPN12 interaction might participate to PTPN12 targeting to specific subcellular domains. Indeed, as shown in Figure 4B, P637Q (and FlnA-G288R not shown) cells exhibited persistent and long trailing tails compared to FlnA-WT cells. Puzzling enough, this feature was reminiscent of the observation made by Sastry and colleagues according to which PTPN12 knock down fibroblasts also “develop long, thin tails in the rear” [29]. One can speculate that altered FlnA-PTPN12 interaction impairs PTPN12 targeting to the trailing tails of migrating cells and that locally impair p190RhoGAP tyrosine status, RhoA activity, and focal adhesion retraction.

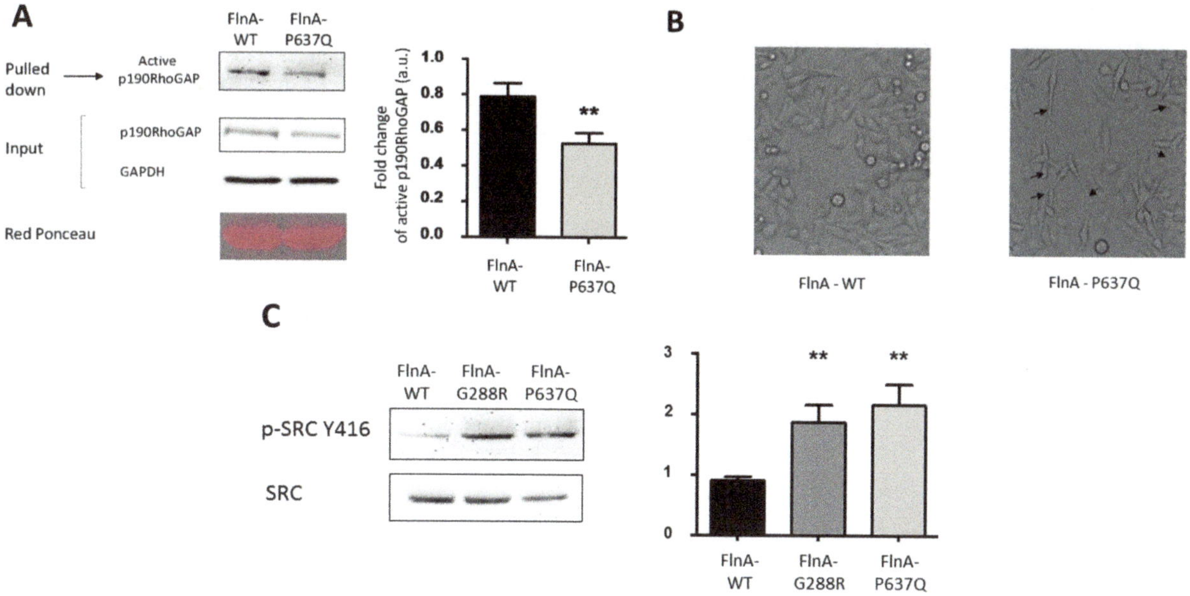

Figure 4. FlnA mutations increase p190RhoGAP activation and Src phosphorylation. (**A**) Active RhoA activating proteins were pulled down using GST-RhoA-Q63L constructs from melanoma cells expressing FlnA-WT or P637Q and the amount of p190RhoGAP retained, quantified by Western blotting. The upper blot shows less p190RhoGAP was retained from FlnA-P637Q cells. ** indicates significant differences in the amount of retained p190RhoGAP in FlnA-P637Q *vs.* FlnA-WT cells ($p < 0.01$, $n = 4$); (**B**) phase contrast images of migrating FlnA-WT and P637Q transfected melanoma cells. Note the long and persistent trailing tails observed in FlnA-P637Q cells (arrow heads); and (**C**) phosphorylation of tyrosine Y416 of Src (phospho-Src-Y416) was significantly increased in FlnA-G288R and P637Q transfected cells *vs.* FlnA-WT cells. ** indicates significant differences *vs.* FlnA-WT ($p < 0.01$, $n = 4$).

Phosphorylated tyrosine (Y416) of Src, which participates in focal adhesion maturation and signaling, is another known target of PTPN12 [31]. We, thus, analyzed Src phosphorylation status in mutant FlnA-expressing cells. As shown on Figure 4C, phosphorylated Src-Y146 levels detected in FlnA-G288R and P637Q cells using pSrc-Y416 antibody almost doubled compared to FlnA-WT expressing cells ($p < 0.01$, $n = 5$).

4. Discussion

The tyrosine phosphatase PTPN12/PTP-PEST was previously shown to interact with FlnA through one of its proline-rich domains but the counterpart binding domain on FlnA remained undefined [28]. Here, we have uncovered that the first eight repeats of FlnA constitute a binding site for PTPN12/PTP-PEST and showed that the FlnA mutations associated to mitral valve prolapse that specifically target this region disrupt PTPN12/FlnA interaction.

PTPN12 is a ubiquitously-expressed phosphatase which has been implicated in immune response and vascular development in part because of its roles in cell-ECM interaction, cell migration, and small GTPases signaling pathways. Considering the large crossover of these pathways with those in which FlnA also participates, it is inciting to speculate that the disruption of their interaction could have a role in the development of MVP in FlnA mutation carriers. The fact that the three mutations tested here all knock down FlnA/PTPN12 interaction suggests, in addition, that similar molecular and cellular mechanisms are at work in the pathology. This is also consistent with the strong homogeneity of the physio-pathological traits observed in the patients, including the poly-valvular damages, the echographic features of the mitral valve prolapse, the early onset of the disease, and the absence of any other symptom. Additionally, not surprising and consistent with the shared, but specific, phenotype, all the mutations target the same narrow region (Igl-1–8 repeats) localized between the two actin binding domains of FlnA [15].

Previous studies identified Ras GTPase, SyK tyrosine kinase, PKC epsilon, and vimentin as binding partners of FlnA N-terminal Igl domains [18,19,32]. However, we did not detect these binding partners in our experiments (not shown). On the other hand, we showed that FlnA-WT does interact with PTPN12, whereas FlnA-G288R, P637Q, and H743P mutations knocked down the PTPN12/FlnA interactions in our two-hybrid assay. In addition, we confirmed this loss of interaction for FlnA-P637Q in both GST pulldown assay and co-immunoprecipitation experiments. The detailed molecular mechanisms of FlnA/PTPN12 interaction remain to be unveiled, but yeast two-hybrid assays strongly suggest a direct interaction between the two partners. Obviously, because of the large crossover in the signaling pathways in which both FlnA and PTPN12 participate they also probably interact through long-range indirect interactions, in large signaling protein complexes. As far as "direct" interaction is concerned, it is tempting to speculate that it specifically involves the N-terminal region of FlnA. Indeed, on one hand, sequence-based classification of FlnA repeats indicated the Igl-4 (targeted by P637Q), and Igl-1 and 5 (targeted by G288R, V711D, and H743P mutations, respectively) belong to distinct repeat subgroups containing other repeats (e.g., subclass C contains Igl repeats one, two, three, and five, while subclass A contains Igl-4 in addition to Igl-9, 12, 17, 19, 21, 23) suggesting PTPN12 may bind other FlnA domains [33]. On the other hand, recent studies showed Igl-3–5 repeats constitute a peculiar three-domain interaction module whose structure is most probably impeded by the mutations. Glycine-288 (G288) is located in Igl-1 at the end of the first β-strand (the A strand) and is the first residue of a GPG motif that makes a helical turn in most Filamin Igl domains (e.g., Igl-16, 18, and 21). Interestingly, in three Filamin Igl domains where this motif is missing, the A-strand is not folded with the rest of the domain [34]. Thus, it is possible that the G288R mutation changes the conformation of Igl-1. Proline-637 (P637) and V711 are residues that point towards the hydrophobic core of Igl-4 and Igl-5, respectively. Substitution of these aliphatic residues with charged side chains in the P637Q and V711D mutations may change the stability of individual domains and also affect the function of the closely-interacting Igl-3–5 triplet [35,36]. Together, these clues suggest FlnA Igl-1–8 constitute a peculiar interaction domain on Filamin A and the major binding site of PTPN12. Future studies will be necessary to ascertain this hypothesis and determine whether the mutations affect the structure and/or mechanosensitivity of this interaction module.

PTP-PEST is a cytosolic ubiquitous protein tyrosine phosphatase (PTP) that contains, in addition to its catalytic domain, several protein-protein interaction domains that allow it to interface with several signaling pathways. Among others, PTP-PEST was shown to be recruited to the EFG receptor signaling complex [20]. However, previous studies essentially pointed to PTPN12 as a key regulator of cellular motility and cytoskeleton dynamics involved in immunity [21], cancer [20], and development [37]. PTPN12 invalidation is embryologically lethal in mice due to important vascular defects and un-successful liver formation [37]. In fact, PTPN12 is not required for endothelial cell differentiation and proliferation, nor the regulation of endothelial permeability, but is required for integrin-mediated adhesion and migration of endothelial cells [38]. This is in agreement with previous studies showing that PTPN12 substrates include the focal adhesion associated proteins Src kinase, p130Cas, and paxillin, as well as small GTPase regulators [22,29,39]. Importantly, FlnA is known to also be intimately associated with focal adhesion signaling pathway regulation and, indeed, we showed previously that MVP-FlnA mutations deregulate Rho/Rac1 balance and affect cellular spreading and migration resulting from an increased RhoA activity [24]. This is consistent with the lower activity of p190RhoGAP we detected in FlnA-P637Q-expressing cells in the present study. On the other hand, we also noticed that migrating mutant FlnA-expressing cells exhibited long trailing tails typically observed in PTPN12-depleted cells where p190RhoGAP activity is increased [29]. To reconcile these apparent discrepancies, one can speculate that FlnA/PTPN12 interaction participate to the targeting of PTPN12 to specific membrane domains and. thus. to the polarized GTPase regulation in migrating cells. as was recently demonstrated for the PTPN12/β8 integrin complex [22]. Consistent with this idea, such targeting properties to specific membrane domains were already ascribed to FlnA for one of its binding partner; FilGAP [40].

Interestingly, and coherent with the remarkable restriction of the FlnA mutations' associated defects to cardiac valves that are submitted to intense hemodynamic stresses, the mechanical stress may also modulate PTPN12/FlnA mutation. In fact, the local tension applied to the actin cytoskeleton was shown to modulate FlnA affinity for its binding partners FilGAP and β7 integrin [41,42]. Whether the mechanical stress also impacts the structure, the binding interface of Igl repeats (1–8) and FlnA/PTPN12 interactions remains to be elucidated [35,36].

5. Conclusions

In conclusion, we have identified here PTPN12 as a specific binding partner of the FlnA domain targeted by the MVP-associated FlnA mutations and showed the later impede FlnA/PTPN12 interaction. The key role of PTPN12 in the regulation of focal adhesion, ECM/cell crosstalk and cellular mechanical stress response signaling pathway make PTPN12 an interesting candidate involved in the physiological processes of FlnA-associated MVP.

Acknowledgments

We thank Steven Nedellec and Philippe Hulin for their technical expertise and assistance in the time lapse experiments that were performed at the core microscopic facility MicroPICell SFR Bonamy in Nantes. This work was funded by The Foundation Leducq, Transatlantic Mitral Network (grant 07CVD04, Paris, France), Clinical Research Hospital Program (PHRC) from the French Ministry of Health (PHRC-I RC12-0143 in 2012), the Fédération Française de Cardiologie, Grant R11065NN/ RAK1193NNA (TLT, JM) and the Fondation Coeur et Recherche (FCR PVM-Fed, Paris, France). T le Tourneau is supported by Inserm (Inserm Translational Research Program 2012–2016). The work at

MUSC was performed in a facility constructed with support from the National Institutes of Health, Grant Number C06 RR018823 from the Extramural Research Facilities Program of the National Center for Research Resources. Other funding sources: National Heart Lung and Blood Institute: R01-HL33756 (RRM), COBRE 1P30 GM103342 (RRM, RAN), 8P20 GM103444 (RRM and RAN); American Heart Association: 11SDG5270006 (RAN); National Science Foundation: EPS-0903795 (RRM); NHLBI K24 HL67434 and HL109506 (RAL).

Author Contributions

J.J.S. and J.M. conceived and designed the experiments; D.D., P.L., L.B., T.L.T. performed the experiments, D.D, P.L., L.B., T.L.T., R.A.N., R.R.M., R.L., J.J.S. and J.M. analyzed the data; J.M. wrote the paper.

Conflicts of Interest

The authors declare no conflict of interest.

References

1. Delling, F.N.; Rong, J.; Larson, M.G.; Lehman, B.; Osypiuk, E.; Stantchev, P.; Slaugenhaupt, S.A.; Benjamin, E.J.; Levine, R.A.; Vasan, R.S. Familial clustering of mitral valve prolapse in the community. *Circulation* **2015**, *131*, 263–268.
2. Lee, B.; Godfrey, M.; Vitale, E.; Hori, H.; Mattei, M.G.; Sarfarazi, M.; Tsipouras, P.; Ramirez, F.; Hollister, D.W. Linkage of marfan syndrome and a phenotypically related disorder to two different fibrillin genes. *Nature* **1991**, *352*, 330–334.
3. Singh, K.K.; Rommel, K.; Mishra, A.; Karck, M.; Haverich, A.; Schmidtke, J.; Arslan-Kirchner, M. TGFBR1 and TGFBR2 mutations in patients with features of marfan syndrome and loeys-dietz syndrome. *Hum. Mutat.* **2006**, *27*, 770–777.
4. Malfait, F.; Coucke, P.; Symoens, S.; Loeys, B.; Nuytinck, L.; De Paepe, A. The molecular basis of classic ehlers-danlos syndrome: A comprehensive study of biochemical and molecular findings in 48 unrelated patients. *Hum. Mutat.* **2005**, *25*, 28–37.
5. Kyndt, F.; Gueffet, J.P.; Probst, V.; Jaafar, P.; Legendre, A.; Le Bouffant, F.; Toquet, C.; Roy, E.; McGregor, L.; Lynch, S.A.; *et al.* Mutations in the gene encoding filamin a as a cause for familial cardiac valvular dystrophy. *Circulation* **2007**, *115*, 40–49.
6. Kyndt, F.; Schott, J.J.; Trochu, J.N.; Baranger, F.; Herbert, O.; Scott, V.; Fressinaud, E.; David, A.; Moisan, J.P.; Bouhour, J.B.; *et al.* Mapping of X-linked myxomatous valvular dystrophy to chromosome xq28. *Am. J. Hum. Genet.* **1998**, *62*, 627–632.
7. Holm, T.M.; Habashi, J.P.; Doyle, J.J.; Bedja, D.; Chen, Y.; van Erp, C.; Lindsay, M.E.; Kim, D.; Schoenhoff, F.; Cohn, R.D.; *et al.* Noncanonical TGFβ signaling contributes to aortic aneurysm progression in marfan syndrome mice. *Science* **2011**, *332*, 358–361.
8. Lacro, R.V.; Dietz, H.C.; Sleeper, L.A.; Yetman, A.T.; Bradley, T.J.; Colan, S.D.; Pearson, G.D.; Selamet Tierney, E.S.; Levine, J.C.; Atz, A.M.; *et al.* Atenolol versus losartan in children and young adults with marfan's syndrome. *N. Engl. J. Med.* **2014**, *371*, 2061–2071.

9. Robertson, S.P.; Jenkins, Z.A.; Morgan, T.; Ades, L.; Aftimos, S.; Boute, O.; Fiskerstrand, T.; Garcia-Minaur, S.; Grix, A.; Green, A.; *et al.* Frontometaphyseal dysplasia: Mutations in flna and phenotypic diversity. *Am. J. Med. Genet. A* **2006**, *140*, 1726–1736.
10. Sheen, V.L.; Dixon, P.H.; Fox, J.W.; Hong, S.E.; Kinton, L.; Sisodiya, S.M.; Duncan, J.S.; Dubeau, F.; Scheffer, I.E.; Schachter, S.C.; *et al.* Mutations in the X-linked filamin 1 gene cause periventricular nodular heterotopia in males as well as in females. *Hum. Mol. Genet.* **2001**, *10*, 1775–1783.
11. Norris, R.A.; Moreno-Rodriguez, R.; Wessels, A.; Merot, J.; Bruneval, P.; Chester, A.H.; Yacoub, M.H.; Hagege, A.; Slaugenhaupt, S.A.; Aikawa, E.; *et al.* Expression of the familial cardiac valvular dystrophy gene, filamin-a, during heart morphogenesis. *Dev. Dyn.* **2010**, *239*, 2118–2127.
12. Sauls, K.; de Vlaming, A.; Harris, B.S.; Williams, K.; Wessels, A.; Levine, R.A.; Slaugenhaupt, S.A.; Goodwin, R.L.; Pavone, L.M.; Merot, J.; *et al.* Developmental basis for filamin-a-associated myxomatous mitral valve disease. *Cardiovasc. Res.* **2012**, *96*, 109–119.
13. Stossel, T.P.; Condeelis, J.; Cooley, L.; Hartwig, J.H.; Noegel, A.; Schleicher, M.; Shapiro, S.S. Filamins as integrators of cell mechanics and signalling. *Nat. Rev. Mol. Cell. Biol.* **2001**, *2*, 138–145.
14. Feng, Y.; Walsh, C.A. The many faces of filamin: A versatile molecular scaffold for cell motility and signalling. *Nat. Cell. Biol.* **2004**, *6*, 1034–1038.
15. Nakamura, F.; Osborn, T.M.; Hartemink, C.A.; Hartwig, J.H.; Stossel, T.P. Structural basis of filamin a functions. *J. Cell. Biol.* **2007**, *179*, 1011–1025.
16. Nakamura, F.; Stossel, T.P.; Hartwig, J.H. The filamins: Organizers of cell structure and function. *Cell. Adh. Migr.* **2011**, *5*, 160–169.
17. Zhou, A.X.; Hartwig, J.H.; Akyurek, L.M. Filamins in cell signaling, transcription and organ development. *Trends Cell. Biol.* **2010**, *20*, 113–123.
18. Gawecka, J.E.; Griffiths, G.S.; Ek-Rylander, B.; Ramos, J.W.; Matter, M.L. R-ras regulates migration through an interaction with filamin a in melanoma cells. *PLoS ONE* **2010**, *5*, e11269.
19. Kim, H.; Nakamura, F.; Lee, W.; Hong, C.; Perez-Sala, D.; McCulloch, C.A. Regulation of cell adhesion to collagen via β1 integrins is dependent on interactions of filamin a with vimentin and protein kinase c epsilon. *Exp. Cell Res.* **2010**, *316*, 1829–1844.
20. Zheng, Y.; Lu, Z. Regulation of tumor cell migration by protein tyrosine phosphatase (PTP)-proline-, glutamate-, serine-,and threonine-rich sequence (PEST). *Chin. J. Cancer* **2013**, *32*, 75–83.
21. Rhee, I.; Zhong, M.C.; Reizis, B.; Cheong, C.; Veillette, A. Control of dendritic cell migration, t cell-dependent immunity, and autoimmunity by protein tyrosine phosphatase ptpn12 expressed in dendritic cells. *Mol. Cell. Biol.* **2014**, *34*, 888–899.
22. Lee, H.S.; Cheerathodi, M.; Chaki, S.P.; Reyes, S.B.; Zheng, Y.; Lu, Z.; DerMardirossian, C.; Lacy-Hulbert, A.; Rivera, G.M.; McCarty, J.H. Ptp-pest and β8 integrin control spatiotemporal patterns of rhogdi1 activation in migrating cells. *Mol. Cell. Biol.* **2015**, *35*, 1401–1413.
23. Boudin, H.; Doan, A.; Xia, J.; Shigemoto, R.; Huganir, R.L.; Worley, P.; Craig, A.M. Presynaptic clustering of mglur7a requires the pick1 pdz domain binding site. *Neuron* **2000**, *28*, 485–497.
24. Duval, D.; Lardeux, A.; Le Tourneau, T.; Norris, R.A.; Markwald, R.R.; Sauzeau, V.; Probst, V.; Le Marec, H.; Levine, R.; Schott, J.J.; *et al.* Valvular dystrophy associated filamin a mutations reveal a new role of its first repeats in small-gtpase regulation. *Biochim. Biophys. Acta* **2014**, *1843*, 234–244.

25. Fromont-Racine, M.; Rain, J.C.; Legrain, P. Toward a functional analysis of the yeast genome through exhaustive two-hybrid screens. *Nature Genet.* **1997**, *16*, 277–282.
26. Formstecher, E.; Aresta, S.; Collura, V.; Hamburger, A.; Meil, A.; Trehin, A.; Reverdy, C.; Betin, V.; Maire, S.; Brun, C.; *et al.* Protein interaction mapping: A drosophila case study. *Genome Res.* **2005**, *15*, 376–384.
27. Nakamura, F.; Heikkinen, O.; Pentikainen, O.T.; Osborn, T.M.; Kasza, K.E.; Weitz, D.A.; Kupiainen, O.; Permi, P.; Kilpelainen, I.; Ylanne, J.; *et al.* Molecular basis of filamin a-filgap interaction and its impairment in congenital disorders associated with filamin a mutations. *PLoS ONE* **2009**, *4*, e4928.
28. Playford, M.P.; Lyons, P.D.; Sastry, S.K.; Schaller, M.D. Identification of a filamin docking site on ptp-pest. *J. Biol. Chem.* **2006**, *281*, 34104–34112.
29. Sastry, S.K.; Rajfur, Z.; Liu, B.P.; Cote, J.F.; Tremblay, M.L.; Burridge, K. Ptp-pest couples membrane protrusion and tail retraction via VAV2 and p190RhoGAP. *J. Biol. Chem.* **2006**, *281*, 11627–11636.
30. Guilluy, C.; Dubash, A.D.; Garcia-Mata, R. Analysis of rhoa and rho gef activity in whole cells and the cell nucleus. *Nat. Protoc.* **2011**, *6*, 2050–2060.
31. Zheng, Y.; Yang, W.; Xia, Y.; Hawke, D.; Liu, D.X.; Lu, Z. Ras-induced and extracellular signal-regulated kinase 1 and 2 phosphorylation-dependent isomerization of protein tyrosine phosphatase (ptp)-pest by pin1 promotes fak dephosphorylation by ptp-pest. *Mol. Cell. Biol.* **2011**, *31*, 4258–4269.
32. Falet, H.; Pollitt, A.Y.; Begonja, A.J.; Weber, S.E.; Duerschmied, D.; Wagner, D.D.; Watson, S.P.; Hartwig, J.H. A novel interaction between flna and syk regulates platelet itam-mediated receptor signaling and function. *J. Exp. Med.* **2010**, *207*, 1967–1979.
33. Ithychanda, S.S.; Hsu, D.; Li, H.; Yan, L.; Liu, D.D.; Das, M.; Plow, E.F.; Qin, J. Identification and characterization of multiple similar ligand-binding repeats in filamin: Implication on filamin-mediated receptor clustering and cross-talk. *J. Biol. Chem.* **2009**, *284*, 35113–35121.
34. Heikkinen, O.K.; Ruskamo, S.; Konarev, P.V.; Svergun, D.I.; Iivanainen, T.; Heikkinen, S.M.; Permi, P.; Koskela, H.; Kilpelainen, I.; Ylanne, J. Atomic structures of two novel immunoglobulin-like domain pairs in the actin cross-linking protein filamin. *J. Biol. Chem.* **2009**, *284*, 25450–25458.
35. Sethi, R.; Ylanne, J. Small-angle x-ray scattering reveals compact domain-domain interactions in the N-terminal region of filamin c. *PLoS ONE* **2014**, *9*, e107457.
36. Sethi, R.; Seppala, J.; Tossavainen, H.; Ylilauri, M.; Ruskamo, S.; Pentikainen, O.T.; Pentikainen, U.; Permi, P.; Ylanne, J. A novel structural unit in the N-terminal region of filamins. *J. Biol. Chem.* **2014**, *289*, 8588–8598.
37. Sirois, J.; Cote, J.F.; Charest, A.; Uetani, N.; Bourdeau, A.; Duncan, S.A.; Daniels, E.; Tremblay, M.L. Essential function of ptp-pest during mouse embryonic vascularization, mesenchyme formation, neurogenesis and early liver development. *Mech. Dev.* **2006**, *123*, 869–880.
38. Souza, C.M.; Davidson, D.; Rhee, I.; Gratton, J.P.; Davis, E.C.; Veillette, A. The phosphatase ptp-pest/ptpn12 regulates endothelial cell migration and adhesion, but not permeability, and controls vascular development and embryonic viability. *J. Biol. Chem.* **2012**, *287*, 43180–43190.

39. Angers-Loustau, A.; Cote, J.F.; Charest, A.; Dowbenko, D.; Spencer, S.; Lasky, L.A.; Tremblay, M.L. Protein tyrosine phosphatase-pest regulates focal adhesion disassembly, migration, and cytokinesis in fibroblasts. *J. Cell. Biol.* **1999**, *144*, 1019–1031.
40. Ohta, Y.; Hartwig, J.H.; Stossel, T.P. Filgap, a rho- and rock-regulated gap for rac binds filamin a to control actin remodelling. *Nat. Cell. Biol.* **2006**, *8*, 803–814.
41. Ehrlicher, A.J.; Nakamura, F.; Hartwig, J.H.; Weitz, D.A.; Stossel, T.P. Mechanical strain in actin networks regulates filgap and integrin binding to filamin A. *Nature* **2011**, *478*, 260–263.
42. Razinia, Z.; Makela, T.; Ylanne, J.; Calderwood, D.A. Filamins in mechanosensing and signaling. *Annu. Rev. Biophys.* **2012**, *41*, 227–246.

16

Evidence of Aortopathy in Mice with Haploinsufficiency of *Notch1* in *Nos3*-Null Background

Sara N. Koenig [1,2], Kevin M. Bosse [1], Holly A. Nadorlik [1,2], Brenda Lilly [1,2] and Vidu Garg [1,2,3,*]

1 The Center for Cardiovascular and Pulmonary Research and Heart Center, Nationwide Children's Hospital, 700 Children's Drive, Columbus, OH 43205, USA;
E-Mails: Sara.Koenig@nationwidechildrens.org (S.N.K.); Kevin.Bosse@nationwidechildrens.org (K.M.B.); Holly.Nadorlik@nationwidechildrens.org (H.A.N.); Brenda.Lilly@nationwidechildrens.org (B.L.)

2 Department of Pediatrics, The Ohio State University, 700 Children's Drive, Columbus, OH 43205, USA

3 Department of Molecular Genetics, The Ohio State University, 484 West 12th Avenue, Columbus, OH 43210, USA

* Author to whom correspondence should be addressed
E-Mail: Vidu.Garg@nationwidechildrens.org

Academic Editor: Christine B. Kern

Abstract: Thoracic aortic aneurysms (TAA) are a significant cause of morbidity and mortality in humans. While the exact etiology is unknown, genetic factors play an important role. Mutations in *NOTCH1* have been linked to bicuspid aortic valve (BAV) and aortopathy in humans. The aim of this study was to determine if haploinsufficiency of *Notch1* contributes to aortopathy using *Notch1*$^{+/-}$; *Nos3*$^{-/-}$ mice. Echocardiographic analysis of *Notch1*$^{+/-}$; *Nos3*$^{-/-}$ mice reveals effacement of the sinotubular junction and a trend toward dilation of the aortic sinus. Furthermore, examination of the proximal aorta of *Notch1*$^{+/-}$; *Nos3*$^{-/-}$ mice reveals elastic fiber degradation, a trend toward increased matrix metalloproteinase 2 expression, and increased smooth muscle cell apoptosis, features characteristic of aneurysmal disease. Although at a lower penetrance, we also found features consistent with aortopathic changes in *Notch1* heterozygote mice and in *Nos3*-null mice. Our findings implicate a novel role for Notch1 in aortopathy of the proximal aorta.

Keywords: ascending aortic dilation; Notch; endothelial nitric oxide; sinotubular junction effacement; smooth muscle cell lineage

1. Introduction

Dissection and rupture of thoracic aortic aneurysms has an incidence of approximately 7 in 100,000 people per year [1]. Thoracic aortic aneurysms (TAA) are often asymptomatic, leading to the high rate of dissection and rupture. Aortic aneurysms are defined as dilation of the aorta to 50% greater than its normal. Histological examination of an aneurysmal aorta demonstrates vascular smooth muscle cell apoptosis and disorganization of the extracellular matrix (ECM) with increased collagen deposition, elastin degradation and increased levels of matrix metalloproteinases.

Aneurysms of the thoracic aorta can occur in the following four main locations—aortic root, ascending, transverse, and descending aorta (Figure 1). Aneurysms of the aortic root can be further localized to the aortic annulus, sinuses of Valsava and the sinotubular junction (STJ) (Figure 1). The clinical phenotype of TAA in genetic syndromes suggests that aneurysms located at varying sites of the thoracic aorta may have different etiologic mechanisms [2], and this may be dictated by contributing embryonic cell lineages (Figure 1). Aneurysms involving the sinuses of Valsava and the STJ are typical for patients with Marfan syndrome [3], who harbor mutations in *FIBRILLIN1* [4–7], and in individuals with familial mutations in *ACTA2* [8] and *MYH11* [9]. While in Fabry disease (α Galactosidase A deficiency), patients present with aortic dilation of the sinuses of Valsava and/or the ascending aorta [10]. Individuals with vascular Ehlers-Danlos syndrome [11] (*COL3A1*) and Loeys-Dietz syndrome (mutations in *TGFBR1*, *TGFBR2*, and *SMAD3*) [12] present with aneurysms throughout the thoracic aorta. Patients with non-syndromic bicuspid aortic valve (BAV) [13,14] usually have aneurysms of the ascending aorta and uncommonly, will have dilation of the aortic annulus, sinuses of Valsava and STJ [15,16]. In BAV that is associated with Turner syndrome, aneurysms are consistently found in the sinuses, STJ and ascending aorta [17–19].

Mutations in *NOTCH1* were first reported in familial BAV and calcific aortic valve disease, and interestingly, a subset of these patients also had dilation of the ascending aorta [20], which is referred to as bicuspid aortopathy [15]. Bicuspid aortopathy is associated with histological changes similar to those observed with TAA [15]. NOTCH1 encodes a transmembrane receptor that signals through cell-cell contact and is essential for cardiovascular development [21]. Notch1 is critical for normal vascular development, as homozygote knock-out mice die at embryonic day 10.5 due to vascular endothelial defects [22,23]. Notch1 is also expressed throughout the cardiac outflow tract and has been shown to be required for proper valve development [20,24,25]. Alterations in Notch1 signaling have been reported in BAV patients with TAA [26–28]; however, the role of Notch1 signaling in TAAs of patients with tricuspid aortic valves is unclear [29].

We recently reported a new highly penetrant mouse model for BAV by backcrossing $Notch1^{+/-}$ into an endothelial nitric oxide synthase (*Nos3)*-null background [30]. The development of ascending aortic dilation has not been investigated in this murine model of BAV. Here, we show that $Notch1^{+/-}$; $Nos3^{-/-}$ adult mice develop aortic dilation specifically with early effacement of the STJ, defined as a loss of a distinct border between the aortic sinus and proximal ascending aorta. This dilation is accompanied by histologic features of aortic aneurysms, including elastic fiber degeneration and an increase in apoptosis and a trend toward increased matrix metalloproteinase 2 (MMP2) expression in aortic smooth muscle cells. Furthermore, we find that the aortic root dilation is independent of hemodynamically significant aortic valve disease consistent with an embryologic origin for BAV-associated aortopathy. Additionally, we have found some features consistent with aortopathy in both *Nos3*$^{-/-}$ and *Notch1*$^{+/-}$ mice. *Nos3*$^{-/-}$ mice display effacement of STJ, albeit at a significantly lower frequency than *Notch1*$^{+/-}$; *Nos3*$^{-/-}$ mice. Alternatively, histological and molecular abnormalities exist within the aorta of *Notch1*$^{+/-}$ mice, including irregular elastin fibers. These data suggest that Notch1 signaling plays a role in the development of aortopathic changes in the ascending aorta.

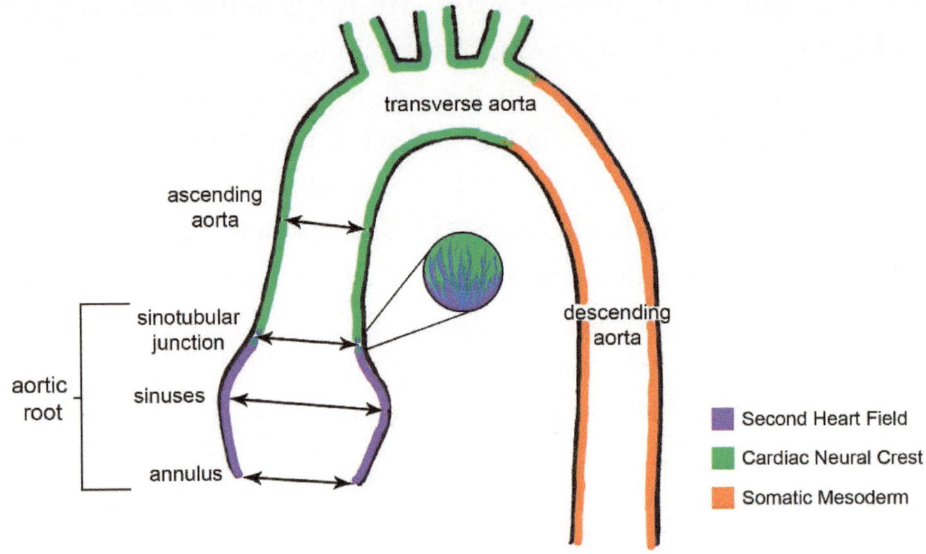

Figure 1. Cell lineages that contribute to the smooth muscle cells lining the ascending, transverse and descending regions of thoracic aorta are shown in schematic [31–34]. Location of echocardiographic measurements of annulus, sinus, and sinotubular junction, and ascending aorta are also shown.

2. Experimental Section

2.1. Mice

All experiments were approved by the Institutional Animal Care and Use Committee at the Research Institute at Nationwide Children's Hospital. *Nos3*$^{-/-}$ and *Notch1*$^{+/-}$ mice were genotyped as originally described [22,35]. *Nos3*$^{-/-}$ mice were bred to *Nos3*$^{-/-}$*; Notch1*$^{+/-}$ mice to obtain wildtype, *Notch1*$^{+/-}$, *Nos3*$^{-/-}$, and *Notch1*$^{+/-}$; *Nos3*$^{-/-}$ littermates.

2.2. Echocardiography

Transthoracic echocardiography was performed using a VEVO 2100 Ultrasound System as previously described [30]. Briefly, mice were sedated briefly with 3% isoflurane, and then titrated to 1%–2% isoflurane to maintain heart rate between 400 and 500 beats per minute. Aortic diameters were measured from parasternal long axis B-mode images (Figure 2) during systole at designated locations (Figure 1). Aortic flow velocity was measured with pulse-wave Doppler across the aortic valve. STJ angle was measured using the STJ as the vertex with arms extending to the sinus and ascending aorta. The greatest angle of the left or right side was chosen. All data points are an average of three measurements.

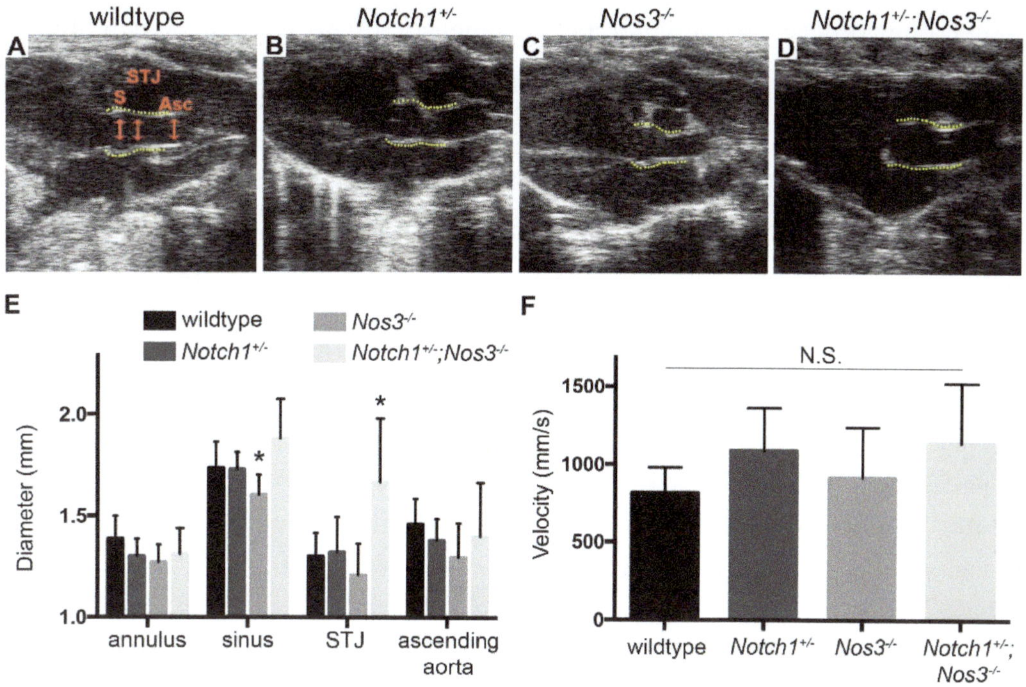

Figure 2. Loss of sinotubular junction in *Notch1*$^{+/-}$; *Nos3*$^{-/-}$ mice. Representative echocardiographic images of ascending aorta at 3 months of age are shown in (**A**–**D**); S, sinus; STJ, sinotubular junction; Asc, ascending aorta. The aortic annulus, aortic sinus, STJ, and ascending aorta are outlined in yellow; (**E**) Aortic diameters at 6 months of age showing a trend of aortic sinus dilation and a significant increase in diameter of STJ in *Notch1*$^{+/-}$; *Nos3*$^{-/-}$ mice compared to wildtype, *Notch1*$^{+/-}$, and *Nos3*$^{-/-}$ mice. * *p*-value < 0.05 (**F**) Velocity (mean and standard deviation) across aortic valve at 6 months of age for each genotype is shown. No evidence of stenosis (defined as velocity > 2000 mm/s) was noted.

2.3. Tissue Fixation and Histology

Experimental animals were euthanized and mouse hearts were perfused in a consistent manner with 1 mL of 10% formalin using a 5 mL syringe into the left ventricle. Serial sections were stained with hematoxylin and eosin, elastin stain kit (Sigma HT25A), Masson's trichrome, and immunohistochemistry (Santa Cruz ImmunoCruz sc-2018 or Cell Signaling 8114, 8125, 8112, and 8059) with primary antibodies against MMP2 (Abcam, ab37150, 1:500), Caspase-3 (Cell Signaling, 9661, 1:300), activated Notch1 (abcam, ab8925, 1:500), and α-Smooth Muscle Actin (Sigma Aldrich, A2547, 1:500). Integrated density was determined using the IHC Toolbox plugin for ImageJ [36].

2.4. Elastin Quantification and Basic Morphometrics

Images of elastin stained tissue sections were measured (3 images per animal), and measurements were repeated 5 times in different areas of each image. (n = 3 wildtype, 3 *Notch1*$^{+/-}$, 3 *Nos3*$^{-/-}$, and 4 *Notch1*$^{+/-}$; *Nos3*$^{-/-}$ mice). Gross images of the aorta were measured at the aortic root, ascending aorta, aortic arch, and descending aorta (n = 4 per genotype). All measurements were made in a blinded fashion in regards to the genotype.

2.5. TGF-β1 ELISA

Blood was collected from the left ventricle prior to perfusion fixation at the time of euthanasia, and platelet-poor plasma was isolated from the blood. The ELISA kit was purchased from R&D systems (MB100B). TGF-β1 was activated in plasma (according to instructions) prior to assay.

2.6. Statistics

Statistical analysis was performed using Student's t-tests and one-way ANOVA for echocardiographic and gross diameter measurements and basic morphometrics, and Fisher's exact test for incidence of STJ effacement. Statistical significance was determined based on a p-value < 0.05.

3. Results and Discussion

3.1. Effacement of Sinotubular Junction and Aortic Root Dilation in Notch1$^{+/-}$*; Nos3*$^{-/-}$ *Mice*

In order to determine if *Notch1*$^{+/-}$; *Nos3*$^{-/-}$ mice develop aneurysms of the ascending aorta, we bred *Nos3*$^{-/-}$ mice to *Nos3*$^{-/-}$; *Notch1*$^{+/-}$ compound heterozygotes to obtain wildtype, *Notch1*$^{+/-}$, *Nos3*$^{-/-}$ and *Notch1*$^{+/-}$; *Nos3*$^{-/-}$ littermates. As expected, Notch1 expression was decreased in *Notch1*$^{+/-}$ and *Notch1*$^{+/-}$; *Nos3*$^{-/-}$ mice by immunohistochemistry (Supplemental Figure 1). Echocardiographic measurement of the ascending aorta of *Notch1*$^{+/-}$; *Nos3*$^{-/-}$ mice at 3 months of age revealed effacement of the STJ in 5 out 5 animals (100%) (Table 1, Figure 2D). Interestingly, effacement of the STJ was also seen in a subset of *Notch1*$^{+/-}$ and *Nos3*$^{-/-}$ mice but at a statistically significant lower frequency (Table 1, Figure 2). At this time point, there was no difference in mean aortic diameter between genotypes [37]. Follow up echocardiographic examination at 6 months of age demonstrated a similar frequency of STJ effacement (Table 1, Supplementary Figure 2) except for one additional *Nos3*$^{-/-}$ mouse had developed STJ effacement. Consistent with this, the aortic sinus-ascending aortic angle was increased in *Notch1*$^{+/-}$; *Nos3*$^{-/-}$ mice at 6 months of age (Supplementary Figure 2Q). At 6 months, the diameter of the STJ was significantly higher in *Notch1*$^{+/-}$; *Nos3*$^{-/-}$ mice than controls (Figure 2E). The aortic sinus significantly larger in the *Notch1*$^{+/-}$; *Nos3*$^{-/-}$ mice than the *Nos3*$^{-/-}$ mice (p value = 0.0016), but this trend was not statistically significant in wildtype or *Notch1*$^{+/-}$ mice (p value > 0.1). The velocity across the aortic valve was not statistically different among all four genotypes (Figure 2F).

Table 1. Effacement of Sinotubular Junction by Genotype. Fraction of mice with STJ effacement is shown at 3 and 6 months of age, * p value <0.05.

	Wildtype	*Notch1*$^{+/-}$	*Nos3*$^{-/-}$	*Notch1*$^{+/-}$; *Nos3*$^{-/-}$
3 months	0/8 (0%)	1/8 (12.5%)	3/11 (27.3%)	5/5 (100%) *
6 months	0/8 (0%)	1/8 (12.5%)	4/11 (36.4%)	5/5 (100%) *

3.2. *Notch1*$^{+/-}$; *Nos3*$^{-/-}$ *Mice Display Gross and Histologic Evidence of Aortopathy*

Gross examination of the proximal ascending aorta at 8 months of age demonstrated a trend toward dilation of the aortic root (mean diameter = 2.03 ± 0.121 mm) in *Notch1*$^{+/-}$; *Nos3*$^{-/-}$ mice (Figure 3A–E), but this was not statistically significant when compared to littermate controls. Measurements did reveal one out of four *Notch1*$^{+/-}$ mice with a grossly dilated aortic root (2.7 mm in diameter). Histologic examination of the aorta in all four genotypes was performed (Figure 3F–M). It demonstrated aortic wall abnormalities reminiscent of medial degeneration (as reviewed in [38]) in *Notch1*$^{+/-}$; *Nos3*$^{-/-}$ mice, indicated by increased "empty" space between cells presumably where smooth muscle cell loss has occurred (Figure 3M, arrowheads). This phenotype was not observed in wildtype, *Nos3*$^{-/-}$, and *Notch1*$^{+/-}$ littermates. In addition, we observed diffuse elastin staining in the aorta of *Notch1*$^{+/-}$ mice similar to the *Notch1*$^{+/-}$; *Nos3*$^{-/-}$ murine aortas. Additionally, *Notch1*$^{+/-}$; *Nos3*$^{-/-}$ mice had elastic fiber degradation, identified by an overall disorganization of the layers (Figure 3Q). The elastin fibers were normal in *Nos3*$^{-/-}$ and wildtype littermates (Figure 3N–Q).

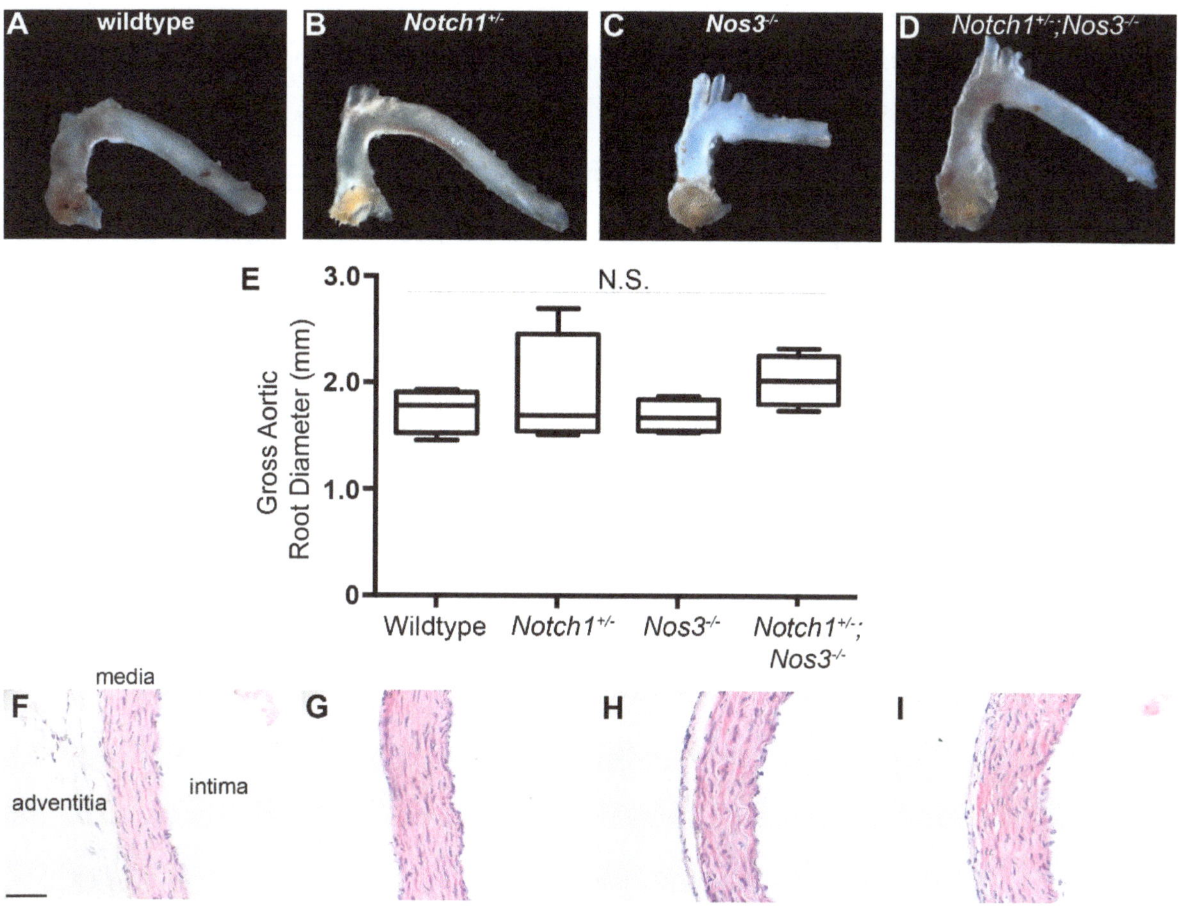

Figure 3. *Cont.*

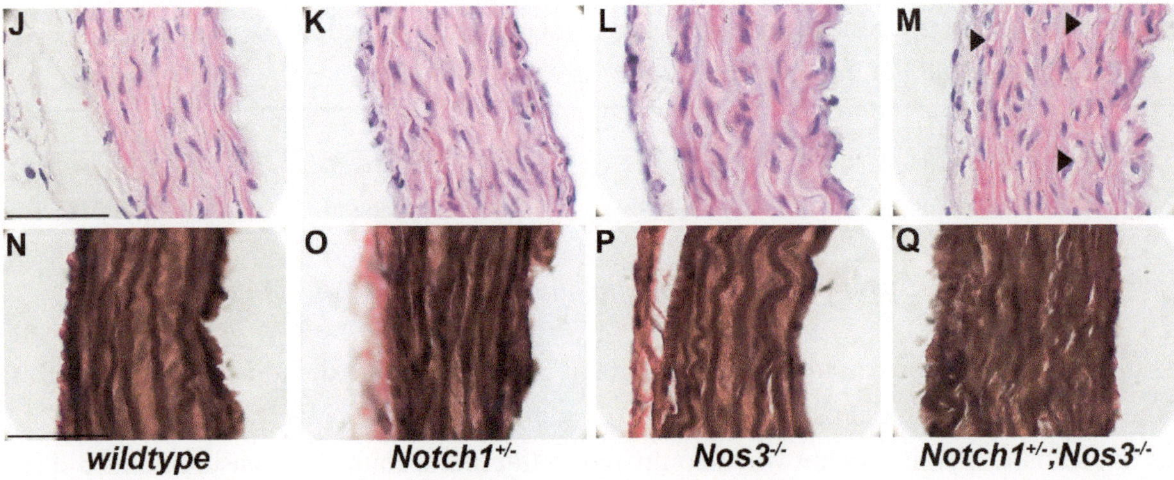

Figure 3. Dilation of proximal ascending aorta in *Notch1*$^{+/-}$; *Nos3*$^{-/-}$ mice. Representative gross images of thoracic aorta at 8 months are shown in (**A–D**); (**E**) Quantification of gross aortic root diameter showing a trend for dilation in *Notch1*$^{+/-}$; *Nos3*$^{-/-}$ mice ($n = 4$ per genotype); N.S., not significant; (**F–M**) Hematoxylin and eosin stained aortic sections at 400x and 1000x, respectively (**F–I**, **J–M**), showing areas of presumed SMC loss in *Notch1*$^{+/-}$; *Nos3*$^{-/-}$ (**M**, arrowheads). (**N–Q**) Representative images of elastin stained aortic cross sections at 1000x, illustrating degraded elastin in the *Notch1*$^{+/-}$ and *Notch1*$^{+/-}$; *Nos3*$^{-/-}$ mice. Scale bar equals 50 microns.

Although evidence of elastin disorganization was observed, there were no quantifiable differences between genotypes in total aorta thickness, medial thickness, elastic layer thickness, distance between elastic layers, and number of elastic layers (Figure 4).

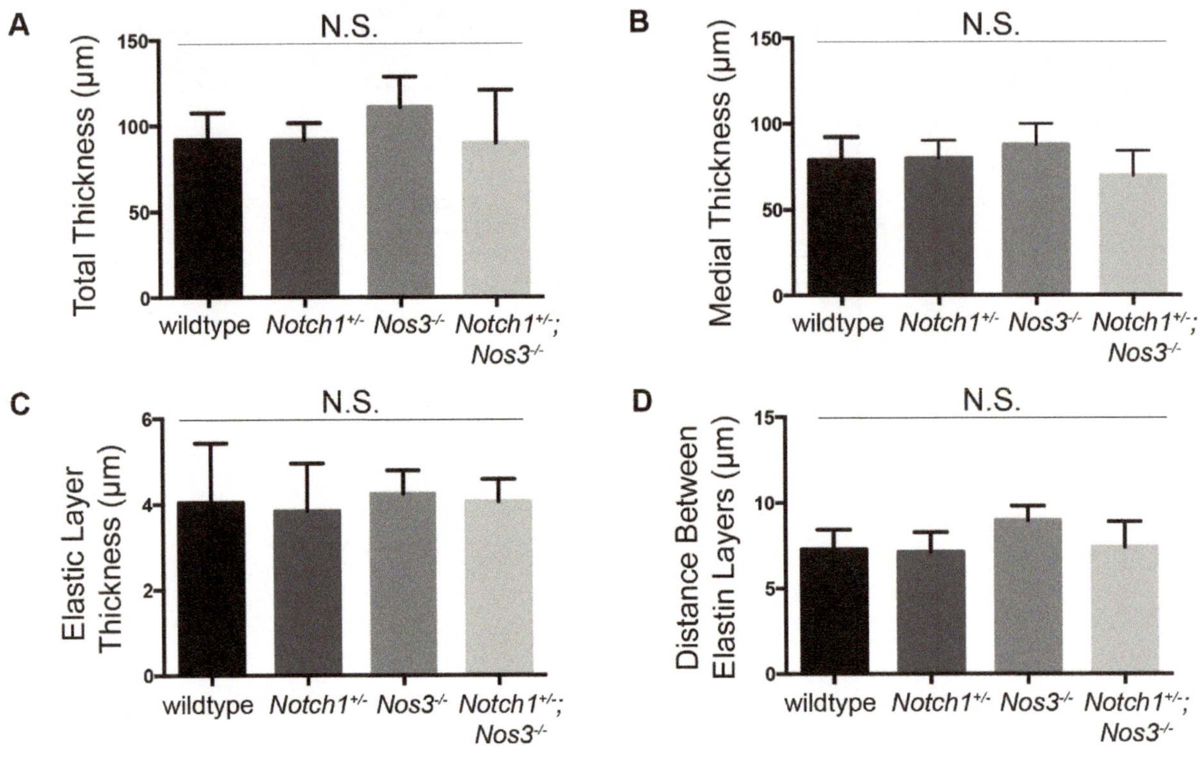

Figure 4. *Cont.*

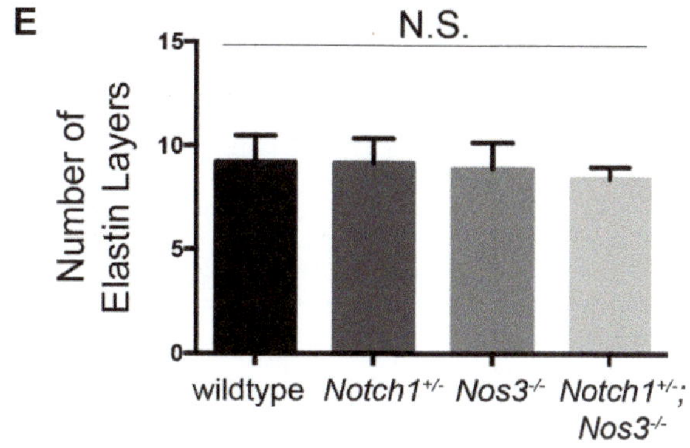

Figure 4. No difference in basic morphometrics of the aortic wall in *Notch1*$^{+/-}$; *Nos3*$^{-/-}$ mice as compared to littermate controls. Quantification of total aortic wall thickness (**A**); medial thickness (**B**); elastic layer thickness (**C**); distance between elastic layers (**D**); and number of elastin layers (**E**). N.S., not statistically significant. N = 3 per for each genotype.

3.3. Notch1$^{+/-}$*; Nos3*$^{-/-}$ *Aortas Display Molecular Evidence of Aortopathy*

To determine if the dilated aorta in *Notch1*$^{+/-}$; *Nos3*$^{-/-}$ mice displayed evidence of ECM degradation, we examined the expression of MMP2, an MMP (matrix metalloproteinase) that is commonly overexpressed in aneurysms [39]. In the aorta, MMP2 expression was found to be increased in *Notch1*$^{+/-}$; *Nos3*$^{-/-}$, and the *Notch1*$^{+/-}$; *Nos3*$^{-/-}$ aortas in comparison to wildtype littermates although it did not reach statistical significance (Figure 5A–D). Another characteristic of aortopathy is smooth muscle cell apoptosis, and therefore, we examined the levels of caspase-3. In the ascending aorta of *Notch1*$^{+/-}$; *Nos3*$^{-/-}$ mice, we found increased expression levels of caspase-3 in comparison to littermates (Figure 5E–H).

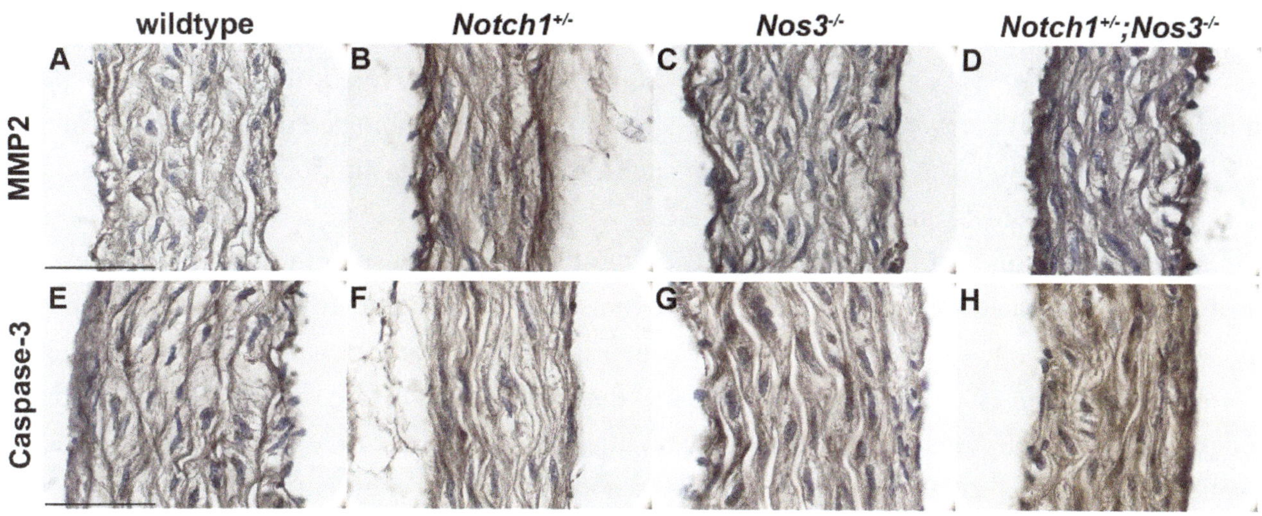

Figure 5. *Cont.*

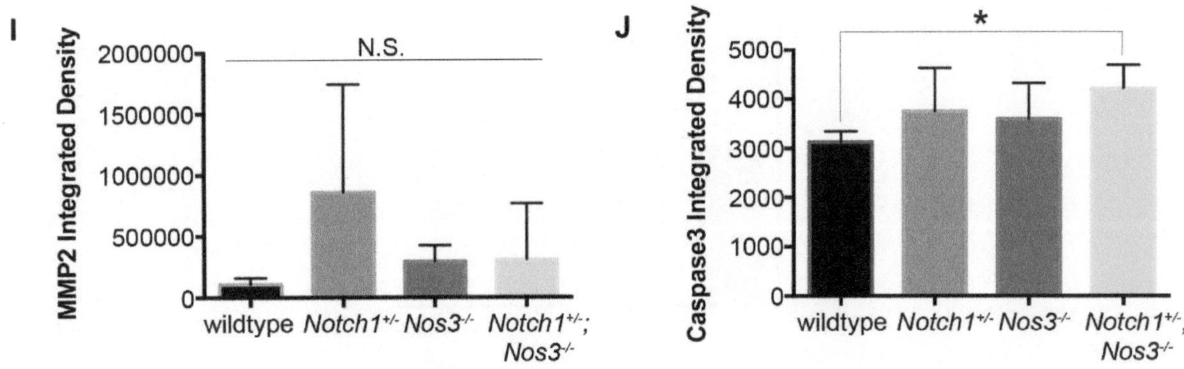

Figure 5. Immunohistochemical evidence of aortopathy in *Notch1*$^{+/-}$; *Nos3*$^{-/-}$ mice. MMP2 protein expression is increased in *Notch1*$^{+/-}$; *Nos3*$^{-/-}$, *Nos3*$^{-/-}$, and *Notch1*$^{+/-}$ in comparison to wildtype (**A–D**, **I**). Caspase-3 protein expression is increased in *Notch1*$^{+/-}$; *Nos3*$^{-/-}$ in comparison to littermates, * p value < 0.05 (**E–H**, **J**). Scale bar equals 50 microns.

3.4. Significance

Thoracic aortic aneurysms are a significant cause of morbidity and mortality in adults, and are particularly prevalent in the BAV population. There is substantial interest in discerning the hemodynamic and genetic influences in aortic aneurysm development in these patients. In this study, we have identified a specific mouse model (*Notch1*$^{+/-}$; *Nos3*$^{-/-}$) which develops dilation of the aortic sinus and effacement of the STJ, characteristics which are proposed to have genetic origins in humans [15]. STJ effacement is usually not an isolated clinical phenomenon, and it is possible that significant aortic dilation would be observed if these mice were further aged. We have also, for the first time, described pathologic changes suggestive of an ascending aortopathy in a subset of *Notch1* heterozygote and *Nos3*-null mice, with effacement of the STJ and a trend toward increased MMP2 expression, although no evidence of dilation was observed in either *Notch1*$^{+/-}$ mice and *Nos3*$^{-/-}$ at 6 months of age. Overall, these findings suggest inherent defects in the aorta of *Notch1*$^{+/-}$ and *Nos3*$^{-/-}$ mice which when combined result in dilation of the aortic root, characterized by classic signs of aneurysm such as medial and elastic fiber degradation and an increased expression of MMP2 and caspase-3.

Effacement of the STJ is noteworthy when considering the embryonic smooth muscle cell lineages that contribute to the thoracic aorta. SMCs in the aortic root are primarily derived from the anterior heart field [32], whereas SMCs in the ascending aorta are primarily derived from the cardiac neural crest [33] (Figure 1). It has been suggested by several investigators that SMCs have different signaling mechanisms that are dependent on their embryonic lineage [31]. While the derivation of the SMCs in the thoracic aorta is split, the endothelial cells are all derived from mesoderm-derived angioblasts (reviewed in [40]). The endothelial lining of the aorta is critical to the maintenance of SMCs and the overall aortic wall. Endothelial cells provide extracellular matrix, inhibit SMC proliferation, and release nitric oxide to aid in vasodilation. Notch1 is predominantly located in endothelial cells throughout the adult cardiovascular system [41]. It is possible that the loss of endothelial nitric oxide and Notch1 specifically affects the STJ because at this point of lineage divergence, SMC response to endothelial cell signals differs. For example, blood flow patterns normally differ between the aortic root and the ascending aorta [42], and endothelial cells signal to SMCs in response to flow patterns [43]. Because the STJ is a heterogeneous population of anterior heart field-derived and cardiac neural-crest derived SMCs (Figure 1) and endothelial cell-SMC signaling is lineage specific, the aortic wall at the STJ could be more susceptible to disrupted endothelial cell signaling than the aortic root or the ascending aorta, both of which have homogenous SMC populations.

TGF-β expression is known to be increased in many TAA patients [44], although its exact mechanism of action in aneurysmal development is unclear [45]. Total (active and inactive) circulating TGF-β1, a transcriptional target of TGF-β signaling, was assayed in the *Notch1*$^{+/-}$; *Nos3*$^{-/-}$ mice, but no clear differences were found (Supplemental Figure 3A). Although MMP2 expression, a transcriptional target of the TGF-β signaling pathway, was increased in our mouse model, we did not find changes in the expression of phosphorylated SMAD2 (Supplemental Figure 3B). It is possible that with age and more severe disease, an increase in circulating TGF-β1 would be more readily measureable.

4. Limitations

While our study is the first to describe an aortopathic phenotype in *Notch1*$^{+/-}$; *Nos3*$^{-/-}$ mice, it has several limitations. First, the mice were only aged to eight months and therefore the identified differences in the compound mutant mice were not dramatic. Additional studies examining the aorta after pharmacologic treatment to induce hypertension (angiotensin II or phenylephrine infusion) of *Notch1*$^{+/-}$ and *Notch1*$^{+/-}$; *Nos3*$^{-/-}$ may give a more definitive picture of the role on Notch1 in this disease. Secondly, it has been suggested that the more common location of aneurysms in BAV patients which are localized to the ascending aorta are due to hemodynamic effects, while those localized to the aortic root are attributed to genetic factors (Figure 1, reviewed in [15]). Consistent with this notion, the *Notch1*$^{+/-}$; *Nos3*$^{-/-}$ mice did not demonstrate abnormal hemodynamics (Figure 2F). We were unable to examine the aortic valve morphology in the *Notch1*$^{+/-}$, *Nos3*$^{-/-}$ and *Notch1*$^{+/-}$; *Nos3*$^{-/-}$ mice, a significant limitation of this study. In our experience, the most reliable method to characterize aortic valve morphology is to dissect the aortic valve with an attached cuff of the proximal aorta as this allows for direct visual inspection and mechanical manipulation to determine cusp fusion [30]. This type of analysis does not allow for histological examination of the diseased portion of the aorta since it was directly adjacent to the valve. Lastly, our model involves the disruption of the Notch1 signaling pathway and therefore these findings may not be relevant to all BAV associated aortopathy.

5. Conclusions

In conclusion, this study describes a new mouse model of aortopathy that includes effacement and dilation of the STJ and a trend toward dilation of the aortic sinus, although this was not significant. Our murine model suggests that STJ effacement may be an early indicator of aortopathy that has embryologic origins and molecular basis. This model has histological and molecular features consistent with ascending aortic aneurysms, including elastin degradation, smooth muscle cell apoptosis, and increased MMP2 expression. Additionally, we have described more subtle and less penetrant pathological changes in the aorta of the *Nos3*$^{-/-}$ and *Notch1*$^{+/-}$ mice.

Acknowledgments

The authors would like to acknowledge Nianyuan Huang for her technical assistance in management of the mouse colony for this project. The project described was supported by Award Number Grant TL1TR001069 from the National Center for Advancing Translational Sciences. The content is solely the responsibility of the authors and does not necessarily represent the official views of the National Center for Advancing Translational Sciences or the National Institutes of Health. This project was also supported by Saving tiny Hearts Society and Nationwide Children's Hospital Research Institute.

Author Contributions

Sara N. Koenig contributed to experimental design, data collection, analysis, and manuscript preparation. Kevin M. Bosse and Brenda Lilly assisted with data interpretation and made critical contributions to the manuscript. Holly A. Nadorlik assisted with echocardiographic analysis. Vidu Garg contributed to experimental design, analysis, and manuscript preparation.

Conflicts of Interest

The authors declare no conflict of interest.

References

1. Clouse, W.D.; Hallett, J.W., Jr.; Schaff, H.V.; Spittell, P.C.; Rowland, C.M.; Ilstrup, D.M.; Melton, L.J., 3rd. Acute aortic dissection: Population-based incidence compared with degenerative aortic aneurysm rupture. *Mayo Clin. Proc.* **2004**, *79*, 176–180.
2. Paterick, T.E.; Humphries, J.A.; Ammar, K.A.; Jan, M.F.; Loberg, R.; Bush, M.; Khandheria, B.K.; Tajik, A.J. Aortopathies: Etiologies, genetics, differential diagnosis, prognosis and management. *Am. J. Med.* **2013**, *126*, 670–678.
3. Romaniello, F.; Mazzaglia, D.; Pellegrino, A.; Grego, S.; Fiorito, R.; Ferlosio, A.; Chiariello, L.; Orlandi, A. Aortopathy in marfan syndrome: An update. *Cardiovasc. Pathol.* **2014**, *23*, 261–266.
4. Kainulainen, K.; Pulkkinen, L.; Savolainen, A.; Kaitila, I.; Peltonen, L. Location on chromosome 15 of the gene defect causing marfan syndrome. *N. Engl. J. Med.* **1990**, *323*, 935–939.
5. Lee, B.; Godfrey, M.; Vitale, E.; Hori, H.; Mattei, M.G.; Sarfarazi, M.; Tsipouras, P.; Ramirez, F.; Hollister, D.W. Linkage of marfan syndrome and a phenotypically related disorder to two different fibrillin genes. *Nature* **1991**, *352*, 330–334.
6. Maslen, C.L.; Corson, G.M.; Maddox, B.K.; Glanville, R.W.; Sakai, L.Y. Partial sequence of a candidate gene for the marfan syndrome. *Nature* **1991**, *352*, 334–337.
7. Dietz, H.C.; Cutting, G.R.; Pyeritz, R.E.; Maslen, C.L.; Sakai, L.Y.; Corson, G.M.; Puffenberger, E.G.; Hamosh, A.; Nanthakumar, E.J.; Curristin, S.M.; *et al.* Marfan syndrome caused by a recurrent *de novo* missense mutation in the fibrillin gene. *Nature* **1991**, *352*, 337–339.

8. Guo, D.C.; Pannu, H.; Tran-Fadulu, V.; Papke, C.L.; Yu, R.K.; Avidan, N.; Bourgeois, S.; Estrera, A.L.; Safi, H.J.; Sparks, E.; *et al.* Mutations in smooth muscle alpha-actin (ACTA2) lead to thoracic aortic aneurysms and dissections. *Nat. Genet.* **2007**, *39*, 1488–1493.
9. Zhu, L.; Vranckx, R.; Khau van Kien, P.; Lalande, A.; Boisset, N.; Mathieu, F.; Wegman, M.; Glancy, L.; Gasc, J.M.; Brunotte, F.; *et al.* Mutations in myosin heavy chain 11 cause a syndrome associating thoracic aortic aneurysm/aortic dissection and patent ductus arteriosus. *Nat. Genet.* **2006**, *38*, 343–349.
10. Barbey, F.; Qanadli, S.D.; Juli, C.; Brakch, N.; Palacek, T.; Rizzo, E.; Jeanrenaud, X.; Eckhardt, B.; Linhart, A. Aortic remodelling in fabry disease. *Eur. Heart J.* **2010**, *31*, 347–353.
11. Pepin, M.; Schwarze, U.; Superti-Furga, A.; Byers, P.H. Clinical and genetic features of ehlers-danlos syndrome type IV, the vascular type. *N. Engl. J. Med.* **2000**, *342*, 673–680.
12. Loeys, B.L.; Schwarze, U.; Holm, T.; Callewaert, B.L.; Thomas, G.H.; Pannu, H.; de Backer, J.F.; Oswald, G.L.; Symoens, S.; Manouvrier, S.; *et al.* Aneurysm syndromes caused by mutations in the tgf-beta receptor. *N. Engl. J. Med.* **2006**, *355*, 788–798.
13. Gurvitz, M.; Chang, R.K.; Drant, S.; Allada, V. Frequency of aortic root dilation in children with a bicuspid aortic valve. *Am. J. Cardiol.* **2004**, *94*, 1337–1340.
14. Cecconi, M.; Manfrin, M.; Moraca, A.; Zanoli, R.; Colonna, P.L.; Bettuzzi, M.G.; Moretti, S.; Gabrielli, D.; Perna, G.P. Aortic dimensions in patients with bicuspid aortic valve without significant valve dysfunction. *Am. J. Cardiol.* **2005**, *95*, 292–294.
15. Verma, S.; Siu, S.C. Aortic dilatation in patients with bicuspid aortic valve. *N. Engl. J. Med.* **2014**, *370*, 1920–1929.
16. Nistri, S.; Sorbo, M.D.; Marin, M.; Palisi, M.; Scognamiglio, R.; Thiene, G. Aortic root dilatation in young men with normally functioning bicuspid aortic valves. *Heart* **1999**, *82*, 19–22.
17. Lopez, L.; Arheart, K.L.; Colan, S.D.; Stein, N.S.; Lopez-Mitnik, G.; Lin, A.E.; Reller, M.D.; Ventura, R.; Silberbach, M. Turner syndrome is an independent risk factor for aortic dilation in the young. *Pediatrics* **2008**, *121*, e1622–e1627.
18. Mortensen, K.H.; Hjerrild, B.E.; Stochholm, K.; Andersen, N.H.; Sorensen, K.E.; Lundorf, E.; Horlyck, A.; Pedersen, E.M.; Christiansen, J.S.; Gravholt, C.H. Dilation of the ascending aorta in turner syndrome—A prospective cardiovascular magnetic resonance study. *J. Cardiov. Magn. Reson.* **2011**, *13*, 24, doi:10.1186/1532-429X-13-24.
19. Olivieri, L.J.; Baba, R.Y.; Arai, A.E.; Bandettini, W.P.; Rosing, D.R.; Bakalov, V.; Sachdev, V.; Bondy, C.A. Spectrum of aortic valve abnormalities associated with aortic dilation across age groups in turner syndrome. *Circul. Cardiovasc. Imaging* **2013**, *6*, 1018–1023.
20. Garg, V.; Muth, A.N.; Ransom, J.F.; Schluterman, M.K.; Barnes, R.; King, I.N.; Grossfeld, P.D.; Srivastava, D. Mutations in Notch1 cause aortic valve disease. *Nature* **2005**, *437*, 270–274.
21. De la Pompa, J.L.; Epstein, J.A. Coordinating tissue interactions: Notch signaling in cardiac development and disease. *Dev. Cell* **2012**, *22*, 244–254.
22. Swiatek, P.J.; Lindsell, C.E.; del Amo, F.F.; Weinmaster, G.; Gridley, T. Notch1 is essential for postimplantation development in mice. *Genes Dev.* **1994**, *8*, 707–719.
23. Krebs, L.T.; Xue, Y.; Norton, C.R.; Shutter, J.R.; Maguire, M.; Sundberg, J.P.; Gallahan, D.; Closson, V.; Kitajewski, J.; Callahan, R.; *et al.* Notch signaling is essential for vascular morphogenesis in mice. *Genes Dev.* **2000**, *14*, 1343–1352.

24. Jain, R.; Rentschler, S.; Epstein, J.A. Notch and cardiac outflow tract development. *Ann. N. Y. Acad. Sci.* **2010**, *1188*, 184–190.
25. Jain, R.; Engleka, K.A.; Rentschler, S.L.; Manderfield, L.J.; Li, L.; Yuan, L.; Epstein, J.A. Cardiac neural crest orchestrates remodeling and functional maturation of mouse semilunar valves. *J. Clin. Investig.* **2011**, *121*, 422–430.
26. McKellar, S.H.; Tester, D.J.; Yagubyan, M.; Majumdar, R.; Ackerman, M.J.; Sundt, T.M., 3rd. Novel Notch1 mutations in patients with bicuspid aortic valve disease and thoracic aortic aneurysms. *J. Thorac. Cardiovasc. Surg.* **2007**, *134*, 290–296.
27. Kent, K.C.; Crenshaw, M.L.; Goh, D.L.; Dietz, H.C. Genotype-phenotype correlation in patients with bicuspid aortic valve and aneurysm. *J. Thorac. Cardiovasc. Surg.* **2013**, *146*, doi:10.1016/j.jtcvs.2012.09.060.
28. Sciacca, S.; Pilato, M.; Mazzoccoli, G.; Pazienza, V.; Vinciguerra, M. Anti-correlation between longevity gene SirT1 and Notch signaling in ascending aorta biopsies from patients with bicuspid aortic valve disease. *Heart Vessels* **2013**, *28*, 268–275.
29. Zou, S.; Ren, P.; Nguyen, M.; Coselli, J.S.; Shen, Y.H.; LeMaire, S.A. Notch signaling in descending thoracic aortic aneurysm and dissection. *PLoS One* **2012**, *7*, e52833.
30. Bosse, K.; Hans, C.P.; Zhao, N.; Koenig, S.N.; Huang, N.; Guggilam, A.; LaHaye, S.; Tao, G.; Lucchesi, P.A.; Lincoln, J.; *et al.* Endothelial nitric oxide signaling regulates Notch1 in aortic valve disease. *J. Mol. Cell Cardiol.* **2013**, *60*, 27–35.
31. Sinha, S.; Iyer, D.; Granata, A. Embryonic origins of human vascular smooth muscle cells: Implications for in vitro modeling and clinical application. *Cell. Mol. Life Sci.* **2014**, *71*, 2271–2288.
32. Verzi, M.P.; McCulley, D.J.; de Val, S.; Dodou, E.; Black, B.L. The right ventricle, outflow tract, and ventricular septum comprise a restricted expression domain within the secondary/anterior heart field. *Dev. Biol.* **2005**, *287*, 134–145.
33. Jiang, X.; Rowitch, D.H.; Soriano, P.; McMahon, A.P.; Sucov, H.M. Fate of the mammalian cardiac neural crest. *Development* **2000**, *127*, 1607–1616.
34. Wasteson, P.; Johansson, B.R.; Jukkola, T.; Breuer, S.; Akyurek, L.M.; Partanen, J.; Lindahl, P. Developmental origin of smooth muscle cells in the descending aorta in mice. *Development* **2008**, *135*, 1823–1832.
35. Shesely, E.G.; Maeda, N.; Kim, H.S.; Desai, K.M.; Krege, J.H.; Laubach, V.E.; Sherman, P.A.; Sessa, W.C.; Smithies, O. Elevated blood pressures in mice lacking endothelial nitric oxide synthase. *Proc. Natl. Acad. Sci. USA* **1996**, *93*, 13176–13181.
36. Shu, J.; Qiu, G.; Ilyas, M. Immunohistochemistry (IHC) image analysis toolbox. Available online: http://rsb.info.nih.gov/ij/plugins/ihc-toolbox/index.html (accessed on 4 March 2015).
37. Koenig, S.N.; Garg, V. Aortic diameter measurements of 3 month old *Notch1*$^{+/-}$; *Nos3*$^{-/-}$ mice. Nationwide Children's Hospital, Columbus, OH, USA. Unpublished data, 2014.
38. Tadros, T.M.; Klein, M.D.; Shapira, O.M. Ascending aortic dilatation associated with bicuspid aortic valve: Pathophysiology, molecular biology, and clinical implications. *Circulation* **2009**, *119*, 880–890.
39. Lindsay, M.E.; Dietz, H.C. Lessons on the pathogenesis of aneurysm from heritable conditions. *Nature* **2011**, *473*, 308–316.

40. Choi, K.; Kennedy, M.; Kazarov, A.; Papadimitriou, J.C.; Keller, G. A common precursor for hematopoietic and endothelial cells. *Development* **1998**, *125*, 725–732.
41. Takeshita, K.; Satoh, M.; Ii, M.; Silver, M.; Limbourg, F.P.; Mukai, Y.; Rikitake, Y.; Radtke, F.; Gridley, T.; Losordo, D.W.; *et al.* Critical role of endothelial Notch1 signaling in postnatal angiogenesis. *Circ. Res.* **2007**, *100*, 70–78.
42. Hope, T.A.; Markl, M.; Wigstrom, L.; Alley, M.T.; Miller, D.C.; Herfkens, R.J. Comparison of flow patterns in ascending aortic aneurysms and volunteers using four-dimensional magnetic resonance velocity mapping. *JMRI* **2007**, *26*, 1471–1479.
43. Chien, S. Mechanotransduction and endothelial cell homeostasis: The wisdom of the cell. *Am. J. Physiol. Heart Circ. Physiol.* **2007**, *292*, H1209–H1224.
44. Hillebrand, M.; Millot, N.; Sheikhzadeh, S.; Rybczynski, M.; Gerth, S.; Kolbel, T.; Keyser, B.; Kutsche, K.; Robinson, P.N.; Berger, J.; *et al.* Total serum transforming growth factor-beta1 is elevated in the entire spectrum of genetic aortic syndromes. *Clin. Cardiol.* **2014**, *37*, 672–679.
45. Gillis, E.; van Laer, L.; Loeys, B.L. Genetics of thoracic aortic aneurysm: At the crossroad of transforming growth factor-beta signaling and vascular smooth muscle cell contractility. *Circ. Res.* **2013**, *113*, 327–340.

17

Takotsubo Cardiomyopathy: A Long Term Follow-up Shows Benefit with Risk Factor Reduction

Koroush Khalighi [1,*], Mohammad Umar Farooq [2,†], Thein Tun Aung [3,†] and Swe Oo [4,†]

[1] Department of Cardiovascular Disease, Easton Hospital Easton, PA Clinical Professor of Medicine, Drexel University, School of Medicine Easton Cardiovascular Associates 2001 Fairview Ave, Easton, PA 18042, USA

[2] Department of Medicine, Easton Hospital, 250 South 21 street, Easton, PA 18042, USA; E-Mail: Mohammad_Farooq@chs.net

[3] Department of Cardiovascular Disease, Wright State University, 921 Wilmington Ave, Apt D, Dayton, OH 45420, USA; E-Mail: theintun.aung@hotmail.com

[4] Department of Medicine, Easton Hospital, 250 South 21 street, Easton, PA 18042, USA; E-Mail: swezin82@gmail.com

† These authors contributed equally to this work.

* Author to whom correspondence should be addressed; E-Mail: koroushkhalighi@gmail.com

Academic Editor: Andy Wessels

Abstract: Only sparse data was available on long-term of Takotusbo Cardiomyopathy (TC). Previous studies suggested prognosis is not necessarily benign. We report the long-term follow-up of 12 TC patients actively managed with risk factor reduction. Retrospective analysis of all patients diagnosed with TC at our hospital between 1998 and 2010. We identified 12 patients with TC among 1651 cases of emergent left heart catheterization over 12 years. Mean follow-up time was 8.3 ± 3.6 years. All were female, 87% had hypertension, 25% had history of Coronary Artery Disease (CAD), 67% had hyperlipidemia, 44% had some preceding emotional trauma, and 44% had some physical/physiological stress. Previous studies have shown that over 50% of TC patients experience future cardiac events, and 10% have a recurrence of TC. Patients were prescribed therapeutic lifestyle changes (TLC) and guideline directed medical therapy

(GDMT) for aggressive risk factor reduction. TLC included diet, exercise, and cardiac rehabilitation. GDMT often included aspirin, beta-blockers, ACE-inhibitors, and statins. Follow-up echocardiograms showed recovery and maintenance of the ejection fraction. There was no cardiac mortality and no recurrences of TC. Aggressive risk factor reduction with TLC and GDMT may be effective in improving the long term outcomes of patients with TC.

Keywords: Takotusbo Cardiomyopathy (TC); Myocardial Infarction with Normal Coronary Arteries (MINCA); stress-induced cardiomyopathy; Coronary Artery Disease (CAD)

1. Introduction

Takotsubo Cardiomyopathy (TC) was first described in 1991 in Japan. It consists of transient systolic dysfunction of the apical and/or mid-segment of the left ventricle, a clinical presentation of that mimics acute myocardial infarction and absence of obstructive coronary artery disease. Sparse data available on long-term outcomes suggests prognosis is not necessarily benign. We report the long-term follow-up of 12 TC patients, and speculate that intensive risk factor modification may account for the good outcomes we observed in this group.

2. Methods

From January 1998 to December 2010, among 1651 who underwent emergent left heart catheterization for acute coronary syndrome (ACS), 12 patients were identified with having TC using the Modified Mayo Criteria. Main components include akinesia of mid-distal LV, non-obstructive Coronary Artery Disease (CAD), new EKG changes, and absence of myocarditis or pheochromocytoma (Table 1).

Table 1. Demographic Characteristics.

Patient Number	Follow up (Years)	Age (Year)	Sex	HTN	DM	CAD	Dyslipidemia	FH CAD
A	13	57	F	No	No	No	Yes	Yes
B	17	36	F	No	No	No	Yes	Yes
C	9	67	F	No	No	No	No	No
D	8	72	F	Yes	No	No	Yes	No
E	7	61	F	No	No	Yes	Yes	No
F	10	89	F	Yes	No	No	No	No
G	6	41	F	Yes	No	No	No	No
H	6	69	F	Yes	No	Yes	Yes	Yes
I	5	69	F	Yes	No	Yes	Yes	Yes
J	5	81	F	Yes	Yes	No	Yes	No
K	5	56	F	Yes	Yes	No	Yes	Yes
L	8	65	F	Yes	No	Yes	Yes	Yes
			100% F	75%	17%	25%	67%	50%

All patients underwent follow-up evaluation of left ventricular function with transthoracic echocardiogram six weeks after the initial event, followed by yearly echocardiograms. We followed these 12 patients, who were actively managed with both lifestyle modification and pharmacologic treatment, over the 5–17 years period after the initial TC event.

Patients were advised regarding therapeutic lifestyle changes (TLC) and prescribed guideline-directed medical therapy (GDMT) for aggressive risk factor reduction. TLC included low-salt, low-fat diet, exercise, and cardiac rehabilitation. GDMT often included anti-platelet agents (aspirin, clopidogrel), beta-blockers (metoprolol or carvedilol), angiotensin converting enzyme inhibitors (ACEI) (lisinopril or ramipril), and statins (atorvastatin). The primary end point was a combination of all-cause death, cardiogenic shock, sudden cardiac death, recurrence of TC, and re-hospitalization for cardiac reasons.

3. Results

All of the patients in our study were female and most were post-menopausal with a median age of 66 years (ranging from 36 to 89 years). Many had risk factors for coronary artery disease (CAD) with 75% (9/12) having hypertension, 67% (9/12) with hyperlipidemia, and 50% (6/12) with a family history of CAD. There were 25% (4/12) who already had a documented history of CAD. On presentation, 58% (7/12) had preceding emotional trauma and 50% (6/12) had physical stress (Tables 1 and 2). All patients presented with chest pain and troponin elevation, while 50% (6/12) had ST elevations on EKG. Coronary angiography revealed no obstructive lesion and left ventriculography revealed apical hypokinesis along with decreased ejection fraction (EF) in all patients (Table 2).

Table 2. Clinical Features.

Patient	Psychological Trauma	Physical Stress	Chest Pain	EKG	Peak Troponin Elevation	Hypokinesis on Ventriculography
A	Yes *	Yes #	Substernal	STE	2.4	Apical
B	Yes ^	No	Substernal	STD-inferior	42	Inferior septal wall
C	Yes	No	Substernal	STE	1.8	Apical
D	Yes	No	Substernal	None	1.4	Infero-apical
E	Yes	Yes	Substernal	None	10	Apical
F	No	Yes	Left Sided	None	1.85	Apical
G	No	Yes	Substernal	STE-inferior	4.13; 1.79	Infero-apical
H	No	Yes	Substernal	STE-anterior	1.39	Infero-apical
I	No	Yes	Left sided	LBBB	1.37	Apical
J	Yes	No	Substernal	STE-anterior	1.45	Apical
K	Yes	No	Substernal	T-inv-inferior	3.34	Infero-apical
L	Yes	No	Substernal	T-inv-inferior	1.5	Infero-apical
				ST elevation = 50%		

* = Argument at work; ^ = Congenital problem in son; # = yard work.

The patients in our study have been followed for 5 to 17 years, with an average follow-up of 8.3 ± 3.6 years. In all patients, echocardiograms performed four weeks after the initial event demonstrated recovery of EF along with normalization of cardiac contraction (Table 3). Further yearly follow-up echocardiograms showed that patients also maintained their ejection fraction for the duration of the study.

Table 3. Management and follow up.

Patient	Initial Ejection Fraction (Percentage)	Follow-up Ejection Fraction (Percentage)	Administered Medications	Follow up (Years)	Chest Pain Recurrence	Documented CAD on Follow-up
A	45	70	Aspirin, Metoprolol, Pravastatin Ramipril	13	Yes	No
B	50	60	Metoprolol, Aspirin	17	No	No
C	25	40	Aspirin, Metoprolol, Clopidogrel, Ramipril	9	No	No
D	35	55	Aspirin, Lisinopril, Metoprolol, Clopidogrel	8	No	No
E	35	55	Metoprolol, Atorvastatin	7	No	No
F	35	61	Lisinopril, Carvedilol	10	Yes	No
G	50	55	Aspirin, Clopidogrel, Valsartan, Atorvastatin	6	Yes	No
H	35	60	Aspirin, Clopidogrel, Metoprolol, Statin	6	No	No
I	25	45	Aspirin, Lisinopril, Metoprolol, Statin,	5	No	No
J	40	55	Aspirin, Statin, Lisinopril, Amlodipine	5	No	No
K	30	50	Aspirin, Metoprolol, Statin, Lisinopril	5	No	No
L	25	60	Aspirin, Statin, Carvedilol, Fosinopril **	8	Yes	Yes

** = Progression of CAD from 30% stenosis of RCA that was later found to be 90%.

There were four patients who experienced recurrences of chest pain. Two patients' symptoms were musculoskeletal in etiology. One patient had a progression of CAD, which was managed conservatively. One patient was found to have a malignant left lung mass. There was no cardiac mortality, and no recurrences of TC.

We followed the blood pressure, heart rate, body weight, and lipid panel results to ensure the patients are following optimal medical therapy and lifestyle modifications. The results are presented in Tables 4 and 5. During the follow up, one patient passed away with lung cancer. Her results will not be updated in the following tables.

After optimal, guideline-directed medical therapy (GDMT), almost all the patients had their blood pressure and heart rate controlled. The majority (8/11) of the patients had maintained or reduced body weight. The majority of the patients (9/11) had well-controlled LDL levels. The LDL level of patient A and patient D had worsened recently. Further review revealed that before these changes, their medical insurances were switched under the new healthcare law. Rosuvastatin was switched to generic Pravastatin and Atorvastatin. Follow up lipid panel results are pending.

Table 4. Changes in blood pressure, heart rate, and body weight with medical management.

Patient	Systolic Blood Pressure at Diagnosis	Most Recent Systolic Blood Pressure	Heart Rate at Diagnosis	Most Recent Heart Rate	Body Weight at Presentation	Most Recent Body Weight
A	122	132	62	60	144	186
B	132	120	83	60	142	135
C	124	120	72	70	156	147
D	193	120	74	66	99	97
E	130	128	68	65	172	190
F	156	104	74	75	130	135

Table 4. *Cont.*

Patient	Systolic Blood Pressure at Diagnosis	Most Recent Systolic Blood Pressure	Heart Rate at Diagnosis	Most Recent Heart Rate	Body Weight at Presentation	Most Recent Body Weight
G	140	111	72	84	115	111
H	116	106	117	98	182	145
I	167	141	85	83	266	266
J	131	128	62	72	149	140
K	135	128	102	80	356	270
L	117	125	90	78	164	175

Table 5. Lipid panel results after medical management.

Patient	Initial Cholesterol	Most Recent Cholesterol	Initial LDL	Most Recent LDL	Initial HDL	Most Recent HDL	Initial Triglycerides	Most Recent Triglycerides
A	169	197	71	112	59	53	124	159
B	164	140	80	60	65	66	91	71
C	159	145	90	73	61	58	76	86
D	164	202	87	127	60	59	85	77
E	212	154	135	95	52	56	168	204
F	153	155	101	93	37	46	72	80
G	168	171	73	79	82	79	61	64
H	172	142	113	63	19	26	202	173
I	168	154	99	81	32	36	187	183
J	151	121	73	59	30	19	238	202
K	154	180	66	74	36	58	258	302
L	119	107	54	37	50	35	75	174

LDL = Low Density Lipoprotein; HDL = High Density Lipoprotein.

4. Discussion

TC is increasingly recognized in the differential diagnosis of acute coronary syndrome (ACS) as a cause of myocardial infarction with normal coronary arteries (MINCA) [1]. Numerous studies document the short-term recovery of TC patients. A meta-analysis of 28 case series by Pilgrim *et al.*, showed complete recovery of EF in 95.9% of patients in 7–37 days, with ejection fraction improving from 20%–49.9% to 59%–76% [2]. Few studies, however, followed the long-term course of these patients.

The few studies following long-term outcomes in TC patients arrive at differing conclusions regarding prognosis. Elesber *et al.*, and Valbusa *et al.*, both tracked overall survival in age and gender-matched TC populations, but found no difference. In contrast, Sharkey *et al.*, and Ionesco *et al.*, found that survival in TC patients was reduced [3–6]. Importantly, all of the aforementioned studies showed high cardiovascular event rates following the initial insult. In the follow-up by Elesber *et al.* during the 4.7 ± 4.8 years follow-up, 17% of patients suffered mortality, 10% of patients suffered recurrence of TC, and 12% of patients suffered re-hospitalization for cardiac reasons, for a total 39% event rate [5]. Ionesco *et al.* also saw this high event rate in their follow-up of 27 TC patients over a mean of 27 ± 16 months. 52% of patients reached a primary end point of a combination of all-cause death, cardiogenic shock, sudden cardiac death, and re-hospitalization for cardiac reasons, with the authors concluding that the long-term outcome of TC is worse than previously reported [3]. In a recent study, spectroscopy and imaging done four months after the initial TC event showed cardiac energetic impairment, adding more evidence of the long term impairment in health and well-being of TC patients [7].

In a recent prospective study by Looi *et al.*, 26% of patients had a complicated hospital course, 4% need circulatory support with an intra-aortic balloon pump, 6% need ventilatory support, 2% in-hospital mortality, and an additional 4% mortality soon after hospital discharge [8].

Meta-analysis by Singh *et al.*, 2014, showed that the in-hospital mortality rate of TC was 4.5%, but only 38% of the mortality was directly related to TC and complications. The remaining 62% of the mortality was due to underlying non-cardiac mortality. It brought the cardiac mortality from TC down to 1.5% [9].

In comparison, we found a trend towards a decrease in morbidity and mortality of TC patients who were prescribed cardiac medical therapy on discharge, indicating a possible benefit from a long-term management strategy (Table 6).

Table 6. Comparing the Data from Previous Studies.

	Ionesco *et al.*	**Elesber *et al.***	**Khalighi *et al.***	**Looi *et al.* 2012**
Number of Patients	27	100	12	100
Mean Age (years)	68 ± 14	66 ± 13	64 ± 15	65 ± 11
Follow/up Duration	2.25 ±1.3 years	4.7 ±4.2 years	8.3 ± 3.6 years	3.0 ±1.7
Patients Antiplatelet agent	33%	50%	83%	90
Patients on BB	33%	51%	83%	65%
Patients on ACE I/ARB	41%	74%	83%	63%
Patients on Statin	30%	32%	67%	69%
Overall patients on optimal medical therapy	34.3%	51.8%	79.0%	
		Results		
Chest pain	2	31	4	78%
Hospitalization for cardiac complaints	8	12	1	26%
Recurrence of TC	2	10	0	7 (7%)
Mortality	4	17	0	4 (4%)
Morbidity/Mortality	14 (52%)	29 (29%) *	1 (8%)	26 (26%)

Morbidity and mortality = hospitalization for cardiac reasons, death from any cause; * event rate is 39% if we include recurrence of TC.

Medical therapy was targeted at preventing the mechanisms believed to cause TC:

(1) Cardioselective beta blockers (carvedilol, metoprolol) to prevent myocardial stunning or microinfarction caused by catecholamine-induced sympathetic overdrive: Wittstein *et al.*, showed that catecholamine levels are 2–4 times higher in patients with stress-induced cardiomyopathy as compared to patients with myocardial infarction. [10] This is the most widely accepted mechanism leading to TC [10,11].

(2) Cardioselective beta-blockers, Calcium channel blockers and/or ACE-I/ARB may prevent coronary artery spasm—Lacy *et al.* [12] showed that stress from public speaking can lead to vasoconstriction of coronary artery segments. Kiuriso *et al.* demonstrated that three of 30 patients with TC had spontaneous multivessel epicardial coronary spasm on angiography, and 10 of 14 patients with TC had coronary spasms on a provocation test using either egonovine or acetylcholine.

(3) Statins and anti-platelet agents to prevent microvascular dysfunction leading to transient thrombosis [2,13]. In a study of 16 patients with TC, Bybee showed that all 16 patients had decreased coronary blood flow in at least one epicardial vessel and 10 patients had this in all three epicardial vessels [14]. In one of the earlier studies of TC, Sadamatsu *et al.* [13] studied the angiography of two patients with TC and found that both had reduced coronary flow reserve.

In cross-analysis with TC patients, followed long-term in other studies, we observed a negative correlation between the percentage of patients on cardiac medications and the subsequent adverse event rate. In contrast to previous studies, most patients in our study were placed on appropriate cardiac medications at the time of discharge (Table 6). They maintained their ejection fraction with only one patient requiring readmission for progression of CAD. Over a long period of follow-up, our patients did well with medical management, including TLC and GDMT. This suggests that aggressive risk factor reduction by medical management might explain the difference in long term prognosis of TC patients seen in these studies.

5. Limitations

This is a single center trial with a limited number of patients without any control group. However, our study has the longest documented follow-up to prove the benefit of long-term medical management. However, due to limited power, we cannot specify which medication produced the greatest benefit.

Our results might also be compounded by selection bias since we followed 12 patients with Takotsubo Cardiomyopathy after discharge from hospital. We selected only the survivors. All of our patients survived the initial hospitalization. The biggest limiting factor to any conclusive statement regarding long-term prognosis and management is the relatively small number of patients available for such an analysis. As the diagnosis becomes more prevalent, future studies may be able to access a larger patient population for greater power.

6. Conclusions

TC patients may be at risk of experiencing long-term cardiovascular events. Following 12 TC patients with TLC and GDMT, we observed recovery and maintenance of the ejection fraction, no cardiac mortality, and an excellent long-term prognosis. Risk factor reduction with TLC and GDMT may be effective in reducing the risk of long-term cardiovascular morbidity and mortality in TC patients.

Acknowledgments

There has been no financial support or assistance for this project.

Author Contributions

Koroush Khalighi MD FACC, FACP, FCCP—involved in conception and design, critical revision of manuscript; Thein Tun Aung MD—involved in acquisition of data, drafting of manuscript and critical revision of manuscript; Swe Oo MD—involved and in acquisition of data; Mohammad Farooq MD—involved in conception and design, acquisition of data, analysis and interpretation of data, drafting of manuscript. Informed consent was taken from all patients to conduct this retrospective chart review. These charts are outpatient records, from the private clinic of the corresponding author.

Conflicts of Interest

The authors declare no conflict of interest.

References

1. Seth, P.S.; Aurigemma, G.P.; Krasnow, J.M.; Tighe, D.A.; Untereker, W.J.; Meyer, T.E. A syndrome of transient left ventricular apical wall motion abnormality in the absence of coronary disease: A perspective from the United States. *Cardiology* **2003**, *100*, 61–66.
2. Pilgrim, T.M.; Wyss, T.R. Takotsubo cardiomyopathy or transient left ventricular apical; ballooning syndrome: A systematic review. *Int. J. Cardiol.* **2008**, *124*, 283–292.
3. Ionescu, C.N.; Aguilar-Lopez, C.A.; Sakr, A.E.; Ghantous, A.E.; Donohue, T.J. Long-term outcome of Tako-tsubo cardiomyopathy. *Heart Lung Circ.* **2010**, *19*, 601–605.
4. Valbusa, A.; Abbadessa, F.; Giachero, C.; Vischi, M.; Zingarelli, A.; Olivieri, R.; Visconti, L.O. Long-term follow-up of Tako-Tsubo-like syndrome: A retrospective study of 22 cases. *J. Cardiovasc. Med.* **2008**, *9*, 805–809.
5. Elesber, A.A.; Prasad, A.; Lennon, R.J.; Wright, R.S.; Lerman, A.; Rihal, C.S. Four-year recurrence rate and prognosis of the apical ballooning syndrome. *J. Am. Coll. Cardiol.* **2007**, *50*, 448–452.
6. Sharkey, S.W.; Windenburg, D.C.; Lesser, J.R.; Maron, M.S.; Hauser, R.G.; Lesser, J.N.; Haas, T.S.; Hodges, J.S.; Maron, B.J. Natural history and expansive clinical profile of stress (tako-tsubo) cardiomyopathy. *J. Am. Coll. Cardiol.* **2010**, *55*, 333–341.
7. Dawson, D.K.; Neil, C.J.; Henning, A.; Cameron, D.; Jagpal, B.; Bruce, M.; Horowitz, J.; Frenneaux, M.P. Tako-Tsubo Cardiomyopathy: A Heart Stressed Out of Energy? *JACC Cardiovasc. Imaging* **2015**, *8*, 985–987.
8. Looi, J.L.; Wong, C.W.; Khan, A.; Webster, M.; Kerr, A.J. Clinical characteristics and outcome of apical ballooning syndrome in Auckland, New Zealand. *Heart Lung Circ.* **2012**, *21*, 143–149.;
9. Singh, K.; Carson, K.; Usmani, Z.; Sawhney, G.; Shah, R.; Horowitz, J. Systematic review and meta-analysis of incidence and correlates of recurrence of takotsubo cardiomyopathy. *Int. J. Cardiol.* **2014**, *174*, 696–701.
10. Wittstein, I.S.; Thiemann, D.R.; Lima, J.A.; Baughman, K.L.; Schulman, S.P.; Gerstenblith, G.; Thiemann, D.R.; Lima, J.A.; Baughman, K.L.; Schulman, S.P.; *et al.* Neurohumoral features of myocardial stunning due to sudden emotional stress. *N. Engl. J. Med.* **2005**, *352*, 539–548.

11. Coupez, E.; Eschalier, R.; Pereira, B.; Pierrard, R.; Souteyrand, G.; Clerfond, G.; Citron, B.; Lusson, J.R.; Mansencal, N.; Motreff, P. A single pathophysiological pathway in Takotsubo cardiomyopathy: Catecholaminergic stress. *Arch. Cardiovasc. Dis.* **2014**, *107*, 245–252.
12. Lacy, C.R.; Contrada, R.J.; Robbins, M.L.; Tannenbaum, A.K.; Moreyra, A.E.; Chelton, S.; Kostis, J.B. Coronary vasoconstriction induced by mental stress (simulated public speaking). *Am. J. Cardiol.* **1995**, *75*, 503–505.
13. Dorfman, T.A.; Iskandrian, A.E. Takotsubo cardiomyopathy: State-of-the-art review. *J. Nucl. Cardiol.* **2009**, *16*, 122–134.
14. Bybee, K.A.; Prasad, A.; Barsness, G.W.; Lerman, A.; Jaffe, A.S.; Murphy, J.G.; Wright, R.S.; Rihal, C.S. Clinical characteristics and thrombolysis in myocardial infarction frame counts in women with transient left ventricular apical ballooning syndrome. *Am. J. Cardiol.* **2004**, *94*, 343–346.

18

Genetic Regulation of Sinoatrial Node Development and Pacemaker Program in the Venous Pole

Wenduo Ye [1,*], Yingnan Song [1,2,3], Zhen Huang [1,2,3], Yanding Zhang [2,3] and Yiping Chen [1,2,*]

1 Department of Cell and Molecular Biology, Tulane University, New Orleans, LA 70118, USA; E-Mails: ysong4@tulane.edu (Y.S.); zhuang3@tulane.edu (Z.H.)
2 Southern Center for Biomedical Research, Fujian Normal University, Fuzhou 350108, China; E-Mail: ydzhang@fjnu.edu.cn
3 Fujian Key Laboratory of Developmental and Neural Biology, College of Life Science, Fujian Normal University, Fuzhou 350108, China

* Authors to whom correspondence should be addressed; E-Mails: wye@tulane.edu (W.Y.); ychen@tulane.edu (Y.C.)

Academic Editors: Robert E. Poelmann and Monique R.M. Jongbloed

---

Abstract: The definitive sinoatrial node (SAN), the primary pacemaker of the mammalian heart, develops from part of pro-pacemaking embryonic venous pole that expresses both Hcn4 and the transcriptional factor Shox2. It is noted that ectopic pacemaking activities originated from the myocardial sleeves of the pulmonary vein and systemic venous return, both derived from the *Shox2*$^{+}$ pro-pacemaking cells in the venous pole, cause atrial fibrillation. However, the developmental link between the pacemaker properties in the embryonic venous pole cells and the SAN remains largely uncharacterized. Furthermore, the genetic program for the development of heterogeneous populations of the SAN is also under-appreciated. Here, we review the literature for a better understanding of the heterogeneous development of the SAN in relation to that of the sinus venosus myocardium and pulmonary vein myocardium. We also attempt to revisit genetic models pertinent to the development of pacemaker activities in the perspective of a Shox2-Nkx2-5 epistatic antagonism. Finally, we describe recent efforts in deciphering the regulatory networks for pacemaker development by genome-wide approaches.

Keywords: pacemaker development; venous pole; atrial fibrillation; SAN; pulmonary vein

1. Introduction

The orchestrated contraction of the four-chambered mammalian heart is highly coordinated by the cardiac conduction system (CCS). The matured CCS of mammals contains the sinoatrial node (SAN), atrioventricular node (AVN), AV bundle and ventricle conduction networks [1]. The primary pacemaker, the SAN, is embedded in the junction between the right superior vena cava (RSVC) and the right atrium (RA). The SAN cells maintain highest automaticity and function to provide the primary impulse for each coordinated contraction. Dysregulation of SAN development and homeostasis causes sick sinus syndrome (SSS) [2].

1.1. The SAN Can Be Divided into Subdomains by Anatomical and Genetic Criteria

Initially noted as "a small condensed area of tissue located just where the cava sinks into the auricle" more than 100 years ago [3], the SAN is now recognized as a complex functional unit and the subdomains within the SAN have been defined both anatomically and genetically. Anatomically, a "head" region of the SAN can be identified as a histologically discrete structure that extends superiorly and wraps around the RSVC. The SAN also extends inferiorly toward the inferior vena cava (IVC) to form a "tail" structure [4–7].

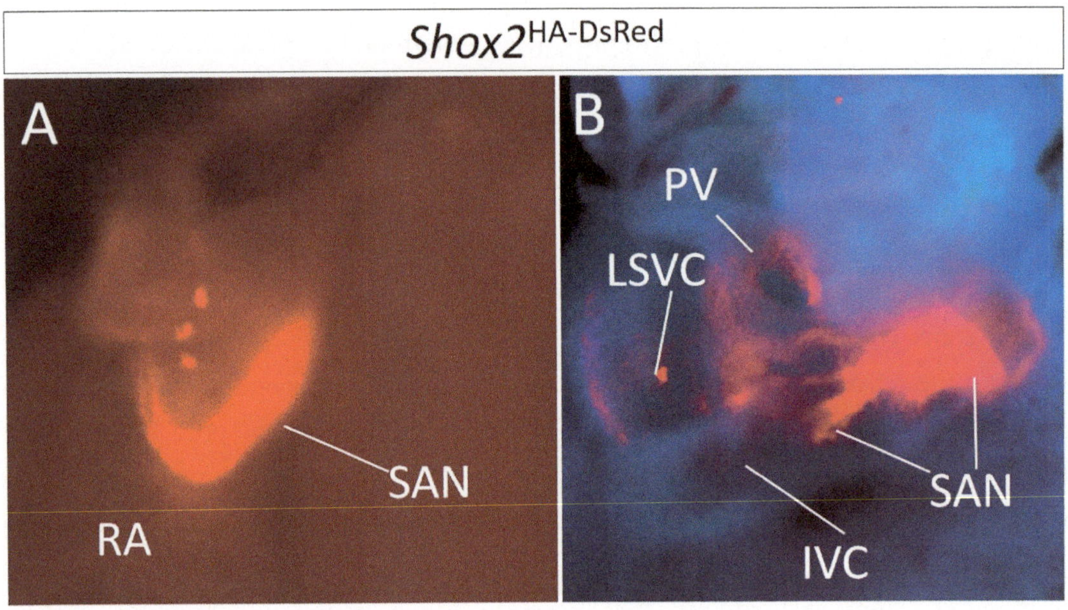

Figure 1. Visualization of *Shox2* expression in the SAN by *Shox2*$^{\text{HA-DsRed}}$ allele. (**A**) Frontal view of *Shox2* expression in the SAN of a mouse carrying a *Shox2*$^{\text{HA-DsRed}}$ allele at Postnatal Day 8 (P8), as revealed by DsRed expression. (**B**) Dorsal view of *Shox2* expression in the same mouse. PV, pulmonary vein; RA, right atrium; IVC, inferior vena cava; SAN, Sinoatrial node; LSVC, left superior vena cava.

Genetically, in the mouse, the SAN can be divided into a *Tbx18*$^{+}$/*Nkx2-5*$^{-}$ head domain and a *Tbx18*$^{-}$/*Nkx2-5*$^{+}$ tail/peripheral domain. In addition, the entire SAN can be identified by the expression of *Shox2*, as shown in Figure 1, as well as *Tbx3*, *Isl1*, and *Hcn4* [8–11]. A number of reporters/markers were also used to identify the developing SAN, such as the *CCS-LacZ* transgene [12] and the surface marker HNK-1 [13], though their specific SAN localization was not indicated. While the distinct functions of the SAN head and SAN tail/peripheral domain have not been well characterized, a recent study indicates that the *Nkx2-5*$^{+}$ SAN tail/peripheral domain is essential for normal SAN function [9].

1.2. Lineage Development of the SAN in Relation to Other Venous Pole Structures

During early development, after the formation of a linear heart tube through bilateral cardiogenic plate fusion (the first heart field, FHF), additional progenitor cells are continuously recruited from the surrounding mesenchyme to the outflow tract and the venous pole (inflow tract) where the SAN resides [14–17]. A morphologically distinct SAN structure can be identified as early as Embryonic Day 9.5 (E9.5) in the mouse. The initial function of the SAN was thought to start at around E12.5 [18] in the mouse, with typical SAN-like action potential (AP) configurations being identified at E14.5 [9,19]. Although the SAN is the dominant pacemaker in the venous pole, cells with pacemaking activities can be found not only in the SAN, but also in the myocardial sleeves of the systemic venous return and the pulmonary vein (PV) myocardium. It was proposed that these cells with pacemaking activities can act as ectopic pacemaker to trigger atrial fibrillation (A-Fib) [20,21], making the characterization of the lineage origin of these sites in relation to the SAN an interesting subject. Multiple lineages have been shown to contribute to the development of the venous pole based on marker expression and genetic fate mapping studies, such as the *Tbx18*$^{+}$/*Nkx2-5*$^{-}$ sinus venosus (SV) cells that develop into the myocardial sleeves of the systemic venous return [14,22], the posterior second heart field (SHF) cells mapped by *Mef2C-AHF-Cre* that develop into the primary atrial septum [16,23], and the cells labeled by *Hcn4Cre*$^{\mathrm{ERT2}}$ induced from E9.5 onward [24]. Based on the observation that *Tbx18*$^{+}$ lineage also maps to the SAN, it was assumed that the SAN is derived mainly from the *Tbx18*$^{+}$/*Nkx2-5*$^{-}$ SV myocardial cells [14,22]. Interestingly, the lineage and genetic attribution of the myocardial sleeves around the PV have been under heavy debate regarding whether it is a SV-like lineage. Similar to the SV myocardium, the PV myocardial cells are *CCS-LacZ* positive and HNK-1 positive as well [25,26]. However, unlike the SV myocardium, the PV myocardium is derived from a *Tbx18*$^{-}$/*Nkx2-5*$^{+}$ lineage [27], arguing against the hypothesis that the PV myocardium and SV myocardium share a common origin. Our recent study showed that the PV myocardium, SV myocardium, as well as SAN are all derived from *Shox2*$^{+}$ cells [9], offering a new perspective for understanding the lineage attribution of the PV myocardium. Interestingly, by using the expression of *Shox2* and *cTnT* as a marker for myocardial cells, a *Shox2*$^{+}$/*cTnT*$^{+}$/*Hcn4*$^{+}$ myocardial continuation was clearly identified in the proximal junction of the left superior vena cava (LSVC) and the PV as early as E10.5, supporting a common origin of the SV and PV myocardium [9]. In adult mice, this group of cells remains positive for *Hcn4* (Figure 2), suggesting a potential etiology for A-fib if the counterpart of these cells is present in humans. Moreover, *Shox2* is expressed in the PV side of the left atrial-PV structural continuum [9], providing a molecular marker for distinguishing the PV derived structure from the atrial-PV confluence structural continuum. Thus, although some genes, such as *Tbx3* and *Isl1*, are the SAN specific markers, other genes that mark the SAN also serve as lineage markers for the venous pole such as *Tbx18* that labels the SV myocardium and *Shox2* that labels the SV myocardium along with the PV myocardium. Such correlation coincides with the knowledge that the SV and PV myocardial cells are prone to develop foci induced A-Fib [20,21], and that the *Shox2*$^{+}$ SV and PV myocardial cells display pacemaker-like characteristics at early embryonic stages [9,20,21]. Given that pacemaker properties are shared among *Shox2*$^{+}$ cells at early developmental stages regardless of the expression of *Tbx3* and *Isl1* that are predominantly expressed in the SAN [9,18], an interesting questions is raised: is the genetic program that controls pacemaker properties in the venous pole independent from the one that controls the development of the histologically discrete SAN?

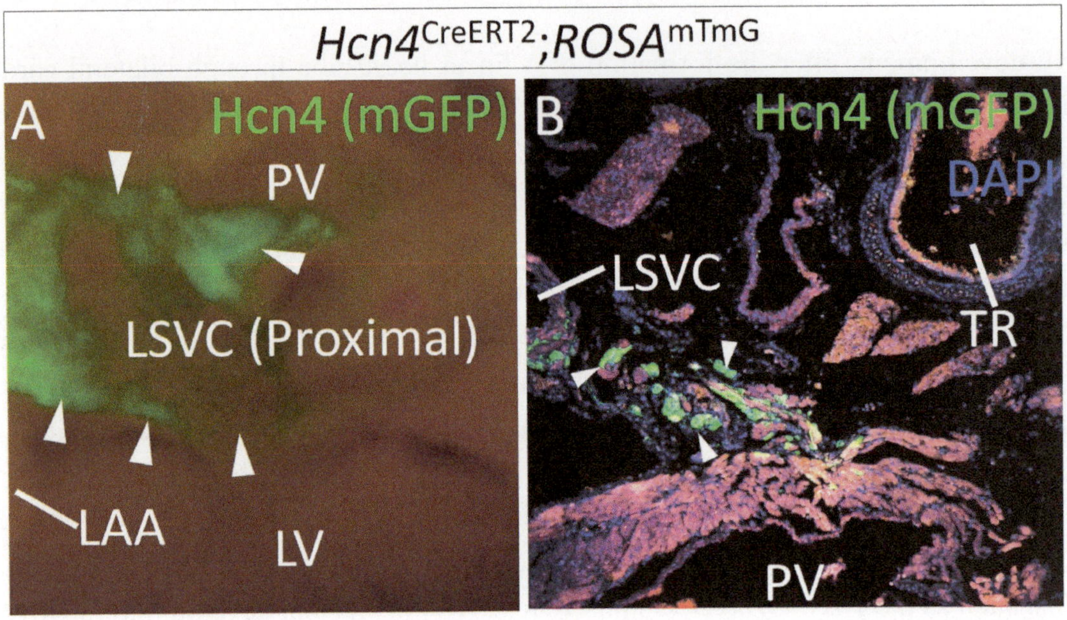

Figure 2. *Hcn4* expression in the proximal junction of the PV and LSVC myocardium of an adult mice. (**A**) Dorsal view of EGFP expression (arrowheads) in an adult *Hcn4*^{CreERT2}; *ROSA*^{mTmG} mouse seven days after tamoxifen induction. (**B**) *Hcn4* positive cells (arrowheads) in the junction between the PV and LSVC of the same mouse. LV, left ventricle; PV, pulmonary vein; TR, Trachea; LAA, left atrial appendage; LSVC, left superior vena cava.

2. Genetic Models for SAN Development

To further understand SAN development in relation to the SV and PV myocardium, we sought to revisit literature describing mouse models generated for studying SAN development. We categorized these models by whether or not mutations would cause phenotypes in both the venous pole and SAN.

2.1. Genes and Genetic Models for SAN Dysgenesis without Complications in the SV and PV Myocardium

Tbx3: *Tbx3*, encoding a T-Box transcription factor, has been well characterized for its essential role in embryonic development and postnatal function of the SAN and AVN. Null mutation or hypomorphism of *Tbx3* causes sick sinus syndrome and atrial-ventricular (A-V) conduction block [8,28–32]. Tbx3 acts predominantly as a molecular repressor on the expression of working myocardial specific genes in the SAN [1,33]. It has been proposed that Tbx3 functions to compete with Tbx5 for binding with Nkx2-5, thus repressing the activation of the target genes of *Nkx2-5* and *Tbx5* such as *Scn5α* (encoding Nav1.5) and *Gja5* (encoding Cx40) [1,33]. Tbx3 may also repress *Nkx2-5* expression directly as conditional inactivation of *Tbx3* elicits ectopic activation of *Nkx2-5* in the adult SAN [32]. Interestingly, although it has been established that *Hcn4* is a repressive target of *Nkx2-5* [9,34], null mutation of *Tbx3* does not cause downregulation of *Hcn4*, suggesting that *Tbx3* is only partially required for the maintenance of the SAN program. The fact that *Tbx3* is expressed in a manner more restricted than that of *Shox2* (Figure 3) in the SAN region at E10.5 when the dominant pacemaker activity is not yet confined to the SAN [18] suggests that the definitive SAN cells are already specified before the establishment of the dominant pacemaker activity and require a distinctive genetic program likely centering around *Tbx3*.

Isl1: *Isl1* encodes a LIM-domain homeodomain transcription factor. Although *Isl1-Cre* maps to the whole SHF derivatives of the mouse heart, *Isl1* is expressed later on only in a small subpopulation of cells in the heart including the SAN [35,36]. Recently, the essential function of *Isl1* in the development and function of the SAN was revealed by genetic and transcriptome studies in an *Isl1*$^{F/F}$; *Hcn4*$^{ERT2Cre/+}$ model in which the deletion of *Isl1* is induced at stages beyond E10.5 at which point the role of *Isl1* in maintaining the progenitor state of SHF cells becomes relatively limited and its deletion is less likely to complicate the analysis of *Isl1* function in the SAN [10,11]. As it was expected, inactivation of *Isl1* causes bradycardia associated with reduced size of the SAN and down-regulation of a number of SAN specific genes including *Hcn4*, *Shox2*, and *Tbx3* [10,11].

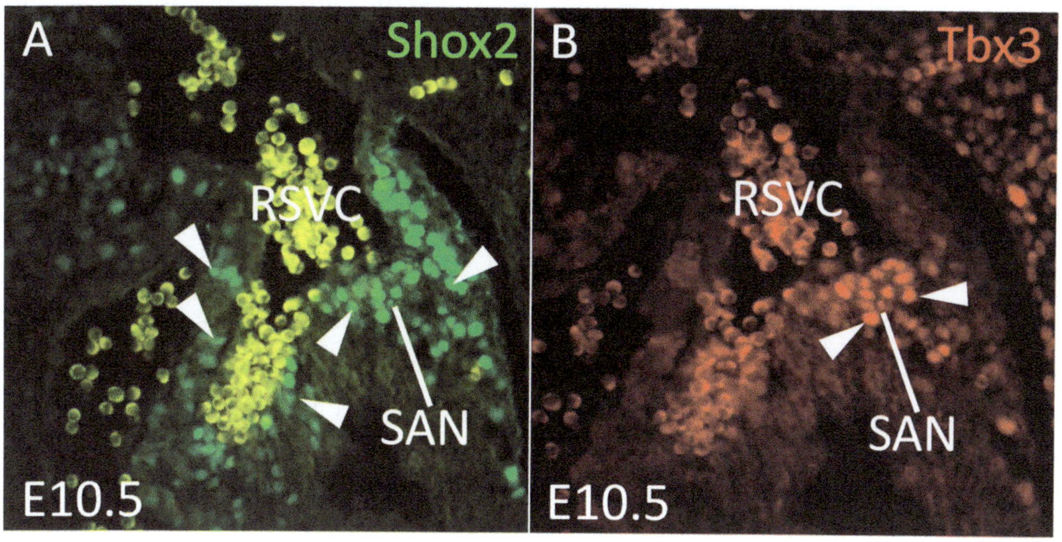

Figure 3. Expression of *Shox2* and *Tbx3* in the SAN at E10.5. Immunofluorescence shows the expression of *Shox2* (arrowheads) in the SAN and other tissues around the SAN (**A**) and the restricted expression of *Tbx3* (**B**) (arrowheads) in the SAN. SAN, sinoatrial node; RSVC, right superior vena cava.

2.2. Gene and Genetic Models Affecting Both the SAN and Other Venous Pole Components

Tbx18: *Tbx18* is the first gene that was shown to be able to convert non-pacemaker cardiomyocytes into pacemaker-like cells when it was forcedly expressed [37,38]. *Tbx18* is expressed in the pro-epicardial organ (PEO), developing SV myocardium, and SAN head in the venous pole [39]. *Tbx18-Cre* could also map to part of the SAN tail/peripheral domain, but not to the PV myocardium [39].

Accordingly, inactivation of *Tbx18* causes dysgenesis of both the SAN head and the SV myocardium [39]. Interestingly, *Tbx18* is never expressed in the PV myocardium, arguing for a different lineage origin of the PV myocardium *versus* the SV myocardium. Although the SAN head undergoes severe dysgenesis in *Tbx18* mutants, a functional SAN tail/peripheral domain is retained, implying the existence of an unidentified mechanism that controls pacemaker development in the SAN tail/peripheral domain and possibly in the PV myocardium as well.

Shox2: Shox2 belongs to the family of short stature homeobox genes and is expressed in the developing SV and PV myocardium, and the SAN in both mice and humans [9], as well as in a small subdomain of the dorsal mesenchymal protrusion [19]. Previous studies showed that *Shox2* is essential for SAN development partially by preventing *Nkx2-5* expression in the SAN head [40,41]. Interestingly, *Tbx3* is also essential for repressing the *Nkx2-5* expression in the SAN head [32], raising the possibility that *Shox2* and *Tbx3* repress *Nkx2-5* synergistically to ensure normal SAN development. This hypothesis is supported by the observation that mice carrying compounded *Shox2* and *Tbx3* hypomorphic alleles have significant higher level of *Nkx2-5* in the SAN compared to the littermate controls [42]. Actually, *Shox2* and *Nkx2-5* are co-expressed extensively in the SAN tail/peripheral region that is also *Tbx3* positive and in a group of cells surrounding the SAN. In addition, *Shox2* and *Nkx2-5* are also co-expressed in the other venous pole components, such as the PV myocardium that is *Hcn4* positive in early embryonic stages and possesses pacemaker properties, suggesting an unidentified mechanism for *Shox2* to control pacemaker development [9]. It was proposed that the *Shox2-Bmp* pathway may function to regulate SAN development [19,43]. However, *Shox2-Cre* mediated site specific inactivation of either *Bmp4*, the major BMP ligand that is highly expressed in the SV and SAN myocardium, or *Smad4*, which is required for the execution of canonical BMP signaling, results in a normal functional SAN [44]. These observations indicate that although *Shox2* is required for the developmental expression of *Bmp4* in the venous pole, the *Shox2-Bmp4* pathway does not sufficiently account for the function of *Shox2* in SAN development.

Nkx2-5: Numerous studies have pinpointed to the importance of *Nkx2-5* in early cardiac development, maturation of cardiomyocytes, and A-V conduction axis. The role of *Nkx2-5* in the venous pole, however, was underappreciated, partially due to embryonic lethality of *Nkx2-5* null mice around E10.5, precluding functional analysis of *Nkx2-5* at later stage of venous pole morphogenesis. *Nkx2-5* is initially absent from the SV myocardium and the SAN head [9,20] but is acquired in the SV myocardium at around E14.5. The PV myocardium is *Nkx2-5*$^{+}$ and expresses a relatively weak level of *Hcn4* expression compared to the SV myocardium [9,45]. In an *Nkx2-5* hypomorphism model in which the expression level of *Nkx2-5* is reduced to about 25% of wide type level [45,46], the PV myocardium acquires strong *Hcn4* expression and losses the expression of *Gja5* (*Cx40*) partially, mimicking the SV myocardial phenotype [45]. Furthermore, hypomorphism of *Nkx2-5* also results in an “invasion” of SAN phenotype to the surrounding atrial tissue, suggesting that the PV myocardium and the atrial tissues peripheral to the SAN are “default” to a pacemaker-like cell fate and such a “default” fate is suppressed by the presence of *Nkx2-5* [45]. It was reported recently that this pacemaker “default” fate is primed and sustained by the presence of *Shox2* [9]. Nevertheless, it is generally accepted that *Nkx2-5* exerts a repressive effect on pacemaker program by facilitating the maturation of cardiomyocytes in the developing venous pole. Such notion is further supported by the observation that venous pole specific deletion of *Nkx2-5* in the *Sln-Cre*; *Nkx2-5*$^{F/F}$ mouse model results in an enlarged SAN [47].

Pitx2: Components of the four-chambered heart, including venous pole structures, undergo left-right asymmetric development at early stage. It has been demonstrated that *Pitx2*, encoding a homeodomain transcription factors, confers left sided patterning information [48–50]. It is noted that the myocardial sleeves of the LSVC and PV are positive for *Pitx2* and were considered "left sided" structures [51,52]. *Pitx2* deficiency leads to the emergence of right-sided structures including the SAN and venous valves (VV) in the left-side SV-atrial junction [18]. Moreover, it was shown that haploinsufficiency of *Pitx2* caused A-Fib and ectopic expression of SAN program including *Tbx3* and *Shox2* in the left-side of the heart [53,54]. Although the loss of either *Nkx2-5* or *Pitx2* results in the ectopic pacemaker phenotype, inactivation of *Pitx2* leads to an acquirement of the complete pacemaker program in the left SV-atrial junction, whereas haploinsufficiency of *Nkx2-5* causes only an upregulation of *Hcn4* in the *Pitx2*$^{+}$ left sided structure, suggesting that these two genes repress pacemaker program through independently functional mechanisms [53,54]. Such hypothesis is further supported by an observation that in some *Pitx2*$^{-}$ right sided structures such as left venous valve, haploinsufficiency of *Nkx2-5* elicits an activation of a relatively complete SAN program including *Tbx3* and *Hcn4* [42].

3. *Shox2-Nkx2-5* Antagonistic Mechanism in the Regulation of Pacemaker Properties

3.1. Shox2-Nkx2-5 Antagonistic Mechanism

To date, genetic, biochemical, and electrophysiological studies have suggested that pacemaker cells retain properties that are common for the early primitive cardiomyocytes such as poorly organized sarcomere and the expression of *Hcn4* that is partially responsible for the high automaticity [55]. Thus it is reasonable to assume that rather than taking a positive acquiring process for pacemaker phenotype, SAN development may undergo a preventive process from maturation towards working myocardial cell fate. Such assumption is well in line with the fact that many machineries required for the maintenance of pacemaker properties are also utilized for sustaining progenitor state of the anterior SHF cells. A good example is that *Isl1*, which is essential for maintaining the undifferentiated state of the SHF cells, is also crucial for SAN development [10,11]. Moreover, similar to its function in the differentiation of the anterior SHF cells, *Nkx2-5* also promotes cardiomyocyte maturation in the venous pole, and *Tbx3* was shown to act as a transcription repressor in the SAN for the working myocardial program that is enforced by *Nkx2-5* and *Tbx5* [28]. However, these transcriptional machineries do not account sufficiently for the pacemaking activities in the SV myocardium and PV myocardium where *Tbx3* and *Isl1* are not expressed. Given that the derivatives of the SV and PV myocardium are prone to acting as triggers for A-Fib [20], characterization of the molecular mechanism that enforces pacemaker properties in these sites would be important for developing gene based therapeutic approaches for A-fib.

Based on the fact that *Shox2* is co-expressed with *Hcn4* in the PV and SV myocardium where *Isl1* and *Tbx3* are not expressed, and that the *Shox2*$^{+}$ PV myocardium cells display pacemaker-like properties, *Shox2* was believed to be a good candidate responsible for the potential pacemaker properties in the SV and PV myocardium independent of the SAN program genes *Tbx3* and *Isl1* [9]. Since hypomorphism of *Nkx2-5* causes augmentation of *Hcn4* expression in the *Nkx2-5*$^{+}$/*Shox2*$^{+}$ PV myocardium [9], and that the *Shox2*$^{+}$/*Hcn4*$^{+}$ SV myocardium is negative for *Nkx2-5*, it was proposed that *Nkx2-5* inhibits pacemaker properties that belong to a primitive cell phenotype, and such effect is counter-balanced by

Shox2. By genetic approaches, it was established that a *Shox2-Nkx2-5* antagonistic mechanism controls pacemaker *versus* working myocardial cell phenotype in the PV myocardium, SV myocardium, and part of the SAN [9]. Consistent with the observation that hypomorphism of *Nkx2-5* results in an "invasion" of SAN phenotype to the surrounding atrial tissue [45], we have recently observed that the tissues being preferentially "invaded" by SAN phenotype are all primed by *Shox2* expression [42], suggesting the balance between *Shox2* and *Nkx2-5* transcription output is critically maintained to restrict the size of the SAN.

3.2. Heterogeneous Development Model of the SAN and the Essential Physiological Function of the $Shox2^{+}/Nkx2\text{-}5^{+}$ *SAN Tail/Peripheral Domain*

Similar to that in the PV myocardium, *Shox2* and *Nkx2-5* are also co-expressed in the developing peripheral SAN and function to regulate the development of this SAN domain by their antagonistic action [9]. The development of the SAN tail/peripheral domain appears to be independent of the SAN head, as the deletion of *Shox2* in the SAN peripheral domain by *Nkx2-5-Cre* ($Shox2^{Nkx2\text{-}5Cre}$) led to virtual absence of the SAN tail/peripheral region but an unaffected SAN head [9]. In line with this notion is the fact that null mutation in *Tbx18* results in a severely hypoplastic SAN head but leaves the SAN tail/periphery unaffected [8]. The physiological importance of the peripheral region of the SAN was initially implied by *Scn5a* heterozygous mutants that exhibit sick sinus syndrome associated with SAN exit block [56]. *Scn5a* encodes a sodium channel protein (Nav1.5) and is expressed in the developing heart including the peripheral region of the SAN but not the SAN head. However, direct evidence supporting an essential role of the peripheral SAN in normal SAN function and S-A conduction was not available, primarily due to the lack of tools or genetic models to inactivate genes specifically in the peripheral SAN domain. In $Shox2^{Nkx2\text{-}5Cre}$ model, a severe sick sinus syndrome was observed associated with the absence of the peripheral SAN [9], providing the first line of direct evidence for the functional importance of the peripheral SAN as an integrated part of the SAN. Furthermore, although previous studies have supported the notion that *Nkx2-5* plays an inhibitory role in general on pacemaker program in the venous pole, the conserved expression of *Nkx2-5* in the SAN tail/periphery in both mice and humans suggests an underappreciated unique role for *Nkx2-5* in SAN development and function. The fact that Nkx2-5 binds directly to a verified enhancer downstream of *Scn5a*, revealed by Nkx2-5 ChIP-Seq results [9,57,58], suggests that *Nkx2-5* regulates *Scn5a* expression directly in the peripheral SAN domain to confer a unique electrophysiological property to the SAN tail/periphery. This hypothesis is supported by our recent observation that mice bearing the deletion of *Nkx2-5* in the SAN peripheral domain also exhibited sick sinus syndrome [42]. We therefore propose a model that the $Shox2^{+}/Nkx2\text{-}5^{+}/Hcn4^{+}/Scn5a^{+}$ SAN peripheral cells possess electrophysiological property intermediate of the $Nkx2\text{-}5^{-}/Shox2^{+}/Hcn4^{+}/Scn5a^{-}$ SAN head and the $Shox2^{-}/Nkx2\text{-}5^{+}/Hcn4^{-}/Scn5a^{+}$ atrial cells. Such property enables the $Shox2^{+}/Nkx2\text{-}5^{+}$ SAN tail/peripheral domain to play a unique role in the S-A conduction in addition to its impulse generation capability. Consistent with this model are: (1) $Shox2^{Nkx2\text{-}5Cre}$ mice exhibit sick sinus syndrome associated with a virtual absence of the SAN tail/peripheral domain [9]; (2) mice lacking *Tbx18* in the heart exhibit normal sinus rhythm regardless the lack of the SAN head [8]; and (3) a computational modeling predicts that the peripheral SAN cells possess higher maximum depolarization slope and higher AP amplitude than the SAN head cells to potentially function as a signal amplifier [59].

4. Genome-Wide Studies on Transcription Regulatory Networks and Chromatin Landscape in the Pro-Pacemaker Cells

It has been established that the SAN and pro-pacemaker cells in the venous pole possess a unique set of cellular properties and genetic features. This notion has been recently elaborated by transcriptome studies that demonstrate the possession of a distinct transcriptome profile by the SAN cells as compared with that in working myocardial cells [10]. It was further demonstrated that such unique SAN cell profile is at least in part maintained by the expression of *Isl1*, as deletion of *Isl1* by *Hcn4-CreER*^{T2} led to in the SAN an upregulation of working myocardial genes such as *Gja5* and *Gja1*, and a downregulation of pacemaker genes including *Tbx3*, *Shox2* and *Hcn4.* As abovementioned, *Shox2* and *Tbx3* are also responsible for the correct expression level of some of these genes in the SAN including *Isl1* itself. Such correlation suggests an epistatic link between *Shox2*, *Tbx3* and *Isl1* in SAN development. These genetic interactions, if tested by compounded allelic serial mutations of *Shox2*, *Tbx3*, and *Isl1*, will provide instrumental insights for a better understanding of the genetic cascades governing the unique pacemaker properties for the SAN and other pacemaker cells in the venous pole.

Furthermore, by ChIP-Seq, the molecular mechanisms involved in maintaining the particular properties of the pacemaker cells are being unveiled. Earlier studies of Tbx3 ChIP-Seq on adult heart using a *Tbx3* gain-of-function allele revealed a mechanism by which Tbx3 directly competes with Tbx5 to repress the working myocardial cell fate [58]. Similarly, a recent ChIP-Seq study on E12.5 mouse embryonic hearts unraveled an extensive genome-wide co-occupation of Shox2 and Nkx2-5, supporting the *Shox2-Nkx2-5* antagonistic mechanism by which Shox2 inhibits the transcription output of Nkx2-5 [9]. These lines of evidence together suggest the importance of transcription repressors in maintaining the pacemaker cell fate in a primitive state. Recent studies have shown that distal acting regulatory elements often reveal crucial information on the lineage specific chromatin landscape and reflect lineage specific transcription events as well as that transcription factor co-occupancy can be used to predict functional enhancers [60]. Our recent in-depth analyses of our published and unpublished ChIP-Seq data further identified co-occupation of Shox2 and Nkx2-5 on distal enhancers of a set of genes. Gene ontology (OG) analysis indicates that A-Fib related biological terms are highly enriched in the Shox2/Nkx2-5 co-occupied sites (Figure 4), suggesting that the co-occupation of Shox2 and Nkx2-5 can serve as a useful criterion for identifying A-Fib related *cis*-regulatory elements.

Interestingly, many of these elements discovered in the embryonic heart are also occupied by Shox2 in other developmental contexts. For example, a co-occupied site by Shox2 and Nkx2-5 in the intron-1 of *Arid1a* (*Baf250a*) in the embryonic heart [9] is also bound by Shox2 in the developing limb, suggesting that this site is accessible in both the developing heart and limb. Indeed, the orthologous region of this site in humans (HS569) [61] was characterized to have enhancer activity in the developing heart and limb in mice (Figure 4B,C). Furthermore, integrative interrogation of the distal regulatory elements identified by Islet1 ChIP-Seq in the postnatal SAN and that by Shox2 ChIP-Seq on the developing limb also unveils that a significant proportion of distal regulatory elements (~1/3) occupied by Islet1 is also bound by Shox2, indicating these regulatory elements are utilized in the development of both heart and limb [62]. Notably, a predominant proportion of these chromatin domains is not in an accessible configuration in the Encode heart DNasesHS dataset generated from working myocardium cells [63], suggesting that the pacemaker cells adopt *cis*-regulatory elements and associated transcription regulatory machinery that are also functioning in other developmental contexts to acquire the cellular phenotype distinct from working myocardial cells. Thus, integrative analysis of transcription factor binding profiles in other developmental context will aid for unraveling the transcriptional machineries operating in the developing SAN and pro-pacemaking cells in the venous pole.

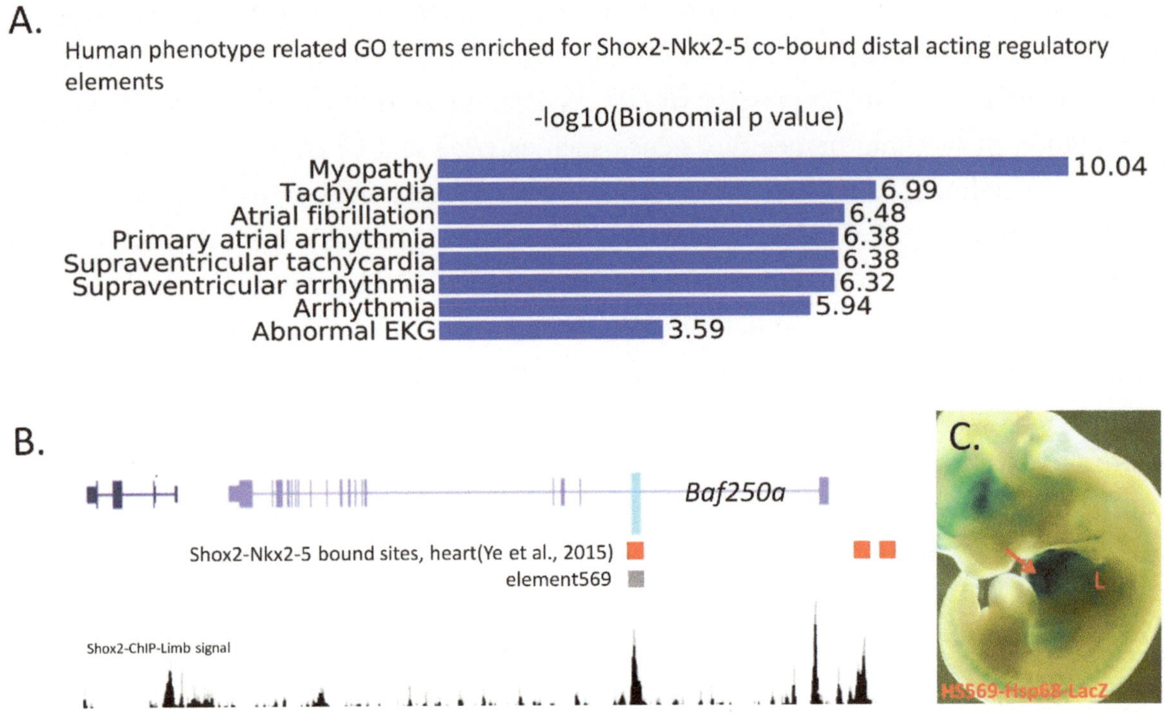

Figure 4. (**A**) Gene-ontology analysis reveals highly enriched atrial fibrillation related function in the Shox2-Nkx2-5 co-bound distal acting regulatory elements. (**B**) Signal track of Shox2-binding in the developing limb at E12.5 in relation to HS569, an enhancer of *Baf250a*, and Shox2-Nkx2-5 co-bound sites in the embryonic heart. (**C**) An E11.5 transgenic embryo carrying a reporter construct driven by Shox2-bound distal acting regulatory element (HS569) shows *LacZ* expression in the heart (arrow) and limb (L).

Recent advance and deepened understanding on regulatory chromatin landscape point towards the possibility that based on the accessibility or particular histone modification on tissue/lineage specific *cis*-regulatory elements, the developmental competence of cells toward the lineage of desire can be predicted. This possibility was nicely exemplified by the studies on human embryonic stem cell derived pancreatic beta cells [64]. It would be important and interesting to explore the features of chromatin landscape in pacemaker cells that are responsible for the specific pacemaker properties including the distinctive sets of gene expression profiles. Such studies on pacemaker cells will similarly benefit the generation of biological pacemakers by providing readouts for the developmental and differentiation competence of precursors toward pacemaker cells. However, technically, it will be very difficult to profile the chromatin landscapes of pacemaker cells directly by DNase-HS, FAIRE-Seq or by ChIP-Seq on various histone modification markers that are predictive of active enhancer/promoter activity. This is due to the relatively scarce SAN cells and that the pro-pacemaker cells in the venous pole are patched with surrounding atrial myocardial cells, precluding accurate isolation of sufficient amount of pacemaker cells in an undisturbed *in vivo* state. Currently, most of the SAN markers, such as Tbx3 and Hcn4, also label other conduction components, including the AVN. A *Shox2* knock-in allele that expresses the *Shox2a* isoform and *DsRed* (*Shox2*$^{\text{HA-DsRed}}$) and allows live imaging of *Shox2* expression in the venous pole and the developing SAN [9] would offer a unique tool for FACS isolation of venous pole pacemaker cells. In conjunction with open chromatin sequencing techniques that were designed for rare population of cells such as ATAC-Seq [65], it would be quite possible to characterize the accessible chromatin landscape of pacemaker cells comprehensively. Nevertheless, current ChIP-Seq studies on transcription factors closely related to pacemaker development in the venous pole provide a glimpse into the chromatin landscape of pacemaker cells.

5. Conclusions

In this review we summarize the previous studies in the perspective of SAN and pro-pacemaking venous pole development (Figure 5). In light of these comprehensive sets of studies, we propose that a delayed maturation towards working myocardium phenotype underpins the pacemaker properties of the *Shox2*$^{+}$ pro-pacemaker cells in the developing SV, PV and SAN. Moreover, a converged repressive transcription output of *Isl1*, *Tbx3*, *Tbx18*, and *Shox2* for working myocardial program appears essential for the solidification of a morphologically distinct SAN. Additional transcription activators that are expressed in the venous pole, such as *Gata4*/6 and CoupTFII, may play crucial role to enforce the *in vivo* developmental program in the SAN.

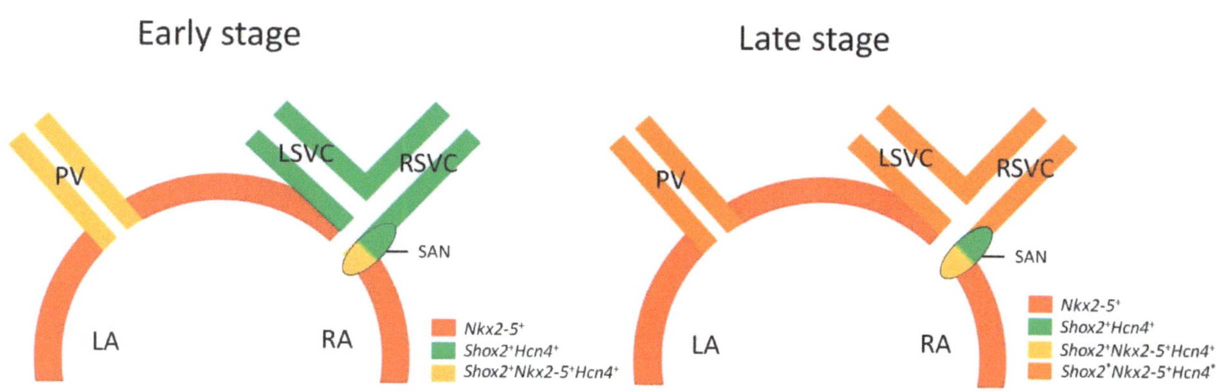

Figure 5. A schematic illustration summarizing the fate decision of cells in the developing venous pole. In the early developing venous pole, *Shox2* is expressed in the SAN head domain as well as the myocardium of the LSVC and RSVC, which are all positive for *Hcn4*. In addition, the SAN tail/peripheral domain and the PV myocardium are positive for *Shox2*, *Nkx2-5*, and *Hcn4*. At the late developmental stage and adult, the myocardium of the PV, LSVC, and RSVC becomes matured and largely adopts working myocardial phenotype, with potential to reacquire pacemaking activities.

Acknowledgments

The work conducted in the authors' laboratories and cited in this review article was supported by an American Heart Association Predoctoral Fellowship (13PRE1375003 to Wenduo Ye), and by the NIH as well as by a grant from the National Health and Family Planning Commission of China (No. WKJ-FJ-24) and an International Collaboration Grant from the Science and Technology Department of Fujian Province, China (No. 2015I0011). The HS569 transgenic embryo shown in Figure 4 was kindly provided by the laboratory of L.A. Pennacchio in the Genome Sciences Department at Lawrence Berkeley National Laboratory.

Author Contributions

Y.C. and W.Y. conceived and outlined the manuscript. W.Y. performed most of the experiments described in the manuscript and wrote the manuscript. Y.S. helped in immunohistochemistry experiments. Z.H. and Y.Z. helped in drawing figures for illustration. Y.C. conducted final revision and editing of the manuscript.

Conflicts of Interest

The authors declare no conflict of interest.

References

1. Christoffels, V.M.; Smits, G.J.; Kispert, A.; Moorman, A.F. Development of the pacemaker tissues of the heart. *Circ. Res.* **2010**, *106*, 240–254.
2. Anderson, J.B.; Benson, D.W. Genetics of sick sinus syndrome. *Card. Electrophysiol. Clin.* **2010**, *2*, 499–507.
3. Keith, A.; Flack, M. The Form and Nature of the Muscular Connections between the Primary Divisions of the Vertebrate Heart. *J. Anat. Physiol.* **1907**, *41*, 172–189.
4. Dobrzynski, H.; Boyett, M.R.; Anderson, R.H. New insights into pacemaker activity: Promoting understanding of sick sinus syndrome. *Circulation* **2007**, *115*, 1921–1932.
5. Herrmann, S.; Fabritz, L.; Layh, B.; Kirchhof, P.; Ludwig, A. Insights into sick sinus syndrome from an inducible mouse model. *Cardiovasc. Res.* **2011**, *90*, 38–48.
6. Morris, G.M.; Monfredi, O.; Boyett, M.R. Not so fast! Sick sinus syndrome is a complex and incompletely understood disease that might prove hard to model in animals. *Cardiovasc. Res.* **2011**, *92*, 178, doi:10.1093/cvr/cvr205.
7. Silverman, M.E.; Hollman, A. Discovery of the sinus node by Keith and Flack: On the centennial of their 1907 publication. *Heart* **2007**, *93*, 1184–1187.
8. Wiese, C.; Grieskamp, T.; Airik, R.; Mommersteeg, M.T.; Gardiwal, A.; de Gier-de Vries, C.; Schuster-Gossler, K.; Moorman, A.F.; Kispert, A.; Christoffels, V.M. Formation of the sinus node head and differentiation of sinus node myocardium are independently regulated by Tbx18 and Tbx3. *Circ Res* **2009**, *104*, 388–397.

9. Ye, W.; Wang, J.; Song, Y.; Yu, D.; Sun, C.; Liu, C.; Chen, F.; Zhang, Y.; Wang, F.; Harvey, R.P.; *et al.* A common Shox2-Nkx2-5 antagonistic mechanism primes the pacemaker cell fate in the pulmonary vein myocardium and sinoatrial node. *Development* **2015**, *142*, 2521–2532.
10. Vedantham, V.; Galang, G.; Evangelista, M.; Deo, R.C.; Srivastava, D. RNA sequencing of mouse sinoatrial node reveals an upstream regulatory role for Islet-1 in cardiac pacemaker cells. *Circ. Res.* **2015**, *116*, 797–803.
11. Liang, X.; Zhang, Q.; Cattaneo, P.; Zhuang, S.; Gong, X.; Spann, N.J.; Jiang, C.; Cao, X.; Zhao, X.; Zhang, X.; *et al.* Transcription factor ISL1 is essential for pacemaker development and function. *J. Clin. Investig.* **2015**, *125*, 3256–3268.
12. Rentschler, S.; Vaidya, D.M.; Tamaddon, H.; Degenhardt, K.; Sassoon, D.; Morley, G.E.; Jalife, J.; Fishman, G.I. Visualization and functional characterization of the developing murine cardiac conduction system. *Development* **2001**, *128*, 1785–1792.
13. Blom, N.A.; Gittenberger-de Groot, A.C.; DeRuiter, M.C.; Poelmann, R.E.; Mentink, M.M.; Ottenkamp, J. Development of the cardiac conduction tissue in human embryos using HNK-1 antigen expression: Possible relevance for understanding of abnormal atrial automaticity. *Circulation* **1999**, *99*, 800–806.
14. Gittenberger-de Groot, A.C.; Mahtab, E.A.; Hahurij, N.D.; Wisse, L.J.; Deruiter, M.C.; Wijffels, M.C.; Poelmann, R.E. Nkx2.5-negative myocardium of the posterior heart field and its correlation with podoplanin expression in cells from the developing cardiac pacemaking and conduction system. *Anat. Rec.* **2007**, *290*, 115–122.
15. Christoffels, V.M.; Mommersteeg, M.T.; Trowe, M.O.; Prall, O.W.; de Gier-de Vries, C.; Soufan, A.T.; Bussen, M.; Schuster-Gossler, K.; Harvey, R.P.; Moorman, A.F.; *et al.* Formation of the venous pole of the heart from an Nkx2-5-negative precursor population requires Tbx18. *Circ. Res.* **2006**, *98*, 1555–1563.
16. Xie, L.; Hoffmann, A.D.; Burnicka-Turek, O.; Friedland-Little, J.M.; Zhang, K.; Moskowitz, I.P. Tbx5-hedgehog molecular networks are essential in the second heart field for atrial septation. *Dev. Cell* **2012**, *23*, 280–291.
17. Snarr, B.S.; Wirrig, E.E.; Phelps, A.L.; Trusk, T.C.; Wessels, A. A spatiotemporal evaluation of the contribution of the dorsal mesenchymal protrusion to cardiac development. *Dev. Dyn.* **2007**, *236*, 1287–1294.
18. Ammirabile, G.; Tessari, A.; Pignataro, V.; Szumska, D.; Sutera Sardo, F.; Benes, J., Jr.; Balistreri, M.; Bhattacharya, S.; Sedmera, D.; Campione, M. Pitx2 confers left morphological, molecular, and functional identity to the sinus venosus myocardium. *Cardiovasc. Res.* **2012**, *93*, 291–301.
19. Sun, C.; Yu, D.; Ye, W.; Liu, C.; Gu, S.; Sinsheimer, N.R.; Song, Z.; Li, X.; Chen, C.; Song, Y.; *et al.* The short stature homeobox 2 (Shox2)-bone morphogenetic protein (BMP) pathway regulates dorsal mesenchymal protrusion development and its temporary function as a pacemaker during cardiogenesis. *J. Biol. Chem.* **2015**, *290*, 2007–2023.
20. Jensen, B.C.; Boukens, B.J.; Wang, T.; Moorman, A.F.; Christoffels, V.M. Evolution of the Sinus Venosus from Fish to Human. *J. Cardiovasc. Dev. Dis.* **2014**, *1*, 14–28.
21. Mommersteeg, M.T.; Christoffels, V.M.; Anderson, R.H.; Moorman, A.F. Atrial fibrillation: A developmental point of view. *Heart Rhythm* **2009**, *6*, 1818–1824.

22. Mommersteeg, M.T.; Dominguez, J.N.; Wiese, C.; Norden, J.; de Gier-de Vries, C.; Burch, J.B.; Kispert, A.; Brown, N.A.; Moorman, A.F.; Christoffels, V.M. The sinus venosus progenitors separate and diversify from the first and second heart fields early in development. *Cardiovasc. Res.* **2010**, *87*, 92–101.
23. Aanhaanen, W.T.; Mommersteeg, M.T.; Norden, J.; Wakker, V.; de Gier-de Vries, C.; Anderson, R.H.; Kispert, A.; Moorman, A.F.; Christoffels, V.M. Developmental origin, growth, and three-dimensional architecture of the atrioventricular conduction axis of the mouse heart. *Circ. Res.* **2010**, *107*, 728–736.
24. Liang, X.; Wang, G.; Lin, L.; Lowe, J.; Zhang, Q.; Bu, L.; Chen, Y.; Chen, J.; Sun, Y.; Evans, S.M. HCN4 dynamically marks the first heart field and conduction system precursors. *Circ. Res.* **2013**, *113*, 399–407.
25. Gittenberger-de Groot, A.C. The development of the pulmonary vein revisited. *Int. J. Cardiol.* **2011**, *147*, 463–464.
26. Douglas, Y.L.; Jongbloed, M.R.; Deruiter, M.C.; Gittenberger-de Groot, A.C. Normal and abnormal development of pulmonary veins: State of the art and correlation with clinical entities. *Int. J. Cardiol.* **2011**, *147*, 13–24.
27. Moorman, A.F.M.; Anderson, R.H. Development of the pulmonary vein. *Int. J. Cardiol.* **2011**, *147*, 182, doi:10.1016/j.ijcard.2010.12.034.
28. Hoogaars, W.M.; Tessari, A.; Moorman, A.F.; de Boer, P.A.; Hagoort, J.; Soufan, A.T.; Campione, M.; Christoffels, V.M. The transcriptional repressor Tbx3 delineates the developing central conduction system of the heart. *Cardiovasc. Res.* **2004**, *62*, 489–499.
29. Bakker, M.L.; Boukens, B.J.; Mommersteeg, M.T.; Brons, J.F.; Wakker, V.; Moorman, A.F.; Christoffels, V.M. Transcription factor Tbx3 is required for the specification of the atrioventricular conduction system. *Circ. Res.* **2008**, *102*, 1340–1349.
30. Hoogaars, W.M.; Engel, A.; Brons, J.F.; Verkerk, A.O.; de Lange, F.J.; Wong, L.Y.; Bakker, M.L.; Clout, D.E.; Wakker, V.; Barnett, P.; *et al.* Tbx3 controls the sinoatrial node gene program and imposes pacemaker function on the atria. *Genes Dev.* **2007**, *21*, 1098–1112.
31. Frank, D.U.; Carter, K.L.; Thomas, K.R.; Burr, R.M.; Bakker, M.L.; Coetzee, W.A.; Tristani-Firouzi, M.; Bamshad, M.J.; Christoffels, V.M.; Moon, A.M. Lethal arrhythmias in Tbx3-deficient mice reveal extreme dosage sensitivity of cardiac conduction system function and homeostasis. *Proc. Natl. Acad. Sci. USA* **2012**, *109*, E154–E163.
32. Wu, M.; Peng, S.; Yang, J.; Tu, Z.; Cai, X.; Cai, C.L.; Wang, Z.; Zhao, Y. Baf250a orchestrates an epigenetic pathway to repress the *Nkx2.5*-directed contractile cardiomyocyte program in the sinoatrial node. *Cell Res.* **2014**, *24*, 1201–1213.
33. Arnolds, D.E.; Liu, F.; Fahrenbach, J.P.; Kim, G.H.; Schillinger, K.J.; Smemo, S.; McNally, E.M.; Nobrega, M.A.; Patel, V.V.; Moskowitz, I.P. TBX5 drives Scn5a expression to regulate cardiac conduction system function. *J. Clin. Investig.* **2012**, *122*, 2509–2518.
34. Mommersteeg, M.T.; Hoogaars, W.M.; Prall, O.W.; de Gier-de Vries, C.; Wiese, C.; Clout, D.E.; Papaioannou, V.E.; Brown, N.A.; Harvey, R.P.; Moorman, A.F.; *et al.* Molecular pathway for the localized formation of the sinoatrial node. *Circ. Res.* **2007**, *100*, 354–362.

35. Weinberger, F.; Mehrkens, D.; Friedrich, F.W.; Stubbendorff, M.; Hua, X.; Muller, J.C.; Schrepfer, S.; Evans, S.M.; Carrier, L.; Eschenhagen, T. Localization of Islet-1-positive cells in the healthy and infarcted adult murine heart. *Circ. Res.* **2012**, *110*, 1303–1310.
36. Tessadori, F.; van Weerd, J.H.; Burkhard, S.B.; Verkerk, A.O.; de Pater, E.; Boukens, B.J.; Vink, A.; Christoffels, V.M.; Bakkers, J. Identification and functional characterization of cardiac pacemaker cells in zebrafish. *PLoS ONE* **2012**, *7*, e47644.
37. Kapoor, N.; Liang, W.; Marban, E.; Cho, H.C. Direct conversion of quiescent cardiomyocytes to pacemaker cells by expression of Tbx18. *Nat. Biotechnol.* **2013**, *31*, 54–62.
38. Munshi, N.V.; Olson, E.N. Translational medicine. Improving cardiac rhythm with a biological pacemaker. *Science* **2014**, *345*, 268–269.
39. Christoffels, V.M.; Grieskamp, T.; Norden, J.; Mommersteeg, M.T.; Rudat, C.; Kispert, A. Tbx18 and the fate of epicardial progenitors. *Nature* **2009**, *458*, E8–E9.
40. Blaschke, R.J.; Hahurij, N.D.; Kuijper, S.; Just, S.; Wisse, L.J.; Deissler, K.; Maxelon, T.; Anastassiadis, K.; Spitzer, J.; Hardt, S.E.; *et al*. Targeted mutation reveals essential functions of the homeodomain transcription factor Shox2 in sinoatrial and pacemaking development. *Circulation* **2007**, *115*, 1830–1838.
41. Espinoza-Lewis, R.A.; Yu, L.; He, F.; Liu, H.; Tang, R.; Shi, J.; Sun, X.; Martin, J.F.; Wang, D.; Yang, J.; Chen, Y. Shox2 is essential for the differentiation of cardiac pacemaker cells by repressing Nkx2-5. *Dev. Biol.* **2009**, *327*, 376–385.
42. Ye, W.; Chen, Y. Revealing the default pacemakers in the venous pole. **2016**, to be submitted for publication.
43. Puskaric, S.; Schmitteckert, S.; Mori, A.D.; Glaser, A.; Schneider, K.U.; Bruneau, B.G.; Blaschke, R.J.; Steinbeisser, H.; Rappold, G. Shox2 mediates Tbx5 activity by regulating Bmp4 in the pacemaker region of the developing heart. *Hum. Mol. Genet.* **2010**, *19*, 4625–4633.
44. Ye, W.; Chen, Y. Department of Cell and Molecular Biology, Tulane University, New Orleans, LA, USA. Unpublished Observation, 2015.
45. Mommersteeg, M.T.; Brown, N.A.; Prall, O.W.; de Gier-de Vries, C.; Harvey, R.P.; Moorman, A.F.; Christoffels, V.M. *Pitx2c* and *Nkx2-5* are required for the formation and identity of the pulmonary myocardium. *Circ. Res.* **2007**, *101*, 902–909.
46. Prall, O.W.; Menon, M.K.; Solloway, M.J.; Watanabe, Y.; Zaffran, S.; Bajolle, F.; Biben, C.; McBride, J.J.; Robertson, B.R.; Chaulet, H.; *et al*. An Nkx2-5/Bmp2/Smad1 negative feedback loop controls heart progenitor specification and proliferation. *Cell* **2007**, *128*, 947–959.
47. Nakashima, Y.; Yanez, D.A.; Touma, M.; Nakano, H.; Jaroszewicz, A.; Jordan, M.C.; Pellegrini, M.; Roos, K.P.; Nakano, A. Nkx2-5 suppresses the proliferation of atrial myocytes and conduction system. *Circ. Res.* **2014**, *114*, 1103–1113.
48. Ai, D.; Liu, W.; Ma, L.; Dong, F.; Lu, M.F.; Wang, D.; Verzi, M.P.; Cai, C.; Gage, P.J.; Evans, S.; *et al.* Pitx2 regulates cardiac left-right asymmetry by patterning second cardiac lineage-derived myocardium. *Dev. Biol.* **2006**, *296*, 437–449.
49. Franco, D.; Campione, M. The role of Pitx2 during cardiac development. Linking left-right signaling and congenital heart diseases. *Trends Cardiovasc. Med.* **2003**, *13*, 157–163.

50. St Amand, T.R.; Ra, J.; Zhang, Y.; Hu, Y.; Baber, S.I.; Qiu, M.; Chen, Y. Cloning and expression pattern of chicken Pitx2: A new component in the SHH signaling pathway controlling embryonic heart looping. *Biochem. Biophys. Res. Commun.* **1998**, *247*, 100–105.
51. Campione, M.; Ros, M.A.; Icardo, J.M.; Piedra, E.; Christoffels, V.M.; Schweickert, A.; Blum, M.; Franco, D.; Moorman, A.F. Pitx2 expression defines a left cardiac lineage of cells: Evidence for atrial and ventricular molecular isomerism in the iv/iv mice. *Dev. Biol.* **2001**, *231*, 252–264.
52. Franco, D.; Campione, M.; Kelly, R.; Zammit, P.S.; Buckingham, M.; Lamers, W.H.; Moorman, A.F. Multiple transcriptional domains, with distinct left and right components, in the atrial chambers of the developing heart. *Circ. Res.* **2000**, *87*, 984–991.
53. Wang, J.; Bai, Y.; Li, N.; Ye, W.; Zhang, M.; Stephanie, B.G.; Tao, Y.; Chen, Y.; Wehrens, X.; Martin, J. Pitx2-microRNA pathway that delimits sinoatrial node development and inhibits predisposition to atrial fibrillation. *Proc. Natl. Acad. Sci. USA* **2014**, *111*, 9181–9186.
54. Wang, J.; Klysik, E.; Sood, S.; Johnson, R.L.; Wehrens, X.H.; Martin, J.F. Pitx2 prevents susceptibility to atrial arrhythmias by inhibiting left-sided pacemaker specification. *Proc. Natl. Acad. Sci. USA* **2010**, *107*, 9753–9758.
55. Bakker, M.L.; Christoffels, V.M.; Moorman, A.F. The cardiac pacemaker and conduction system develops from embryonic myocardium that retains its primitive phenotype. *J. Cardiovasc. Pharmacol.* **2010**, *56*, 6–15.
56. Butters, T.D.; Aslanidi, O.V.; Inada, S.; Boyett, M.R.; Hancox, J.C.; Lei, M.; Zhang, H. Mechanistic links between Na^+ channel (SCN5A) mutations and impaired cardiac pacemaking in sick sinus syndrome. *Circ. Res.* **2010**, *107*, 126–137.
57. He, A.; Kong, S.W.; Ma, Q.; Pu, W.T. Co-occupancy by multiple cardiac transcription factors identifies transcriptional enhancers active in heart. *Proc. Natl. Acad. Sci. USA* **2011**, *108*, 5632–5637.
58. Van den Boogaard, M.; Wong, L.Y.; Tessadori, F.; Bakker, M.L.; Dreizehnter, L.K.; Wakker, V.; Bezzina, C.R.; Hoen, P.A.; Bakkers, J.; Barnett, P.; *et al*. Genetic variation in T-box binding element functionally affects SCN5A/SCN10A enhancer. *J. Clin. Investig.* **2012**, *122*, 2519–2530.
59. Lei, M.; Zhang, H.; Grace, A.A.; Huang, C.L. SCN5A and sinoatrial node pacemaker function. *Cardiovasc. Res.* **2007**, *74*, 356–365.
60. Attanasio, C.; Nord, A.S.; Zhu, Y.; Blow, M.J.; Li, Z.; Liberton, D.K.; Morrison, H.; Plajzer-Frick, I.; Holt, A.; Hosseini, R.; *et al.* Fine tuning of craniofacial morphology by distant-acting enhancers. *Science* **2013**, *342*, doi:10.1126/science.1241006.
61. Visel, A.; Minovitsky, S.; Dubchak, I.; Pennacchio, L.A. VISTA Enhancer Browser—A database of tissue-specific human enhancers. *Nucleic Acids Res.* **2007**, *35*, D88–D92.
62. Ye, W.; Chen, Y. *Shox2* functions as a patterning factor in limb development. **2016**, to be submitted for publication.
63. Yue, F.; Cheng, Y.; Breschi, A.; Vierstra, J.; Wu, W.; Ryba, T.; Sandstrom, R.; Ma, Z.; Davis, C.; Pope, B.D.; *et al.* A comparative encyclopedia of DNA elements in the mouse genome. *Nature* **2014**, *515*, 355–364.
64. Wang, A.; Yue, F.; Li, Y.; Xie, R.; Harper, T.; Patel, N.A.; Muth, K.; Palmer, J.; Qiu, Y.; Wang, J.; *et al.* Epigenetic priming of enhancers predicts developmental competence of hESC-derived endodermal lineage intermediates. *Cell Stem Cell* **2015**, *16*, 386–399.

65. Pott, S.; Lieb, J.D. Single-cell ATAC-seq: Strength in numbers. *Genome Biol.* **2015**, *16*, 172, doi:10.1186/s13059-015-0737-7.

Permissions

All chapters in this book were first published in JCDD, by MDPI; hereby published with permission under the Creative Commons Attribution License or equivalent. Every chapter published in this book has been scrutinized by our experts. Their significance has been extensively debated. The topics covered herein carry significant findings which will fuel the growth of the discipline. They may even be implemented as practical applications or may be referred to as a beginning point for another development.

The contributors of this book come from diverse backgrounds, making this book a truly international effort. This book will bring forth new frontiers with its revolutionizing research information and detailed analysis of the nascent developments around the world.

We would like to thank all the contributing authors for lending their expertise to make the book truly unique. They have played a crucial role in the development of this book. Without their invaluable contributions this book wouldn't have been possible. They have made vital efforts to compile up to date information on the varied aspects of this subject to make this book a valuable addition to the collection of many professionals and students.

This book was conceptualized with the vision of imparting up-to-date information and advanced data in this field. To ensure the same, a matchless editorial board was set up. Every individual on the board went through rigorous rounds of assessment to prove their worth. After which they invested a large part of their time researching and compiling the most relevant data for our readers.

The editorial board has been involved in producing this book since its inception. They have spent rigorous hours researching and exploring the diverse topics which have resulted in the successful publishing of this book. They have passed on their knowledge of decades through this book. To expedite this challenging task, the publisher supported the team at every step. A small team of assistant editors was also appointed to further simplify the editing procedure and attain best results for the readers.

Apart from the editorial board, the designing team has also invested a significant amount of their time in understanding the subject and creating the most relevant covers. They scrutinized every image to scout for the most suitable representation of the subject and create an appropriate cover for the book.

The publishing team has been an ardent support to the editorial, designing and production team. Their endless efforts to recruit the best for this project, has resulted in the accomplishment of this book. They are a veteran in the field of academics and their pool of knowledge is as vast as their experience in printing. Their expertise and guidance has proved useful at every step. Their uncompromising quality standards have made this book an exceptional effort. Their encouragement from time to time has been an inspiration for everyone.

The publisher and the editorial board hope that this book will prove to be a valuable piece of knowledge for researchers, students, practitioners and scholars across the globe.

List of Contributors

Georg Vogler and Rolf Bodmer
Development, Aging and Regeneration Program, Sanford-Burnham Medical Research Institute, 10901 N. Torrey Pines Road, La Jolla, CA 92037, USA

Daniel P. Judge
Faculté de Médecine, Université Paris Descartes, Sorbonne Paris Cité, Paris 75005 France
Division of Cardiology, Johns Hopkins University, Baltimore, MD 21287, USA

Hany Neamatalla
Paris Cardiovascular Research Center, INSERM U970, Paris 75016 France
Department of Cardiology, Assistance Publique-Hôpitaux de Paris, Hôpital Européen Georges Pompidou, Paris 75016 France

Russell A. Norris, Annemarieke de Vlaming and Roger Markwald
Department of Regenerative Medicine and Cell Biology, Medical University of South Carolina, Charleston, SC 29403, USA

Robert A. Levine
Cardiac Ultrasound Laboratory, Massachusetts General Hospital and Harvard Medical School, Boston, MA 02114 USA

Jonathan T. Butcher and Kevin H. Kang
Department of Biomedical Engineering, Cornell University, Ithaca, NY 14853 USA

Nicolas Vignier
INSERM U582, University Pierre et Marie Curie-Paris 6, IFR14, Paris 75005 France

Quangtung Nguyen
Department of Cardiology, Assistance Publique-Hôpitaux de Paris, Hôpital Européen Georges Pompidou, Paris 75016 France

Patrick Bruneval
Faculté de Médecine, Université Paris Descartes, Sorbonne Paris Cité, Paris 75005 France
Institut de recherche des Cordeliers, INSERM U652, Paris 75005, France

Marie-Cécile Perier
Paris Cardiovascular Research Center, INSERM U970, Paris 75016 France

Emmanuel Messas
Faculté de Médecine, Université Paris Descartes, Sorbonne Paris Cité, Paris 75005 France
Paris Cardiovascular Research Center, INSERM U970, Paris 75016 France

Xavier Jeunemaitre
Faculté de Médecine, Université Paris Descartes, Sorbonne Paris Cité, Paris 75005 France
Paris Cardiovascular Research Center, INSERM U970, Paris 75016 France

Lucie Carrier
Institute of Experimental and Clinical Pharmacology and Toxicology, University Medical Center Hamburg-Eppendorf, Hamburg 20246, Germany

Albert A. Hagège
Faculté de Médecine, Université Paris Descartes, Sorbonne Paris Cité, Paris 75005 France
Paris Cardiovascular Research Center, INSERM U970, Paris 75016 France
Department of Cardiology, Assistance Publique-Hôpitaux de Paris, Hôpital Européen Georges Pompidou, Paris 75016 France

Robert B. Hinton and Teresa A. Smolarek
Divisions of Cardiology and Genetics, Cincinnati Children's Hospital Medical Center, Cincinnati, OH 45229, USA

Kim L. McBride and Vidu Garg
Center for Cardiovascular and Pulmonary Research and Heart Center, Nationwide Children's Hospital and Department of Pediatrics, Ohio State University, Columbus, OH 43205, USA

Steven B. Bleyl and Neil E. Bowles
Division of Pediatric Cardiology, University of Utah School of Medicine, Salt Lake City, UT 84132, USA

William L. Border
Division of Cardiology, Children's Healthcare of Atlanta, Atlanta, GA 30322, USA

Seema R. Lalani
Department of Molecular and Human Genetics, Baylor College of Medicine, Houston, TX 77030, USA

Stephanie M. Ware
Departments of Pediatrics and Medical and Molecular Genetics, Indiana University School of Medicine, Indianapolis, IN 46202, USA

Yang Lei, Masaya Iwashita, Jung Choi, Masanori Aikawa and Elena Aikawa
Center for Interdisciplinary Cardiovascular Sciences, Division of Cardiovascular Medicine, Brigham and Women's Hospital, Harvard Medical School, Boston, MA 02115, USA

Maëlle Perrocheau, Soto Romuald Kiando, Déwi Vernerey and Nabila Bouatia-Naji
Paris Cardiovascular Research Center, INSERM UMR970, 56 rue Leblanc, Paris F-75015, France Paris Descartes University, Sorbonne Paris Cité, 12 rue de l'école de medicine, Paris F-75006, France

Christian Dina
INSERM UMR1087, CNRS UMR 6291, Institut du Thorax, 8 Quai Moncousu, Nantes F-44007, France
Centre Hospitalier Universitaire (CHU) Nantes, Université de Nantes, 8 Quai Moncousu,

Pilar Galan
Equipe de Recherche en Epidémiologie Nutritionnelle (EREN), Centre d'Epidémiologie et Statistiques Sorbonne Paris Cité, Inserm (U1153), Inra (U1125), Cnam, Université Paris 13, COMUE Sorbonne Paris Cité, Bobigny F-93017, France

Albert Hagege,
Paris Cardiovascular Research Center, INSERM UMR970, 56 rue Leblanc, Paris F-75015, France Paris Descartes University, Sorbonne Paris Cité, 12 rue de l'école de medicine, Paris F-75006, France
Department of Cardiology, Hôpital Européen Georges Pompidou, Assistance publique-Hôpitaux de Paris (AP-HP), 20 rue Leblanc, Paris F-75015, France

Xavier Jeunemaitre
Paris Cardiovascular Research Center, INSERM UMR970, 56 rue Leblanc, Paris F-75015, France Paris Descartes University, Sorbonne Paris Cité, 12 rue de l'école de medicine, Paris F-75006, France Nantes F-44007, France
Department of genetics, Hôpital Européen Georges Pompidou, Assistance publique-Hôpitaux de Paris (AP-HP), 20 rue Leblanc, Paris F-75015, France

Allen J. Yiu and Razia Sultana
Calcium Signaling Laboratory, Research Service, Veterans Affairs Medical Center, 50 Irving Street, NW, Washington, DC 20422, USA

Daniel Callaghan
Calcium Signaling Laboratory, Research Service, Veterans Affairs Medical Center, 50 Irving Street, NW, Washington, DC 20422, USA
Department of Pharmacology and Physiology, Georgetown University, 3900 Reservoir Road, NW, Washington, DC 20007, USA

Bidhan C. Bandyopadhyay
Calcium Signaling Laboratory, Research Service, Veterans Affairs Medical Center, 50 Irving Street, NW, Washington, DC 20422, USA
Department of Pharmacology and Physiology, Georgetown University, 3900 Reservoir Road, NW, Washington, DC 20007, USA
Department of Pharmacology and Physiology, School of Medicine, George Washington University, Ross Hall 2300 Eye Street, NW, Washington, DC 20037, USA

Vinal Menon
Department of Cell Biology and Anatomy, School of Medicine, University of South Carolina, Columbia, SC 29209, USA

John F. Eberth and Jay D. Potts
Department of Cell Biology and Anatomy, School of Medicine, University of South Carolina, Columbia, SC 29209, USA
Biomedical Engineering Program, College of Engineering and Computing, University of South
Carolina, Columbia, SC 29208, USA

Richard L. Goodwin
Biomedical Sciences, School of Medicine, University of South Carolina, Greenville, SC 29605, USA

Kerryanne Johnson, Stacey Neilson, Andrew To, Nezar Amir, Andrew Cave, Tony Scott, Mia Parata and Victoria Day
North Shore hospital, Waitemata District Health Board, Takapuna, 0620 Auckland, New Zealand

Martin Orr
North Shore hospital, Waitemata District Health Board, Takapuna, 0620 Auckland, New Zealand
Clinical Informatics Systems Group, North Shore Hospital, Waitemata District Health Board, Takapuna, 0620 Auckland, New Zealand

Patrick Gladding
North Shore hospital, Waitemata District Health Board, Takapuna, 0620 Auckland, New Zealand
Theranostics Laboratory, North Shore Hospital, Waitemata District Health Board, Takapuna, 0620 Auckland, New Zealand
Auckland Bioengineering Institute, University of Auckland, 0620 Auckland, New Zealand

Robert B. Hinton and Amy M. Opoka
The Heart Institute, Division of Cardiology, Cincinnati Children's Hospital Medical Center, Cincinnati, OH 45208, USA

Obah A. Ojarikre
Mill Hill Laboratory, Francis Crick Institute, London NW7 1AA, UK

Lawrence S. Wilkinson and William Davies
MRC Centre for Neuropsychiatric Genetics and Genomics and Institute of Psychological Medicine and Clinical Neurosciences, School of Medicine, Cardiff University, Cardiff CF24 4HQ, UK
Neuroscience and Mental Health Research Institute, Schools of Medicine and Psychology, Cardiff University, Cardiff CF24 4HQ, UK

Ronen Durst and Dan Gilon
Heart Institute, Ein Kerem Campus, Hadassah Hebrew University Medical Center, POB 12000, 92110 Jerusalem, Israel

Vaia D. Raikou
Department of Medicine—Propaedaetic, National and Kapodistrian University of Athens, School of Medicine, Athens, 11527, Greece

Despina Kyriaki
Department of Nuclear Medicine, General Hospital "LAÏKO", Athens, 11527, Greece

Peter S. Martin, Benjamin Kloesel and Simon C. Body
Department of Anesthesiology, Perioperative and Pain Medicine, Brigham and Women's Hospital, Harvard Medical School, 75 Francis St., Th724, Boston, MA 02115, USA

Russell A. Norris
Department of Regenerative Medicine and Cell Biology, Children's Research Institute, Medical University of South Carolina, 173 Ashley St, Charleston, SC 29403, USA

Mark Lindsay and David Milan
Cardiovascular Research Center, Richard B. Simches Research Center, Massachusetts General Hospital, 185 Cambridge Street, Boston, MA 02114, USA

Tori E. Horne, Matthew VandeKopple, Sara N. Koenig and Lindsey J. Anstine
Center for Cardiovascular and Pulmonary Research and The Heart Center at Nationwide Children's Hospital Research Institute, 575 Children's Drive, Research Building III, WB4239, Columbus, OH 43215, USA

Kimberly Sauls and Russell A. Norris
Department of Regenerative Medicine and Cell Biology, Medical University of South Carolina, Charleston, SC 29425, USA

Vidu Garg and Joy Lincoln
Center for Cardiovascular and Pulmonary Research and The Heart Center at Nationwide Children's Hospital Research Institute, 575 Children's Drive, Research Building III, WB4239, Columbus, OH 43215, USA
Department of Pediatrics, The Ohio State University, Columbus, OH 43215, USA

Kimberly Sauls, Katelynn Toomer, Katherine Williams, Amanda J. Johnson, Roger R. Markwald and Russell A. Norris
Department of Regenerative Medicine and Cell Biology, Children's Research Institute, Medical University of South Carolina, 171 Ashley Ave, Charleston, SC 29425, USA

Zoltan Hajdu
Department of Bioengineering, Clemson University, 200 C Patewood Drive, Greenville, SC 29615, USA

Damien Duval, Pauline Labbé, Léa Bureau, Thierry Le Tourneau, Jean-Jacques Schott and Jean Mérot
Institut du thorax, Inserm UMR 1087, CNRS UMR 6291, 8 Quai Moncousu, Nantes F-44007, France

Russell A. Norris and Roger R. Markwald
Department of Cell Biology and Anatomy, Medical University of South Carolina, Charleston, SC 29425, USA

Robert Levine
Harvard Medical School, Massachusetts General Hospital, Boston, MA 02114-2696 USA

Sara N. Koenig, Holly A. Nadorlik and Brenda Lilly
The Center for Cardiovascular and Pulmonary Research and Heart Center, Nationwide Children's Hospital, 700 Children's Drive, Columbus, OH 43205, USA
Department of Pediatrics, The Ohio State University, 700 Children's Drive, Columbus, OH 43205, USA

Vidu Garg
The Center for Cardiovascular and Pulmonary Research and Heart Center, Nationwide Children's Hospital, 700 Children's Drive, Columbus, OH 43205, USA
Department of Pediatrics, The Ohio State University, 700 Children's Drive, Columbus, OH 43205, USA
Department of Molecular Genetics, The Ohio State University, 484 West 12th Avenue, Columbus, OH 43210, USA

Kevin M. Bosse
The Center for Cardiovascular and Pulmonary Research and Heart Center, Nationwide Children's Hospital, 700 Children's Drive, Columbus, OH 43205, USA

Koroush Khalighi
Department of Cardiovascular Disease, Easton Hospital Easton, PA Clinical Professor of Medicine, Drexel University, School of Medicine Easton Cardiovascular Associates 2001 Fairview Ave, Easton, PA 18042, USA

Mohammad Umar Farooq
Department of Medicine, Easton Hospital, 250 South 21 street, Easton, PA 18042, USA

Thein Tun Aung
Department of Cardiovascular Disease, Wright State University, 921 Wilmington Ave, Apt D, Dayton, OH 45420, USA

Swe Oo
Department of Medicine, Easton Hospital, 250 South 21 street, Easton, PA 18042, USA

Wenduo Ye
Department of Cell and Molecular Biology, Tulane University, New Orleans, LA 70118, USA

Yingnan Song and Zhen Huang
Department of Cell and Molecular Biology, Tulane University, New Orleans, LA 70118, USA
Southern Center for Biomedical Research, Fujian Normal University, Fuzhou 350108, China
Fujian Key Laboratory of Developmental and Neural Biology, College of Life Science, Fujian Normal University, Fuzhou 350108, China

Yanding Zhang
Southern Center for Biomedical Research, Fujian Normal University, Fuzhou 350108, China
Fujian Key Laboratory of Developmental and Neural Biology, College of Life Science, Fujian Normal University, Fuzhou 350108, China

Yiping Chen
Department of Cell and Molecular Biology, Tulane University, New Orleans, LA 70118, USA
Southern Center for Biomedical Research, Fujian Normal University, Fuzhou 350108, China